DATE DUE

SSSP

Springer
Series in
Social
Psychology

SSSP

Compatible and Incompatible Relationships

Edited by
William Ickes

Springer-Verlag
New York Berlin Heidelberg Tokyo

Dr. William Ickes
Department of Psychology
University of Texas—Arlington
Arlington, Texas 76019-0528 U.S.A.

With 13 Figures

Library of Congress Cataloging in Publication Data
Main entry under title:
Compatible and incompatible relationships.
  (Springer series in social psychology)
  Bibliography: p.
  Includes index.
  1. Interpersonal relations. I. Ickes, William John.
II. Series.
HM132.C625   1984   302   84-10651

Typeset by Ampersand, Inc., Rutland, Vermont.
Printed and bound by R.R. Donnelley, Harrisonburg, Virginia.
Printed in the United States of America.

9 8 7 6 5 4 3 2 1

ISBN 0-387-96024-4   Springer-Verlag New York Berlin Heidelberg Tokyo
ISBN 3-540-96024-4   Springer-Verlag Berlin Heidelberg New York Tokyo

Dedicated, with love and pride,
and gratitude for his time with us,
to the memory of William Edward Ickes.

Preface

Several years ago, two of my colleagues and I had the opportunity to interview Fritz Heider—perhaps the most influential theorist in the field of social psychology (Harvey, Ickes, & Kidd, 1976). During our interview, Heider affirmed a belief that had guided his career since the 1920s, the belief that the study of human relationships is the most important task in which social scientists can engage. Although many social scientists would profess to share this belief, it is nonetheless true that the study of human relationships has been one of the most neglected tasks in the history of the social sciences—including psychology.

What Heider found in the 1920s—that most psychologists acknowledged the importance of studying human relationships but at the same time tended to focus their own research on more "tractable" topics such as memory and cognition—is still very much evident in the 1980s. Even within the more specific domain of social psychology, a majority of researchers still choose to address those hybrid topics ("social cognition," "social categorization and stereotyping," "person memory," etc.) that relate most directly to traditional areas of psychological research. Still other researchers, while choosing to study such important interpersonal phenomena as altruism, aggression, conflict, and interpersonal attraction, tend to focus so exclusively on these isolated and abstracted phenomena that they fail to provide a more inclusive view of the relationships in which these phenomena occur. Only a small minority of researchers choose to abandon the security of the relatively well-developed theories and research methodologies in these circumscribed topic areas in order to address the more difficult problems of conceptualizing and documenting the dynamic, interpersonal processes by which relationships begin, intensify, deteriorate, and dissolve. That is why, after nearly a century of psychology's history as a science, the study of compatibility and incompatibility in relationships can still be regarded as a relatively new and emerging area for theory and research.

Fortunately, despite its relatively late start, the study of compatibility and incompatibility in relationships has attracted some of the most active and talented researchers in psychology and other social science disciplines. The present collection of edited chapters represents the theory and research of a distinguished set of contributors, each of them offering a valuable perspective on personal and/or social relationships.

The topic of this volume—compatible and incompatible relationships—sets it apart from other edited works on social interaction or interpersonal relations. This focus on compatibility and incompatibility is important for at least three reasons. First, and most obvious, it provides a unifying theme for the book—a theme whose development is long overdue. Second, it requires the contributors, each in his or her own way, to come to grips with the problems of specifying exactly what it is about relationships that justifies characterizing them as compatible or incompatible. Although the perspectives of the various contributors diverge considerably (e.g., in the kinds of relationships they study, in their definitions of "compatibility" and "incompatibility," and in their emphases on different processes assumed to underlie these two phenomena), a common set of issues and conceptual distinctions emerges from their individual efforts. These issues and distinctions appear to be the ones from which a more general theoretical framework will eventually be constructed.

A third reason why the theme of compatibility and incompatibility is important is that the issues it implicates are of central concern to most, if not all, of the social sciences. These issues have a compelling interest for social scientists in disciplines that include communication, counseling, ethology, psychology, psychiatry, sociology, and social work. Theorists, researchers, and clinical practitioners in all of these disciplines (and in such subdisciplines as clinical, developmental, personality, and social psychology) have all been concerned—both practically and theoretically—with the processes underlying compatible and incompatible relationships. This commonality of interest may not be fully realized, however, because of the diverse theoretical perspectives, points of application, and methodological approaches that have been brought to bear on the study of these processes.

In order both to reflect this diversity and to facilitate a broader theoretical integration, I have solicited chapters that represent a wide range of perspectives on the theme of compatible and incompatible relationships. A major assumption that guided the selection of contributors and the organization of the volume is the assumption that the issue of compatibility is fundamental to all social relationships, both across different species and across the life span of individuals within a particular species. Accordingly, although this collection of chapters emphasizes human relationships in general and adult heterosexual relationships in particular, some care has been taken to ensure that comparative-ethological and developmental perspectives are also represented.

As these considerations suggest, *Compatible and Incompatible Relationships* is intended for a relatively broad audience. Although nearly all of the contributors were trained as clinical, developmental, personality and/or social psychologists, the book should be of interest to professionals in communication, counseling, psychiatry, sociology, and social work as well. It is primarily intended, however, to be used within each of these disciplines as a senior or graduate-level text in courses and seminars that focus on problems in human relationships.

The rewards of having edited this collection of chapters have been many. Over the course of the last two years, I have—through phone calls, correspondence, and face-to-face contacts with the other contributors—enjoyed personal and professional relationships with some of the nicest and most intellectually stimulating people on this planet. I have learned and gained insight from each of them, and I have come to regard many of them as friends as well as colleagues. In addition to helping me prepare this book, many of these people—and others not connected with this project— have helped me to deal with the death of a son in ways that I could not have anticipated but will always remember and appreciate. To all of these people, my sincere thanks.

I would also like to express my appreciation to the staff of Springer-Verlag, with whom I seem to be developing a long and mutually loyal association. Their editorial and production assistance has been exemplary, as in the past, and I look forward to many more years of the compatible relationship I have enjoyed with them.

Arlington, Texas   William Ickes

Contents

Contributors

Margaret S. Clark, Department of Psychology, Carnegie-Mellon University, Pittsburgh, Pennsylvania 15213, USA.

Ellen Berscheid, Department of Psychology, University of Minnesota, Minneapolis, Minnesota 55455, USA.

William C. Follette, Department of Psychology, University of Washington, Seattle, Washington 98195, USA.

Wyndol Furman, Department of Psychology, University of Denver, Denver, Colorado 80208, USA.

Kathleen E. Gilbride, Department of Psychology, University of Utah, Salt Lake City, Utah 84112, USA.

Toni Giuliano, Department of Psychology, University of Texas— Austin, Texas 78712, USA.

Elaine Hatfield, Department of Psychology, University of Hawaii at Manoa, Honolulu, Hawaii 96822, USA.

Julia Hay, Department of Sociology, University of Wisconsin, Madison, Wisconsin 53706, USA.

Cindy Hazan, Department of Psychology, University of Denver, Denver, Colorado 80208, USA.

Paula T. Hertel, Department of Psychology, Trinity University, San Antonio, Texas 78284, USA.

William Ickes, Department of Psychology, University of Texas—Arlington, Texas 76019, USA.

Neil S. Jacobson, Department of Psychology, University of Washington, Seattle, Washington 98195, USA.

Roger M. Knudson, Department of Psychology, Miami University, Oxford, Ohio 45056, USA.

Michael E. Lamb, Department of Psychology, University of Utah, Salt Lake City, Utah 84112, USA.

George Levinger, Department of Psychology, University of Massachusetts, Amherst, Amherst, Massachusetts 01003, USA.

D. W. Rajecki, Department of Psychology, School of Science, Purdue University, Indianapolis, Indiana 46223, USA.

Marylyn Rands, Department of Psychology, Wheaton College, Norton, Massachusetts 02766, USA.

Harry T. Reis, Department of Psychology, University of Rochester, Rochester, New York 14627, USA.

Phillip Shaver, Department of Psychology, University of Denver, Denver, Colorado 80208, USA.

Alan L. Sillars, Department of Communication, Ohio State University, Columbus, Ohio 43210, USA.

Susan Sprecher, Department of Sociology, University of Wisconsin, Madison, Madison, Wisconsin 53706, USA.

Jane Traupmann, Women's Study Center, Wellesley College, Wellesley, Massachusetts 02181, USA.

Daniel M. Wegner, Department of Psychology, Trinity University, San Antonio, Texas 78284, USA.

Mary Utne, National Opinion Research Center, University of Chicago, Chicago, Illinois 60637, USA.

Introduction

William Ickes

What does it mean for relationships to be characterized as compatible versus incompatible? In our everyday discourse, we have no difficulty making this distinction. Compatible relationships are ones in which the members of the relationship "get along" with each other, whereas incompatible relationships are ones in which the members do not "get along" together. These descriptions are very close to those provided by dictionary entries in which compatible is defined as "capable of existing together," and incompatible as "incapable of association because incongruous, discordant, or disagreeing" (Webster's New Collegiate Dictionary, 1974).

The second of these definitions begins to suggest some of the complexity underlying the apparent simplicity of the distinction between compatible and incompatible relationships. If a relationship is incompatible, it is because its members are *incongruous* (they do not "mesh" or "fit together"), *discordant* (they are "out of harmony" or "out of sync" with each other), or *disagreeing* (they do not share common attitudes, goals, feelings, etc.). By implication, if a relationship is compatible, it is because its members are *congruous* (they do "mesh" or "fit together"), *accordant* (they are "in harmony" or "in sync" with each other), or *agreeing* (they share common attitudes, goals, feelings, etc.).

Still more complexity is suggested by an etymological analysis which relates "compatible" to "compassion" through the Latin verb *compati* ("to suffer with, be sympathetic to"). This analysis not only emphasizes the affective or emotional aspect of compatibility, but also hints that the condition may reflect an active, intentional attempt by the members of a relationship to understand and accommodate each other. The true etymology of "compatible" may even help us find some insight in Ogden Nash's pseudoetymological quip that "a man and a woman are incompatible if he has no income and she isn't patible." The rather cynical, selfish, and mutually exploitative relationship suggested by Nash's conception of incompatibility may be contrasted quite meaningfully with the conception of a compatible relationship as one based on the members' mutual willingness to share and suffer together.

The complexity inherent in the semantic definition of compatibility and incompatibility becomes even more evident when one attempts to theorize about the nature and dynamics of compatible versus incompatible relationships. For example, when the editor of this volume was pressed by potential contributors for his "operational definition" of compatibility, he found it difficult to come up with one that was both simple enough to be convenient and accurate enough to be acceptable. Trying to suggest some possible defining attributes that could be readily operationalized, he proposed in a letter to the contributors that:

> Compatibility might be defined in terms of (1) the *stability* of the relationship, (2) the *integrative functioning* of the relationship, and (3) the *perceived quality of and satisfaction with* the relationship. Stability, the first of these three aspects, could be operationally defined in terms of the longevity of the relationship and its resistance to disruption. Integrative functioning could be operationally defined in terms of the individuals' capacity to reach consensus, meet each other's needs, facilitate each other's goals, resolve conflicts, etc. And perceived quality and satisfaction could be assessed by various self-report measures of love, liking, marital satisfaction, etc.

As anticipated, this operational definition did not prove to be acceptable in every respect. All of the contributors seemed to agree that integrative functioning was indeed a defining attribute of compatibility in human (and animal) relationships, but there was somewhat less consensus about the need to include the other two elements. Beyond these concerns, many of the contributors appeared to share the editor's developing sense that the interrelated constructs of "compatibility" and "incompatibility" were too complex and multifaceted to lend themselves to a simple operational definition. What was needed instead was a fully articulated conceptual explication of these constructs that acknowledged their complexity—an explication that was currently lacking in the psychological literature.

To some degree, such an explication can be found in each of the chapters in this volume. Its purest realization, however, is the conceptual analysis proposed in Chapter 6 by Ellen Berscheid. Berscheid's analysis of compatibility and incompatibility is both insightful and compelling, and it may prove to be a definitive one. Drawing upon the general model of dyadic interdependence that Kelley, Berscheid, Christensen, Harvey, Huston, Levinger, McClintock, Peplau, and Peterson (1983) used to analyze the processes occurring in close relationships, Berscheid accounts for compatibility and incompatibility in terms of the interconnected activities of the members of the relationship:

> That portion of the relationship's infrastructure (that is, again, the causal interconnections between the partners' activity chains) that is especially relevant to the relationship's compatibility or incompatibility is that portion that encompasses activities that are intrachained—or, in other words, that portion that represents each partner's organized action sequences and higher-order plans. Thus, whether—and how—the individual's sequences and plans impinge on the partner's sequences and plans (and vice versa) should determine the emotional tenor of the relationship. Where interchain connections between the partners interrupt one or both persons' intrachain activities, negative

emotion should result; where interchain connections facilitate each person's performance of intrachain activities, or where there are no interchain connections to these activities, harmony should prevail. In the beginning of a relationship, both persons bring with them a lifetime of organized behavior sequences as well as current plans in progress. How these two sets of intrachain activities fit together not only helps determine whether the relationship will be compatible or incompatible, close or distant, but also whether it shall live or die. (p. 153)

Interdependence and Compatibility at Different Levels of Analysis

As Berscheid's account makes clear, the causal interconnections between the partners' activity chains are responsible for the interdependence of their dyadic and individual outcomes at different "levels" of analysis. Oversimplifying a bit, one can speak of compatibility or incompatibility within a relationship at (1) the level of its members' *behavior* (e.g., making love versus making "war"; performing versus not performing actions that fulfill each other's needs), (2) the level of their *emotions* (e.g., loving versus hating; experiencing the interaction as gratifying and pleasurable rather than frustrating and painful), and (3) the level of their *cognitions* regarding self, other, and the nature of their relationship (e.g., having expectations confirmed versus disconfirmed).

The need to conceptually distinguish the different "levels of interdependence" within a relationship can be illustrated by an example of the compatibility/incompatibility distinction in its simplest, most fundamental form. Consider the relationships within two sets of gears: In the first set, the two gears are precisely matched to each other; in the second set, the two gears are badly mismated. When the two gears are compatible (i.e., precisely matched), their relationship "works," and they operate together in a smooth, synchronized manner. On the other hand, when the two gears are incompatible (i.e., badly mismated), their relationship does not "work," and, instead of meshing together and integrating their respective movements without unnecessary friction, they grind and grate against each other, producing heat, discordant noise, mutual wear and tear, and—in some cases—a complete mutual inhibition of movement.

The gear example is obviously useful as a metaphor suggesting some of the processes that may characterize compatibility in more complex relationships, such as those involving two people. Of current interest, however, is not the power of this metaphor but a recognition of its limitations. The relationship between two animate and sentient beings, unlike the relationship between two gears, is not limited to events occurring solely at the level of sheer physical behavior. Thus, whereas an adequate account of the "compatibility" or "incompatibility" of two gears need only consider the interdependence of events occurring at the *physical/behavioral* level of analysis, an adequate account of the compatibility or incompatibility of two sentient beings must also consider the interdependence of events occurring at the *psychological* levels of analysis (i.e., events that are defined by the thoughts and feelings of these beings.)

The distinction between these levels of analysis provides the basis for the organization of the chapters in *Compatible and Incompatible Relationships*. The need for this distinction is clearly documented in the three chapters that comprise Part I of this volume. In Chapter 1, D. W. Rajecki offers a comparative-ethological perspective that suggests how—in contrast to the relationship between two inanimate objects—the relationship between two animals may be characterized by both behavioral and cognitive-emotional interdependence. A compatible relationship between two chimpanzees, for example, appears to depend more on their ability to predict each other's behavior than on the harmonious interdependence of the behavior itself. The importance of mutual predictability is further emphasized in Michael Lamb and Kathleen Gilbride's account in Chapter 2 of the origins of compatibility in the relationships of human infants and their parents. Both infants and their caretakers must play an active role in developing and maintaining predictable interaction sequences, and "failures" on the part of either participant may contribute to such disastrously incompatible infant-parent relationships as those in which child abuse occurs. Moreover, because it is not long before children themselves become important caretakers and socializing agents for others, their ability to form compatible relationships is soon manifested in their interactions with siblings and peers. In Chapter 3, Wyndol Furman reviews an extensive body of developmental research in order to document the sources of compatibility and incompatibility at different levels of children's peer and sibling relationships.

The relationships of young and older adults are emphasized in the remaining chapters, which are grouped according to the level at which the interdependence and compatibility of the partners is examined. The focus of the chapters in Part II is on behavioral interdependence and social exchange. In Chapter 4, Elaine Hatfield, Jane Traupmann, Susan Sprecher, Mary Utne, and Julia Hay propose that the capacity of relationship partners to reward or punish each other through their behavior makes equity considerations salient as determinants of compatibility. After considering the question of "whether or not equity considerations *should* apply to intimate relations," Hatfield and her colleagues "summarize the recent evidence indicating that equity principles *do* seem critically important in our most significant relations." The data reviewed by these authors strongly support the claim that, in the long run, the perception by marriage partners that they are equitably rewarded is essential to the compatibility of their intimate relationship. In Chapter 5, however, Margaret Clark suggests an important qualification to this claim. Clark proposes that equity considerations can undermine compatibility in intimate relationships—in the short run, at least—because these considerations are inconsistent with the implicit rules governing the distribution of benefits in intimate/"communal" relationships.

A theme that is introduced in Parts I and II—the emotional implications of the partners' behavioral interdependence—is the major focus of the chapters in Part III. Chapter 6, by Ellen Berscheid, offers both a penetrating conceptual analysis of compatibility and incompatibility and a cogent model of the processes by which emotion in relationships is engendered. For the most part complementing but occasionally taking issue with Berscheid's perspective, Phillip Shaver and Cindy Hazan emphasize the importance of social needs in their analysis of emotion in relationships. In Chapter 7, they propose a stage model to characterize the hypothesized process by which individuals who are isolated or are incompatible with their current partners experience negative, social-need-based emotions that in turn evoke romantic, "limerent" fantasies about potential new partners.

The interdependence of relationship partners at the cognitive level—particularly with regard to their conceptions of self and other—is the theme of the chapters in Part IV. In Chapter 8, William Ickes suggests how one aspect of self-concept—the specific "sex role orientations" that men and women have adopted—can guide and channel their behavior in ways that predictably influence the compatibility of their intimate and nonintimate relationships. Following Ickes' chapter, the role of self-concept in the initiation and course of social interaction is explored in more abstract and general terms by Harry Reis. In Chapter 9, Reis discusses "the different ways in which the self is responsible for constructing the social world in which it participates." These processes by which self-concepts guide and shape the course of relationships are explored in Chapter 10 in the specific context of marital interactions. Roger Knudson reviews theory and data suggesting that marital compatibility may vary according to the degree to which the behavior of each partner confirms and supports the other's self-conceived identity.

The idea that partners in close relationships are cognitively interdependent is taken quite literally by Daniel Wegner, Toni Giuliano, and Paula Hertel in Chapter 11. Drawing upon theory and research in cognitive psychology, these authors update and legitimize the "group mind" concept in order to examine the various ways that relationship partners employ and come to depend on the *transactive memory* that emerges from their interaction together. As a counterpoint to the emphasis in Chapter 11 on cognitive interdependence in relationships, Alan Sillars argues in Chapter 12 that independence—not interdependence—is the rule. Sillars integrates theory and findings from various disciplines to support his conclusion that the interpersonal perceptions of relationship partners are commonly unrelated or incongruent.

The two chapters in Part V provide complementary perspectives on marital interaction. Chapter 13, by George Levinger and Marylyn Rands, characterizes marital compatibility in terms of the same "interconnected event" model employed by Berscheid in Chapter 6. Levinger and Rands apply this model to different stages of the marital relationship in order to explain how variations in compatibility at each of these stages may result in transitions such as those from dating to marriage and from marriage to divorce. The concluding chapter, by William Follette and Neil Jacobson, describes the practical problems that marriage counselors and clinical psychologists confront in their attempts to assess and treat incompatible marital relationships. In Chapter 14, these authors present a comprehensive yet remarkably concise review of the history and current status of marital therapy.

It has been assumed in this introduction that compatibility within relationships may extend over one or more "levels" of interdependence. For heuristic reasons, it may be useful to extend this idea by suggesting that there may be at least a rough correspondence between these levels of interdependence and the levels of Maslow's (1962) hierarchy of human needs.

As depicted in Figure I-1, Maslow's hierarchy segregates and orders different sets of human needs according to the immediacy with which their satisfaction is required. Basic physiological needs are assumed to be the most pressing and fundamental ones, and their satisfaction is seen as prerequisite to seeking the satisfaction of the safety needs at the next higher level. Satisfaction of the safety needs is, in turn, prerequisite to seeking the satisfaction of self-esteem needs, and so on.

Bercheid's analysis (Chapter 6) assumes that compatible and incompatible relationships differ primarily in the degree to which the partners' interaction in the relationship either facilitates or impedes their attempts to obtain satisfaction of their individual needs. If this assumption is correct, then the seemingly *different* bases for compatibility and incompatibility proposed by the various contributors to this volume can be shown, in virtually every case, to have a

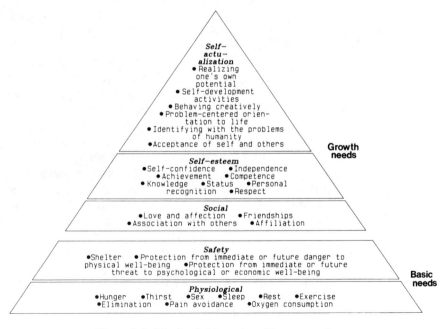

Figure I-1. Maslow's hierarchy of human needs.

conceptually *common* basis in the facilitation versus frustration of a specific type of need or class of needs.

Chapters 1 and 2, for example, are essentially concerned with the mutual fulfillment of the partners' safety needs as a basis for their compatibility (i.e., with their need to be able to predict each other's behavior in order to feel secure and safe in the relationship). Similarly, Chapters 4 and 5 tend to emphasize the safety needs that are fulfilled by ensuring that mutually agreeable "rules" are followed for the distribution of rewards within the relationship. Chapters 3, 6, and 7 are primarily concerned with the partners' attempts to fulfill their social and emotional needs. Chapter 8 explores the outcome of relationships in which fulfillment of the intense social-emotional needs of one partner (a stereotypically feminine woman) is frustrated by and at odds with the attempts by the other partner (a stereotypically masculine man) to fulfill his intense self-esteem needs. Chapters 9 and 10 emphasize such self-esteem needs as the recognition and validation of one's identity and self-conception (i.e., personal recognition, status, respect). Chapter 11 concerns the self-esteem needs of knowledge and competence. And Chapter 12, in a curious sort of way, may reflect another type of self-esteem need—the need of the partners to preserve their independence within their interdependent relationship.

Where do Chapters 13 and 14 fit into this scheme? Quite possibly, they relate to the highest level of Maslow's hierarchy. If, in their marriage relationship, two people are able to integrate their lives in a way that permits the mutual fulfillment of their needs at all of the lower levels, their relationship may become a context in which their self-actualization as individuals and as a couple can occur. If, on the other hand, they fail at this admittedly difficult task, they may have to return to a lower level of Maslow's pyramid and—in too many cases—continue on their journey alone.

Reference

Kelly, H. H., Berscheid, E. S., Christensen, A., Harvey, J., Huston, T. L., Levinger, G., McClintock, E., Peplau, L. A., & Peterson, D. R. (1983). *Close relationships.* San Francisco: Freeman.

Part I

Comparative and Developmental Perspectives

Chapter 1

Predictability and Control in Relationships: A Perspective from Animal Behavior

D. W. Rajecki

The thesis of this chapter is that the predictability or controllability of individuals within certain dyads or more complex relationships—such as in the human nuclear family, between playmates, or between nonhumans living in structured groups—is an important factor in the dynamics of these social units. This idea will be illustrated principally with findings from research on animal behavior. First, the case will be made that dominance and subordinance[1] structures are characteristic of many interindividual behavior patterns, human and nonhuman alike. Next, an argument will be made that one consequence of a dominance relationship between individuals is that it yields and ensures their mutual predictability or controllability, which in turn promotes the functioning and longevity of the global relationship. A corollary will then be drawn that the above principle can be illustrated in the case where two (or more) individuals who are not yet in a dominance relationship encounter one another. That is, reactions to strangers—xenophobia in particular—will be reviewed. Attention will focus on the xenophobic behavior of a variety of nonhuman species, with special reference to the introduction of strangers into primate groups. The relevance of this literature for an understanding of compatible and incompatible human relationships will then be discussed.

Dominance Relations

The phenomenon of dominance and subordinance relations between individuals within groups has been studied at different levels of analysis and from various theoretical orientations. An early view was that human dominance or ascendance is a dimension of personality, thus the basis for the pattern can be

---

[1]It has been suggested that the word "subordinacy" rather than "subordinance" is the correct usage in this context (see the editor's note in Deag, 1977, p. 466). However, I choose to employ subordinance because, even if less correct, it is the better known of the two terms.

traced to traits in the individual (e.g., Allport, 1937). A contrasting view—one held by certain animal behaviorists—is that dominance is not the property of the individual, but is rather an emergent product of the group's social structure such that "one's degree of dominance can be known only in reference to one's place in the structure" (see Zivin, 1983, p. 183). More recently, in developmental psychology, there has been a union or merger of the personality and social structure (animal) formulations, into what Zivin (1983) has termed a "hybrid model" of dominance relations. In the hybrid model, dominance relations are recognized as an essential element of group structure, and one's place in the hierarchy is thought to be due to individual differences (traits).

Another perspective on dominance—that from sociobiology—concentrates on "genetic fitness": an index of the contribution of offspring (hence, genes) to the next generation by one genotype (individual organism) in a population, relative to the contributions of other genotypes (other individual organisms). Because dominant group members presumably have priority of access to food, shelter, and mates, all of which promote reproductive success, dominance is thought to raise their genetic fitness (see Wilson, 1975).

Finally, the notion of dominance emerges as a salient dimension in a "structural analytic model of social behavior" (also called an interpersonal behavioral taxonomy), which has been used as a clinical instrument for describing and quantifying interpersonal styles or difficulties, and the changes in relationships that occur as a result of certain experiences such as psychotherapy (Benjamin, 1977). This model represents the behavior involved in interpersonal relations via two-dimensional planes or charts, each based on the intersections of a horizontal axis labeled "affiliation" and a vertical axis named "inter-dependence." Specific two-dimensional planes of behavior characterize specific members of a dyad. For the so-called parentlike behaviors, the terms "dominate" and "emancipate" are polar opposites on the vertical dimension; for the so-called childlike behaviors, the terms "submit" and "be emancipated" are opposites on this dimension (see Benjamin, 1974, p. 394).

Certainly, the phenomenon of dominance relations has engaged the attention of many researchers and theorists. These writers and their colleagues speak to somewhat different issues when considering human or nonhuman relations, but the reader gets the impression that they would not feel out of place in one another's company. Even Benjamin (1974), the most clinically oriented of the lot, alludes to the resemblance between her scheme and the literature on nonhuman primates (pp. 398, 423), and it is on nonhumans that we will concentrate in the discussion to follow.

While recognizing that the models under consideration are by no means equivalent, it would nonetheless be useful to examine some real-world dominance relations to show why behavioral scientists have become so interested in such affairs. Setting aside for a moment the thorny problems of comparative psychology or ethology, we now turn to an especially thorough and revealing study of relations between members of dyads within a larger group, namely, Deag's (1977) report of a social hierarchy in a troop of wild Barbary macaques *(Macaca sylvanus)* living relatively undisturbed in a cedar forest in the Moroccan Middle Atlas Mountains.

The fact that Deag studied free-ranging monkeys is important because earlier analysts had argued that nonhuman primate dominance hierarchies already seen in laboratories and zoos were merely artifacts of captivity (e.g., Rowell, 1974). The discovery of dominance relations in a "natural" setting would go far to establish such patterns as characteristic of the social life of at least the species under study. For Deag, the dominant member of any given pair (or pairing) of animals within the troop was the one "whose behaviour is not limited by the other." Conversely, the subordinate individual was the one "whose behaviour is limited by the other and which shows submission" (p. 466). To put it another way, a dominant monkey is one who gives to another more dyadic threats than it receives, and receives more dyadic avoidance or submission from the other than it gives. The subordinate animal is defined simply as the opposite of the dominant. These acts of threat, submission, and avoidance in nonhuman primates are amply documented and can be reliably recorded. (For more details on these behaviors, see the review of Rajecki and Flanery, 1981.)

The troop in question contained 25 animals and was quite active socially. In 78 hours of observation, Deag recorded 1,740 social interactions of various sorts, 312 of which were threats within dyads, and 267 of which involved avoidance or submission. Thus, there were more than enough raw data to use as a basis for analyzing dominance relations within the troop, and the hierarchy that emerged is depicted in Figure 1-1. In the upper-left portion of the figure, the statement AM1 > AM2 means that Adult Male #1 was dominant over Adult Male #2. In keeping with the definition provided earlier, this means that AM1

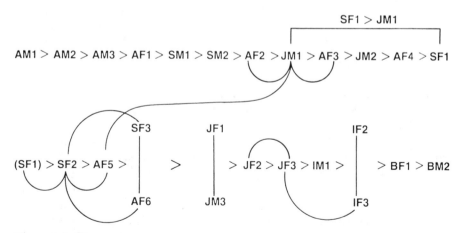

Figure 1-1. The dominance hierarchy in a troop of free-ranging Barbary macaques. M = male, F = female, A = adult, S = subadult, J = juvenile, I = infant, and B = baby. The horizontal line between SF1 and JM1 shows one major reversal; the vertical or curved lines between other individuals show some minor reversals (see text). Reproduced from Figure 1 of Deag (1977), with permission.

was on record as having given AM2 more threats than AM2 returned, or that AM1 received more avoidance and submission from AM2, or both. Indeed, AM1 was dominant over all the other animals in the troop. For his part, AM2 was also a highly dominant monkey, being subordinate only to AM1. Next, AM3 was dominant over most of the other animals except AM1 and AM2, and so on down the hierarchy.

The hierarchy in Figure 1-1 is very nearly linear, but it does contain a few reversals—a pattern which is typical of such structures. A linear hierarchy would be one in which $A > B$, $B > C$, and $A > C$. A reversal in a hierarchy would be such that $A > B$, $B > C$, but $C > A$. Deag describes only one "major" reversal in this particular hierarchy between JM1 (Juvenile Male #1) and SF1 (Subadult Female #1), and some "minor" reversals between other individuals, as seen in Figure 1-1. In this context, a major reversal is one that is permanent or long standing, and minor ones are those that are infrequent or temporary. Nevertheless, reversals accounted for only a trivial 2% of recorded interactions between identified individuals; thus for all practical purposes, this hierarchy can be characterized as being essentially linear.

Several other interesting findings came out of Deag's (1977) analysis. First, when a dominance hierarchy based on threats alone was compared with one based on avoidance and submission alone, it was found that they were mirror images. Moreover, some social interactions began with threats while others consisted only of avoidance. This means that *both* dominant and subordinate animals were active in maintaining the hierarchy. Second, a monkey's rank determined its very style of interaction with the rest of the troop:

> The frequency with which animals avoided others was more closely correlated with the avoided animal's rank than with their own, indicating that the subordinate was "choosing" its partner with greater care for rank. . . . The frequency with which animals threatened others was more closely correlated with their own rank than that of the animal threatened, indicating that the dominant animal was not paying such close attention to the other interactant's rank (Deag, p. 468).

In other words, these patterns are reminiscent of an "attention structure" wherein low-ranking individuals monitor the behavior of high-ranking others more than vice versa (Chance, 1976).

Of course, Deag's dominance study is only one in a large literature on a wide variety of nonhuman animals, both primate and nonprimate. Further, it is of more than passing interest that hierarchies in various human groups are also on record. Social structures based on rank have been seen in groups of children (e.g., Abramovitch & Strayer, 1978; Strayer & Strayer, 1976), female and male adolescents (respectively: Deutsch, Esser, & Sossin, 1978; Savin-Williams, 1976, 1977, 1979), and adult males in captive (prison) circumstances (Austin & Bates, 1974). Although several extensive collections and reviews of dominance research are now available (e.g., Omark, Strayer, & Freedman, 1980; Rajecki & Flanery, 1981; Syme & Syme, 1979; Zivin, 1983), it is not the main purpose of this chapter to provide an extensive review of dominance patterns but rather to examine the social-psychological ramifications of such structures. To do this we now turn to a consideration of the advantages of dominance and the compensations of subordinance.

Advantages and Compensations of Hierarchies

Taking a functional approach, one could ask about the "usefulness" of a dominance heirarchy within, say, a troop of Barbary macaques as studied by Deag. Several replies come to mind. First, inequalities in social status doubtless do increase or maximize the genetic fitness of dominant animals, as mentioned earlier. Second, it also follows that the genetic fitness of even subordinate animals is optimized in a hierarchical situation because exchanges of threats and submissive acts are clearly less dangerous than physical attack and fighting. Furthermore, a hierarchy allows the subordinate to remain with the group, where there are at least some chances of mating. Without such an opportunity to reproduce, genetic fitness would automatically be zero. Finally, the very existence of a group may be made possible by a hierarchy, in that it provides a structure for minimizing conflict and ensuring that animals are more or less tolerant of one another. Insofar as group rather than solitary living is beneficial to the entire membership, hierarchies contribute to the propagation of the species. It should be recognized, however, that the preceding four points are made at a biological (or sociobiological) level of analysis, and are not necessarily germane to an understanding of the *psych*ology of such relationships. To get at the psychological aspects of all of this, one might well pose the question: "What's in it for the individual?"

Deag himself offers a suggestion of what might be going on at the level of individual awareness. He comments on the fact that when groups of captive monkeys are formed there is usually a high incidence of physical aggression early on, but that these flareups are "temporary and wane as new relationships are established" (a finding that we will consider in some detail later).

He further argues that:

> The fact that during group formation in captivity the level of aggression falls as a hierarchical pattern emerges does not mean that the hierarchy has caused a reduction of fighting. It is more accurate to state that fighting has resulted in the formation of the predictable relationships which make up the hierarchy (Deag, p. 472).

For the individual, then, this is what a hierarchy means. To use anthropomorphic language for convenience, each animal can be said to know[2] its place

---

[2]This is not the proper place to raise the issue of animal awareness. However, interest in nonhuman cognition, consciousness, information processing, and mentalism is, in fact, on the increase (see Griffin, 1976; Roitblat, 1982; Sober, 1983). It is enough to say that if monkeys cannot really discriminate between individuals, they at least *act* as if they can.

in the social structure and what to expect from other animals in their respective positions. Dominant animals can predict the behavior of subordinates and can control them with mere threats if need be. On the other hand, even subordinate individuals can, in a real sense, predict and "control" the behavior of higher-ranking members. Submission—sometimes called appeasement—can effectively terminate threats, and avoidance can prevent the occurrence or escalation of threat or physical attack (see Wickler, 1967).

Whereas control implies prediction, prediction in turn aids control. As noted, subordinate monkeys visually monitor dominant members more than the other way around. Even more interesting, it has been observed that as ranks change within a group, the attention structure changes accordingly. Newly dominant monkeys are granted more attention than they got previously, and newly subordinate animals less (Christopher, 1972). This in and of itself argues for individuals' awareness of status differentials within the group, and the need for subordinates to anticipate the actions of higher-ups. In sum, dominant monkeys are predictably troublesome to subordinates, but the controlling effects of submission and avoidance help to keep the situation from getting entirely out of hand. Thus, although subordinates themselves are highly controllable and predictable by those that are dominant, the reverse is also true to some degree.

If this application of the notions of predictability and control is correct, then one can account for the fact that monkeys and other animals can exist in aggregates simply because their species-mates are tolerable due to familiarity. This seems plausible if only because this sort of tolerance or preference for predictable and controllable stimuli finds its counterpart in the human domain. These effects are thought to occur because:

> Life can be viewed as a struggle against randomness—an attempt to acquire the freedom to make choices or exercise control. [Accordingly,] in the current literature on control . . . the term is used to refer to the continual attempt of the human or animal to deal effectively with and to manipulate his environment (Perlmuter & Monty, 1977, p. 759).

Interest in these matters has led researchers of human behavior to study a wide variety of topics, including urban stress (Glass & Singer, 1972), learned helplessness (Seligman, 1975), well-being and survival in the elderly (Langer & Rodin, 1976; Schulz, 1976), and the illusion of control on task performance (Perlmuter & Monty, 1977), among others.

Returning to predictability and control in nonhuman societies, one finds in Marler (1976) a view similar to the position advanced above:

> Perhaps the most subtle and difficult to understand, and yet perhaps ultimately the most important, factor in reducing the probability of aggression is familiarity. If strangeness is such a potent stimulus for aggression, familiarity between habitual companions is probably the most important single factor in reducing the likelihood of aggression between them. . . . The performance of overt behaviors in particular and ritualized form may prove to be reassuring in their reinforcement of familiarity, quite apart from any specific message that they carry. If familiarity is so important, there may be good insurance in conveying it in as many ways as possible, perhaps by several sensory

modalities. I have a suspicion that much of the endless cycle of social ritual in animals is designed to permit companions to expose themselves to each other in many different circumstances, with ample opportunity to know each other's smell and sound as well as how they look, to know how they are likely to behave in a variety of situations (p. 245).

The study of reactions of animals to unfamiliar species-mates would thus seem to offer an interesting avenue by which to explore the idea that more or less amicable relations between group members are due to their mutual control and predictability. To use anthropomorphic language again, when a monkey or another kind of animal encounters or confronts a stranger of the same age and sex, it neither knows with certainty what behavior to expect nor what dominance relation exists between itself and the other. Assuming that the sheer ambiguity is intolerable, and further that most gregarious organisms continuously strive for dominance and exercise it when they have it, the issue of the status relationship between the two strangers should not remain unsettled for long. If the two remain in contact, attempts to establish predictability and control should be made manifest quickly, and perhaps dramatically. Because of the primacy of this process, most of the balance of this chapter will be devoted to a review of xenophobia, with special reference to the introduction of strangers into nonhuman primate groups.

Before we turn to this literature, however, it will be useful to make a slight digression in order to consider certain "rules" in comparative psychology. These "rules" refer to the procedures or criteria for making meaningful behavioral comparisons between humans and other members of the animal kingdom. Once certain rules have been established, the relevance of the subsequent comparative data will be more clearly evident.

Comparative Social Psychology

According to several recent accounts, there are three fundamental categories or classes of behavioral comparison between any two or more species: *homologies, analogies,* and *models* (cf. Eibl-Eibesfeldt, 1983; Rajecki, 1983; Rajecki & Flanery, 1981; Suomi & Immelmann, 1983). Behavioral (or morphological) similarities are *homologies* if they are due to genetic similarities that can be traced—directly or indirectly—to a common ancestor. In biology, homologies of structure can be investigated first-hand or inferred from morphological taxonomies. There are several formal criteria for establishing such inferred homologies, including the so-called criterion of special quality: Similar structures can be considered homologous if they agree in several unusual characteristics. In other words, the greater the complexity and degree of correspondence, the more probable it is that the structures are homologous (see Atz, 1970). For instance, compared with prosimians, certain sensory and anatomical features found across humans, apes, and monkeys (reduced sense of smell; the loss of primitive muzzle, tactile hairs, and mobility of external ears) are probably homologous according to the criterion of special quality

(Washburn & Avis, 1958). This criterion can also be applied to similar behaviors seen in two or more species.

Behavioral similarities are *analogies* if they are a consequence of convergent evolution. If situational demands place extreme selection pressure on a variety of animals living in a given environment, any number of species might evolve along the same structural or behavioral lines regardless of their genetic relatedness. An illustration of this principle is the streamlined shape of many aquatic animals. Dolphins and sharks are quite distinct in terms of genetics, yet they look very much alike. According to the idea of biological analogy, dolphins and sharks both evolved in this fashion because it maximized their efficiency in moving through their watery environment. However, unlike the case for homologies, there are not yet any formal rules for "proving" structural or behavioral analogies, so critics urge conservatism and common sense in applying this idea in comparative psychology (Hodos & Campbell, 1969; Lockard, 1971).

A third way to deal with behavioral comparisons is to seek animal models of human behavior. The meaning of *model* in this context is roughly equivalent to the meaning of *substitute*, as in the usage of Corson, Corson, Arnold, and Knopp (1976): "Some of these animal models (but not all) respond favorably to amphetamine . . . , thus these animal models represent suitable subjects for . . . developing rational diagnostic, pragmatic, and therapeutic criteria which might be applicable to . . . children and adults" (pp. 133–134). From this point of view, models—whatever species happen to be involved—are used as temporary or convenient replacements for humans in research and evaluation programs. The issue here is not whether there are genetic links or evolutionary parallels between the species to be compared, but whether the animals are somehow suitable for resolving particular research issues. For instance, the warning on labels of some dietary foods ("Use of this product may be hazardous to your health. This product contains saccharine which has been determined to cause cancer in laboratory animals") probably stems from a rodent model of human cancers.

What are the implications of these behavioral-comparison categories for a comparative review of xenophobia? Will there be an argument for homologies, analogies, or simply animal models of predictability and control in relationships? Answers to these questions are probably best postponed until we come to the end of the review on xenophobia, but even this short explication on the technical meaning of homologies, analogies, and models will become useful in helping the reader to evaluate the implications of the animal data to follow.

Xenophobia

It was suggested that because of the motivation deriving from uncertainty, xenophobic reactions, or the resolution of behavior and status ambiguities between strangers, might be dramatic. Indeed, reports from laboratories and field settings show this to be the case. Nonhumans often react with considerable violence to unfamiliar species-mates, and examples of these incidents will be forthcoming. For the moment, one can suggest the probable psychological intensity of the experience of encountering a stranger by examining certain physiological and other reactions that reveal the stress of such situations. Table 1-1 provides a short sampler of these types of reactions.

Of course, the most dramatic of these reactions are observed in those cases in which an unfortunate animal, usually in the role of a willing or unwilling intruder into an occupied territory, is traumatized to the point of death. Although strangers are sometimes killed in fights, it is frequently the case that the death of an intruder is due to something like psychological shock. For example, Telle (1966) reports on the introduction of foreign brown rats into an established colony of other brown rats:

> A part of these foreign rats remained in the vicinity of the runs . . . from which they had been driven only a short while earlier; in many cases we found these animals dead in a few days without exhibiting external injuries. . . . We performed autopsies on these specimens. Hematomas or internal injuries were found in no case. Following similar observations, Barnett . . . has mentioned

Table 1-1. Sampler of Physiological and Other Reactions of Strangers

Source	Reaction	Animal
Barnett, Hocking, Munro, and Walker (1975)	renal pathology	rats
Bernstein (1969)	collapse and death	pigtail monkeys
Bernstein (1971)	pulmonary hemorrhage: death	mangabeys
Bernstein, Gordon, and Rose (1974)	heat exhaustion: death	rhesus monkeys
Bronson and Eleftheriou (1965)	corticosterone increase	mice
Campos, Emde, Gaensbauer, and Henderson (1975)	elevated heart rate	human infants
Candland, Bryan, Nazar, Kopf, and Sendor (1970)	elevated heart rate	squirrel monkeys
Candland, Taylor, Dresdale, Leiphart, and Solow (1969)	elevated heart rate	roosters
Goldberg and Welch (1972)	catecholamine increase	mice
Hall (1962)	stress: yawning	patas monkeys
Henry, Meehan, and Stephens (1967)	elevated blood pressure	mice
Lalljee and Cook (1973)	stress: speech patterns	human adults
Luciano and Lore (1975)	gastric ulcers	rats
Rose, Bernstein, and Gordon (1978)	plasma testosterone drop	rhesus monkeys
Rosenblum, Levy, and Kaufman (1968)	stress: autogrooming	squirrel monkeys
Siegel and Siegel (1961)	adrenal hypertrophy	roosters
Southwick (1964)	eosinophil drop	mice
Telle (1966)	collapse and death	rats

the possibility that death might have been due to hypoglycemic shock, as is known from other animals following long-term emotional stress (p. 46 of the translation).

As the reader may have noted, an intruder into another animal's territory has the obvious *double* disadvantage of being a stranger in a strange land. Even so, it can be argued—in the case of rats, at least—that social stress is the lethal agent. In a case in which the element of social stress was absent, Telle (1966, p. 37 of the translation) introduced a group of rats into a foreign territory (i.e., containing burrows and scent-marked runs) from which the former residents had been recently eradicated, and found that the newcomers quickly appropriated the location and seemed to suffer no ill effects. Whatever the specific cause(s) of the effect, Table 1-1 indicates that the collapse and death of strangers is also seen in certain nonhuman primates.

Indeed, nonhuman primates of certain species are widely known for their volatile reactions to strangers. In a field experiment in India, Southwick, Siddiqi, Farooqui, and Pal (1974) introduced captive rhesus monkeys into natural troops in urban and rural settings. Except for some infant strangers,[3] all the rest of the introduced animals were met with intense aggression that included threats, chases, and direct physical attacks. In one instance the researchers released two females into a troop of 65 rhesus near a rural location called Chhatair, with the following result.

> Upon release both were threatened and chased away by the group, but both persisted in trying to return to the group. The younger adult female came directly back into the group despite a tremendous barrage of threats and some direct attacks. She ran back into the center of the group's home range and cowered on the ground in a state of total submission. In this condition she was attacked and bullied by many members of the group, especially juveniles and other adult females. They bit her rump and tail and tugged at her ears and scalp. We fended off some of the most violent attacks to prevent serious wounding. Although there were no bleeding wounds, the female went into a state of shock—her face paled, breathing became shallow, and she became very weak and lost motor coordination. We chased away the other monkeys and took her to a refuge under a bush 200 [yards] away where she recovered some color and strength. She was still there at nightfall 3 [hours] after release (p. 199).

Alas, when the researchers returned to the site the next morning, all they could find of the two new females was one skeleton with "sufficient nyanzol dye on some of the remaining fur to confirm it as one of our releases." Overall, aggression in natural groups such as these increased over baseline by from 42% to 822% as a consequence of the release of strangers in their vicinity. Of the 18 strangers released in the study (again, excluding infants), 100% were either killed or driven completely away!

---

[3]Foreign infants generally elicited exploration of themselves, and parental or protective behavior by troop members. Clearly, there are loopholes in the law of xenophobia in rhesus monkeys. But this exception may prove the rule, as we shall see in a later section on the so-called social template in xenophobic behavior.

Temporal Patterns in Xenophobia

Apart from their frequently dramatic or violent nature, xenophobic responses in monkey groups have another interesting feature: They predictably conform to a certain time-line. That is, things happen quickly in monkey xenophobia, and events unfold in a characteristic temporal pattern. Southwick et al. (1974) noted that all monkey strangers in their field study were recognized as such by the residents within 15 minutes of release, and that in some cases this recognition was instantaneous. The temporal pattern of this xenophobia is made even clearer in studies of the introduction of a strange species-mate to a captive group of monkeys.

For example, Bernstein (1964) introduced a succession of foreign rhesus monkeys into an established group of one adult male and three adult female rhesus that were housed in a large enclosure. The animals' reactions—including those of the strangers—are presented in Table 1-2 in terms of positive, or prosocial, behavior, and aggressive behavior, or behavior seen during bouts of aggression. (As a general category, these aggression-related responses are termed "agonistic.") It is evident from Table 1-2 that the introduction of a stranger had a profound influence on social behavior in the group. During a baseline period prior to the first introduction, the group was peaceful and engaged in prosocial behavior. However, within the first 20 minutes of an introduction, positive behavior was all but eliminated by the eruption of aggression. Aggression, in turn, was greatly reduced by the next day (and thereafter), and the animals' social behavior returned to its more pacific forms.

Table 1-2. Prosocial and Agonistic Behavior (as a Proportion (%) of Total Behavior) as a Consequence of the Introduction of a Stranger into a Group of Captive Monkeys

Response	Baseline	Period following introduction			
		First 20 minutes	24 Hours	48 Hours	168 Hours[a]
Prosocial behavior					
Contact or huddle	3.4	0.5	2.5	5.5	10.3
Groom	8.4	0.9	9.1	4.0	17.6
Agonistic behavior					
Threat	—[b]	2.7	0.5	0.1	0.8
Chase	—	2.2	0.2	0.1	0.6
Fight	—	11.1	0.1	—	—
Fear (expression)	—	0.5	0.1	—	0.4
Scream	—	2.8	—	—	—

(After Bernstein, 1964)

[a]Observations in the last column were made 168 hours after the introduction of the last of a succession of strangers, all of which remained with the group after introduction.

[b]An entry of (—) indicates a value of less than one half of one percent, as in the original table.

Subsequent to the above study, Bernstein reported on various group formation techniques—(1) successive introductions of individuals into established groups, (2) simultaneous release of all individuals involved, (3) the introduction of an established group to another established group—for a variety of nonhuman primate species (pigtail macaques: Bernstein, 1969; mangabeys: Bernstein, 1971; and, again, rhesus monkeys: Bernstein, Gordon, & Rose, 1974; and see also Scruton & Herbert, 1972, and Southwick, 1969). The temporal patterns of xenophobia in all these studies were pretty much the same. Aggression between strangers occurred quickly and then declined over later observations, presumably due to increases in predictability and control between individuals as they became familiar with one another.

By accident, almost, Bernstein et al. (1974) discovered what could result when high rates of aggression do *not* show such declines over time. They formed one group (#3 in their article) by the simultaneous introduction of ten adult rhesus (four male, six female) with no known prior contact. The authors had reason to expect that group formation under these circumstances might be relatively nonviolent, because of an earlier report on the advantages of this particular method (Bernstein, 1964). Unfortunately, things did not work out so well for the ten animals in the 1974 experiment. As usual, rates of aggression were high when the animals first encountered one another, but for some reason the anticipated decline did not occur, with a grim result:

> The high contact aggression scores and the failure of aggressive interactions to decline continued over the next several days. All hopes of stabilizing the group were abandoned as the animals died one by one as a direct or indirect consequence of prolonged serious fighting. The experiment was terminated after the sixth mortality (p. 88).

Social Template in Xenophobia

Despite the capacity of nonhuman primates for violent xenophobic behavior, it was noted in an earlier section that when Southwick et al. (1974) introduced *infant* strangers to established groups, these young animals usually were not met with aggression but rather with parental care. Similar observations are on record elsewhere (Bernstein, 1971). Why were strange infants not attacked like older strangers were? I submit that a solution to this puzzle comes from a consideration of the social hierarchies of the groups under consideration. For a prototype of such a structure we can return to Figure 1-1. Without too much simplification, it can be said of the hierarchy recorded by Deag (1977) that it was headed by adult and subadult males, followed by adult and subadult females, followed by juveniles, followed by infants, with a certain amount of overlap at the margins of any two contiguous (with respect to rank) subgroups.

In a sense, then, there are up to four more or less distinct hierarchies within the total structure seen in Figure 1-1. If we go back to the assumption that monkeys *strive* for dominance (and Deag and others think they do), it follows that any given animal might be most concerned (anthropomorphically speaking) about the predictability and control of specific others within its own age/sex classification. I would wager that juvenile males, for instance, would feel little inclination to seriously challenge the adult males or females in their group, at least not after the first time this sort of foolhardy move was attempted. I would also make this bet in cases in which the adult females are considered vis-à-vis the adult males. The adult males, for their part, are probably not concerned about the female or juvenile hierarchies since virtually all the individuals in these categories will always be subordinate to the males regardless of their status within their respective hierarchies. On the other hand, any given animal is likely to be extremely attentive to its relative position within its own age/sex classification since one's rank—or change in rank—is central in determining the nature (quality) of the social life of that individual.

If the above formulation has merit, it could be used to predict differential reactions among members of a mixed troop of monkeys (consisting of males, females, and juveniles) to strangers or intruders having particular age/sex characteristics, including infants. The prediction would be that there might generally be a correspondence between the attacker and the animal it attacks. A test of this hypothesis would be relatively straightfoward: Simply establish a mixed group in captivity, then successively introduce strangers of the three main age/sex categories and carefully record who aggresses against whom.

This is exactly what Southwick (1969) did. He established a mixed group of rhesus in a large enclosure in Calcutta, then in a varied sequence added male, female, and juvenile strangers. The results of this procedure can be seen in Table 1-3. Sure enough, strangers within particular age/sex classifications received a majority of attacks from their age/sex counterparts in the established group. Southwick labeled this pattern of aggression a "social template," which is a useful shorthand for describing the pattern seen in Table 1-3.

Although the social template is not always observed in cases of xenophobia (see Southwick et al., 1974), it has been recorded in enough places to raise one's confidence in its validity. For example, when Bernstein (1969) introduced two unfamiliar groups to each other, he found that "the two groups formed facing lines with adult and adolescent males clustered together. Adult females faced adult females and juveniles faced juveniles" (p. 10). Given this analysis, one could argue that strange infants would not be attacked by juveniles, females, or males because the babies present no challenge to the status of the individuals in any of these categories. So why bother to attack them?

Table 1-3. Percent (%) Attacks Initiated by Resident Males, Females, and Juveniles on Strange Males, Females, and Juveniles: The Social Template

Age/sex classification of resident	Age/sex classification of stranger		
	Adult male	Adult female	Juvenile
Adult male	80.2	2.8	3.5
Adult female	3.7	66.2	41.2
Juvenile	16.1	31.0	55.3
Total attacks on stranger (%)	100.0	100.0	100.0

(After Southwick, 1969)

The Strangeness of Strangers

Marler (1976) provides an increasingly qualified list of features of "external situations especially liable to provoke aggression" (p. 242):

1. Proximity of an animal.
2. Of one's own kind.
3. A stranger.
4. Behaving aggressively.
5. Inflicting pain.
6. Or otherwise creating frustration.

We have seen that xenophobia as a form of aggression requires only the first three features in this list, and sometimes the aspects of age and sex as well. But what makes for "strangeness" in a strange animal? Deag (1977) was doubtless correct when, as quoted earlier, he asserted that fighting among strangers can result in the formation of the predictable relationships that make up a hierarchy. The probable scenario is that one or both opponents attempt to assert dominance, and that once one of the animals is forced into submission, the conditions of predictability and control are established and the relationship can approach tolerance, if not amicability. Indeed, this scenario fits most of the data that are available from the group-formation literature. It is known that strangers who submit quickly usually receive less abuse than those who attack or retaliate (Bernstein, 1964, p. 62).

Still, there are aspects of xenophobia in nonhuman primates that are not captured by this analysis, because even in the brief review provided above we have encountered major exceptions. Recall the quote from Southwick et al. (1974) regarding the released female in the Chhatair area who was savagely attacked while actually cowering on the ground. Further, male submission and female sexual solicitation were frequent in Bernstein et al.'s (1974) Group #3, but these responses did not prevent the ultimate deaths due to fighting of more than half the group's original members. Exceptions such as these suggest that simple or gross submission may not guarantee the feeling of predictability and control in dominant animals that keeps them from attacking the strange one.

Fortunately, there are clues as to what else might be involved in the evocation of attacks by group members. Southwick et al. (1974) provide a hint in their description of the behavior of certain strangers upon being released in the vicinity of a group. Their impression was that "the aggressive response of the group was very rapid, almost instantaneous, if the stranger cowered with alarm or distress reactions upon release and was then spotted by an aggressive individual," and that "sometimes this recognition was evident by the awkward behavior and fright responses of the introduced animal" (p. 203). To put it in a way that was used earlier, intruders may have the *triple* disadvantage of being strangers in a strange land who may also *behave* strangely. One is tempted to suggest a mathematical model wherein the xenophobic effects of a stranger's sheer physical appearance are perhaps multiplied by its relatively bizarre fear behavior on the occasion.

Anecdotes seem to bear out this contention. First, Bernstein (1969) reports three distinct styles of reaction on the part of certain strangers in his study of pigtail macaques: (1) avoidance and attempts to escape, (2) vigorous defense, and (3) attempts to initiate play or grooming with some of the residents. According to Bernstein (p. 9), "The last named pattern was most successful in that these animals sustained the fewest injuries." In other words, the more "normal" the behavior on the part of the pigtail stranger, the less violent were the xenophobic reactions of the residents.

Second, an even more fascinating account of the consequences of bizarre or unusual behavior comes from van Lawick-Goodall's (1968) description of the fate of several unfortunate members of a chimpanzee society whose behavior suddenly *became* strange:

> Once, aggression was apparently stimulated by fear of injured conspecifics. This was observed during the epidemic which paralysed the limbs of some chimpanzees in 1966. Three mature males all displayed violently at the old male who had lost the use of both legs. One of them actually attacked him, stamping on his back and half rolling him over as he cowered on the ground. A second, when the sick male was in a nest high in a tree, shook the branches violently, hitting the victim on many occasions, until the latter was shaken out of his nest. Two young mature males, who both lost the use of one arm, were repeatedly subjected to quite violent attacks by other adolescent and mature males for the first few weeks after their affliction. That the aggression, in the above examples, was initially motivated by fear, is suggested by the fact that most of the chimpanzees, when they first saw the victims, showed immediate hair erection, and ran to embrace or pat each other with 'grinning' expressions [a form of reassurance]. Why the two young males were attacked again and again was not clear (p. 279).

Although we have compassion for the crippled animals here, we can speculate that they were attacked "again and again" because their relatively abnormal behavior continued to elicit xenophobic reactions on the part of the other chimps. This possibility seems consistent with a similar incident involving free-living mountain gorillas observed by Fossey (1983). In that field study, a young female named Quince contracted malaria, and with increasingly weakened and usual behavior became the target for more and more aggression from other group members. Because the dying animal had always been a gentle individual, her ultimate treatment at the hands of fellow members seemed surprising, and prompted Fossey to argue:

> The weaker Quince became, the more persistent the attempts of the others who were unable to evoke customary conventional reactions from her. In my opinion the concept of "cruelty" could not be ascribed to the treatment Quince received because both her "attackers" and she were acting anomalously during the terminal stages of her illness (p. 101).

Conclusion, Generalization, and Speculation

In this chapter I have tried to establish the importance of predictability and control in nonhuman relationships in connection with patterns of dominance and xenophobic reactions. How far do these ideas and data generalize to the human condition? The answer is that it depends on one's definition of the term "generalize." According to my *Webster's Seventh New Collegiate Dictionary*, one definition of *generalize* is "to give general applicability to" (a law of nature, for example). This is the meaning most social psychologists seem to have in mind when they attempt to extend an interpretation based on a controlled set of conditions (such as in a laboratory) to an uncontrolled set of conditions (such as exist in the real world). In this manner, one infers or extrapolates. But another definition of *generalize* is "to derive or induce (a general conception or principle) from particulars." Here, one is not involved in extension, extrapolation, or inference, because actual points of comparison are available; that is, there are particulars.

Obviously, engaging in either the first or second form of generalization depends entirely on how much data are available. Because, with rare exceptions, social scientists are unable to experiment powerfully in the real world, they are dependent on extensions and extrapolations from the results of their laboratory manipulations (the first meaning of generalize), and, within the bounds of common sense, are therefore warranted in generalizing those findings to our society and culture. Unfortunately, this first form of generalization has historically resulted in many questionable "truths" in comparative psychology and ethology. Depending on what kind of hard data are missing (human or nonhuman), writers can all too easily fall into the trap of anthropomorphism or, in more recent trends, zoomorphism.[4] This is evident in the cases of certain popularizers such as Ardrey (*African Genesis*), Lorenz (*On Aggression*), and Morris (*The Naked Ape*).

Therefore, in comparative psychology one should insist on the second form of generalization noted above. Scientists who aspire to meaningfully compare similar human and nonhuman behavior must base their derivations or inductions on particulars. General concepts or principles have to be based on valid findings from both human and nonhuman sources. Of course, this immediately brings us back to a consideration of homologies, analogies, and animal models in comparative social psychology, for these are the very classes of generalizing concepts available to us.

Using the second form of generalization, I have elsewhere convinced myself that homologies exist between aspects of human and nonhuman dominance behavior (see Rajecki & Flanery, 1981), and that analogies exist in the phenomenon of infant social attachment across a variety of species, including

---

[4]Anthropomorphism involves explaining animal behavior in human terms: "The bitch loves her puppies." Zoomorphism involves explaining human behavior in animal terms: "The mother has a maternal instinct."

humans (see Rajecki, Lamb, & Obmascher, 1978). In terms of one of our current topics—xenophobia—I have already made tentative arguments that certain aspects of this phenomenon may be biologically or psychologically analogous in certain fish, birds, rodents, primates, and humans, principally in terms of the time-dependent profiles described above (see Rajecki, 1983). If homologies or analogies can thus be established, then something fundamental about human nature is revealed.

But even in the unlikely event that these alleged homologies and analogies are eventually discredited, the study of nonhuman behavior, and particularly that of primates, would still be of great value in the development of animal models of human behavior. One should further not lose sight of the intrinsic worth of such information. Still, I have a hunch that with continued study the similarities in xenophobia across humans and nonhumans will become clearer and clearer, until someday the homologous nature of this behavior will be undeniable. Predictability and control—based on dominance or some other factor—are surely involved in compatible and incompatible human relations, and information from animal behavior can only increase our understanding of these matters.

Having said all of this about rigorous rules or restrictions in comparing behavior across species, the temptation remains to make quick comparisons, even if they may seem uncritical or facile. Here I will indulge myself in yielding to this temptation briefly. At present it is not altogether clear if the subjective sense of predictability and control in nonhuman social situations is in any way equivalent to our human experience of such conditions. Even so, I would wager that in subsequent chapters of this book the reader will encounter many accounts of compatible and incompatible relationships that hinge on the same two concepts. In the human domain, predictability and control must surely be involved in the total life-span picture: Parent-infant interactions, sibling relations, children's peer relationships, dating patterns, marital relationships, and all the rest depend in part on how well we are able to mesh our behavior with others, and on the degree to which we can anticipate one another's actions and demands.

This speculation is borne out in the next chapter, "Compatibility in Parent-Infant Relationships: Origins and Processes" (this volume). The authors, Lamb and Gilbride, speak to the development of *in*compatible parent-infant relationships, which sometime lead to the extremes of child abuse. Predictability on the part of *both* parent and child are apparently critical here. With respect to the parent, for example:

> If . . . a parent persistently fails to perceive the infant's distress until it has reached high intensity, and then either selects an inappropriate response or implements an appropriate response poorly, incompatibility is likely to result. In such circumstances, the infant learns that the parent's behavior is neither predictable nor responsive to his or her immediate needs, and consequently, that the parent cannot be relied on as a source of comfort or security. The pattern of interaction that develops is asynchronous in that there is poor intermeshing of parent and infant behaviors (p. 36).

With respect to the infant, for example:

> Socially competent infants, who provide parents with clear signals, behave in a
> predictable fashion, and respond promptly to adult stimulation, foster smooth
> reciprocal interactions in which both parents and infants develop feelings of
> efficacy. . . . By contrast, when infants are unpredictable, unreadable, and
> unresponsive, parents may be "trapped" in cycles of ineffective interaction
> because their feelings of failure predominate. Such "incompetent dyads"
> constitute incompatible relationships in the absence of attempts to compensate
> for the infants' limited skills (p. 44).

Of course, the behavior involved in a human parent-infant interaction bears very little similarity to that between two mature monkeys in a troop. Nevertheless, it is hard to deny that these two cases have something in common. That commonality is that the participants in these relationships might view one another as intolerable, tolerable, or even attractive as a consequence of the amount of predictability or control they experience in the social situation. As noted earlier, it will be fascinating to learn how much of this commonality is due to our genetic or evolutionary relatedness to our nonhuman counterparts.

Acknowledgments. Parts of this chapter were based on an unpublished manuscript ("Xenophobia") written by David R. Nerenz and me while at the University of Wisconsin in 1979.

References

Abramovitch, R., & Strayer, F. (1978). Preschool social organization: Agonistic, spacing, and attentional behaviors. In L. Krames, P. Pliner, & T. Alloway (Eds.), *Aggression, dominance, and individual spacing.* New York: Plenum Press.

Allport, G. W. (1937). *Personality: A psychological interpretation.* New York: Henry Holt.

Ardrey, R. (1967). *African genesis.* New York: Dell.

Atz, J. W. (1970). The application of the idea of homology to behavior. In L. R. Aronson, E. Tobach, D. S. Lehrman, & J. S. Rosenblatt (Eds.), *Development and evolution of behavior.* San Francisco: W. H. Freeman.

Austin, W. T., & Bates, F. L. (1974). Ethological indicators of dominance and territory in a human captive population. *Social Forces, 52,* 447–455.

Barnett, S. A., Hocking, W. E., Munro, K. M. H., & Walker, K. Z. (1975). Socially induced renal pathology of captive wild rats (*Rattus villosissimus*). *Aggressive Behavior, 1,* 123–133.

Benjamin, L. S. (1974). Structural analysis of social behavior. *Psychological Review, 81,* 392–425.

Benjamin, L. S. (1977). Structural analysis of a family in therapy. *Journal of Consulting and Clinical Psychology, 45,* 391–406.

Bernstein, I. S. (1964). The integration of rhesus monkeys introduced to a group. *Folia Primatologica, 2,* 50–63.

Bernstein, I. S. (1969). Introductory techniques in the formation of pigtail monkey troops. *Folia Primatologica, 10,* 1–19.

Bernstein, I. S. (1971). The influence of introductory techniques on the formation of captive mangabey groups. *Primates, 12*, 33–44.

Bernstein, I. S., Gordon, T. P., & Rose, R. M. (1974). Aggression and social controls in rhesus monkey (*Macaca mulatta*) groups revealed in group formation studies. *Folia Primatologica, 21*, 81–107.

Bronson, F. H., & Eleftheriou, B. E. (1965). Adrenal response to fighting in mice: Separation of physcial and psychological causes. *Science, 147*, 627–628.

Campos, J. J., Emde, R. N., Gaensbauer, T., & Henderson, C. (1975). Cardiac and behavioral interrelationships in the reactions of infants to strangers. *Developmental Psychology, 11*, 589–601.

Candland, D. K., Bryan, D. C. Nazar, B. L., Kopf, K. J., & Sendor, M. (1970). Squirrel monkey heart rate during formation of status orders. *Journal of Comparative and Physiological Psychology, 70*, 417–423.

Candland, D. K., Taylor, D. B., Dresdale, L., Leiphart, J. M., & Solow, S. (1969). Heart rate, aggression, and dominance in the domestic chicken. *Journal of Comparative and Physiological Psychology, 67*, 70–76.

Chance, M. R. A. (1976). Attention structure as the basis of primate rank orders. In M. R. A. Chance & R. R. Larsen (Eds.), *The social structure of attention*. New York: Wiley.

Christopher, S. B. (1972). Social validation of an objective measure of social dominance in captive monkeys. *Behavior Research Methods and Instrumentation, 4*, 19–20.

Corson, S. S., Corson, E. O., Arnold, L. E., & Knopp, W. (1976). Animal models of violence and hyperkinesis: Interaction of psychopharmacological and psychosocial therapy in behavior modification. In G. Serban & A. Kling (Eds.), *Animal models in human psychobiology*. New York: Plenum Press.

Deag, J. M. (1977). Aggression and submission in monkey societies. *Animal Behaviour, 25*, 465–474.

Deutsch, R. D., Esser, A. H., & Sossin, K. M. (1978). Dominance, aggression, and the use of space in institutionalized female adolescents. *Aggressive Behavior, 4*, 313–329.

Eibl-Eibesfeldt, I. (1983). The comparative approach in human ethology. In D. W. Rajecki (Ed.), *Comparing behavior: Studying man studying animals*. Hillsdale, NJ: Lawrence Erlbaum Associates.

Fossey, D. (1983). *Gorillas in the mist*. Boston: Houghton Mifflin.

Glass, D. C., & Singer, J. E. (1972). *Urban Stress*. New York: Academic Press.

Goldberg, A. M., & Welch, B. L. (1972). Adaptation of the adrenal medulla: Sustained increase in choline acetyltransferase by psychosocial stimulation. *Science, 178*, 319–320.

Griffin, D. R. (1976). *The question of animal awareness*. New York: Rockefeller University Press.

Hall, K. R. L. (1962). Behaviour of monkeys towards mirror-images. *Nature, 196*, 1258–1261.

Henry, J. P., Meehan, J. P., & Stephens, P. M. (1967). The use of psychosocial stimuli to induce prolonged systolic hypertension in mice. *Psychosomatic Medicine, 29*, 408–432.

Hodos, W., & Campbell, C. B. G. (1969). *Scala Naturae*: Why there is no theory in comparative psychology. *Psychological Review, 76*, 337–350.

Lalljee, M., & Cook, M. (1973). Uncertainty in first encounters. *Journal of Personality and Social Psychology, 26*, 137–141.

Langer, E. J., & Rodin, J. (1976). The effects of choice and enhanced personal responsibility for the aged: A field experiment in an institutional setting. *Journal of Personality and Social Psychology, 34*, 191–198.

Lockard, R. B. (1971). Reflections on the fall of comparative psychology: Is there a message for us all? *American Psychologist, 26*, 168–179.

Lorenz, K. (1967). *On aggression.* New York: Bantam.

Luciano, D., & Lore, R. (1975). Aggression and social experience in domesticated rats. *Journal of Comparative and Physiological Psychology, 88,* 917–923.

Marler, P. (1976). On animal aggression. *American Psychologist, 31,* 239–246.

Morris, D. (1967). *The naked ape.* New York: McGraw-Hill.

Omark, D., Strayer, F. F., & Freedman, D. G. (Eds.). (1980). *Dominance relations.* New York: Garland STMP Press.

Perlmuter, L. C., & Monty, R. A. (1977). The importance of perceived control: Fact or fantasy? *American Scientist, 65,* 759–765.

Rajecki, D. W. (1983). Animal aggression: Implications for human aggression. In R. G. Geen & E. I. Donnerstein (Eds.), *Aggression: Theoretical and empirical reviews: Vol. 1.* New York: Academic Press.

Rajecki, D. W., & Flanery, R. C. (1981). Social conflict and dominance in children: A case for a primate homology. In M. E. Lamb & A. L. Brown (Eds.), *Advances in developmental psychology: Vol. 1.* Hillsdale, NJ: Lawrence Erlbaum Associates.

Rajecki, D. W., Lamb, M. E., & Obmascher, P. (1978). Toward a general theory of infantile attachment: A comparative review of aspects of the social bond. *Behavioral and Brain Sciences, 1,* 417–464.

Roitblat, H. L. (1982). The meaning of representation in animal memory. *Behavioral and Brain Sciences, 5,* 353–406.

Rose, R. M., Bernstein, I. S., & Gordon, T. P. (1978). Consequences of social conflict on plasma testosterone levels in rhesus monkeys. *Psychosomatic Medicine, 40,* 60–70.

Rosenblum, L. A., Levy, E. J., & Kaufman, I. C. (1968). Social behaviour of squirrel monkeys and the reaction to strangers. *Animal Behaviour, 16,* 288–293.

Rowell, T. E. (1974). The concept of social dominance. *Behavioral Biology, 11,* 131–154.

Savin-Williams, R. C. (1976). An ethological study of dominance formation and maintenance in a group of human adolescents. *Child Development, 47,* 972–979.

Savin-Williams, R. C. (1977). Dominance in a human adolescent group. *Animal Behaviour, 25,* 400–406.

Savin-Williams, R. C. (1979). Dominance hierarchies in groups of early adolescents. *Child Development, 50,* 923–935.

Schulz, R. (1976). Effects of control and predictability on the physical and psychological well-being of the institutionalized aged. *Journal of Personality and Social Psychology, 33,* 563–573.

Scruton, D. M., & Herbert, J. (1972). The reaction of groups of talapoin monkeys to the introduction of male and female strangers of the same species. *Animal Behaviour, 20,* 463–473.

Seligman, M. E. P. (1975). *Helplessness: On depression, development, and death.* San Francisco: W. H. Freeman.

Siegel, H. S., & Siegel, P. B. (1961). The relationship of social competition with endocrine weights and activity in male chickens. *Animal Behaviour, 9,* 151–158.

Sober, E. (1983). Mentalism and behaviorism in comparative psychology. In D. W. Rajecki (Ed.), *Comparing behavior: Studying man studying animals:* Hillsdale, NJ: Lawrence Erlbaum Associates.

Southwick, C. H. (1964). *Peromyscus leucopus*: An interesting subject for studies of socially induced stress. *Science, 143,* 55–56.

Southwick, C. H. (1969). Aggressive behaviour of rhesus monkeys in natural and captive groups. In S. Garattini & E. B. Sigg (Eds.), *Aggressive behaviour.* New York: Wiley.

Southwick, C. H., Siddiqi, M. F., Farooqui, M. Y., & Pal, B. C. (1974). Xenophobia among free-ranging rhesus groups in India. In R. L. Holloway (Ed.), *Primate aggression, territoriality, and xenophobia.* New York: Academic Press.

Strayer, F. F., & Strayer, J. (1976). An ethological analysis of social agonism and dominance relations among preschool children. *Child Development*, *47*, 980–989.

Suomi, S. J., & Immelmann, K. (1983). On the process and product of cross-species generalization. In D. W. Rajecki (Ed.), *Comparing behavior: Studying man studying animals*. Hillsdale, NJ: Lawrence Erlbaum Associates.

Syme, G. J., & Syme, L. A. (1979). *Social structure in farm animals*. New York: Elsevier.

Telle, H.-J. (1966). Bietrag zur Kenntnis der Verhaltenweise von Ratten, vergleichend dargestellt bei *Rattus norvegicus* und *Rattus rattus*. *Zeitschrift fur angewandte Zoologie*, *53*, 129–196. (Available in English as Technical Translation 1608, Translation Section, National Science Library, National Research Council of Canada, Ottawa, Ontario, Canada.)

van Lawick-Goodall, J. (1968). The behaviour of free-living chimpanzees in the Gombe Stream Reserve. *Animal Behaviour Monographs*, *1*, 161–311.

Washburn, S. L. & Avis, V. (1958). Evolution of human behavior. In A. Roe & G. G. Simpson (Eds.), *Behavior and evolution*. New Haven: Yale University Press.

Wickler, W. (1967). Socio-sexual signals and their intra-specific imitation among primates. In D. Morris (Ed.), *Primate ethology*. Chicago: Aldine.

Wilson, E. O. (1975). *Sociobiology*. Cambridge, MA: Belknap Press.

Zivin, G. (1983). Hybrid models: Modifications in models of social behavior that are borrowed across species and up evolutionary grades. In D. W. Rajecki (Ed.), *Comparing behavior: Studying man studying animals*. Hillsdale, NJ: Lawrence Erlbaum Associates.

Chapter 2

Compatibility in Parent-Infant Relationships: Origins and Processes

Michael E. Lamb and Kathleen E. Gilbride

Developmental and clinical theorists have long been interested in the compatibility or incompatibility of infant-parent (usually, infant-mother) relationships. Ever since the first part of this century, when Freud turned attention to early experiences (see Freud, 1940, for a summary of this position), psychoanalysts and their successors have emphasized the formative significance of the infant-caretaker relationship (see Maccoby and Masters, 1970, for a review). Initially, researchers were chiefly concerned with identification of normative trends and processes (Bowlby, 1969; Rajecki, Lamb, & Obmascher, 1978), but over time they came to recognize the importance of individual differences, and this led to a focus on the compatibility or incompatibility of specific relationships (Ainsworth, Blehar, Waters, & Wall, 1978). As consensus emerged regarding the normative trends and processes—if not concerning their interpretation—so the relative amount of attention paid to individual differences increased to the point that the vast majority of studies concerned with parent-infant relationships now focus on individual differences (Lamb, Thompson, Gardner, Charnov, & Estes, 1984).

Nevertheless, theorists have only recently come to view individual differences in terms of the compatibility or incompatibility of relationships. Consistent with the traditional environmentalist orientation of American behavioral science, the emphasis was initially on maternal characteristics as determinants of variations in the child's development. Within the last decade, this unidirectional focus has been criticized roundly, and both theorists and researchers have come to recognize that influence patterns are usually bidirectional (Bell & Harper, 1977; Chess & Thomas, 1977; Lewis & Rosenblum, 1974). In a further elaboration of this view, many developmental psychologists have adopted a "transactional" perspective, in terms of which the initial characteristics of both adult and infant are believed to shape the course of their interaction as well as the way in which both are affected by their interaction (Sameroff & Chandler, 1975). The assumption is that each individual is affected by each interaction that he or she experiences, and so enters future encounters with slightly different characteristics. The challenge for researchers and theorists alike is to move beyond this truism to researchable hypotheses about the characteristics that are important and the processes by means of which change takes place. Identification of these characteristics and illustration of how these processes influence parent-infant compatibility are the foci of the present chapter.

First, we present a general view of the infant-parent relationship and of the ways in which the quality of interactions or relationships is likely to be affected by the personalities and circumstances of the partners. With this as a background, we then review the factors that we believe to be important determinants of interactional quality and thus of relationship compatibility. We focus on parental characteristics, infant characteristics, and aspects of the dyads' social circumstances (both intra- and extrafamilial). We also speculate about the ways in which these diverse factors interact with one another so as to shape the process or course of interaction. Both characteristics and processes are then illustrated more concretely in the third section, where our focus is on extreme incompatibility of relationships, as defined by the occurrence of child abuse and neglect. Because child maltreatment is popularly viewed as a manifestation of parental incompetence, evidence that the origins are broader and more complex than this is especially persuasive in strengthening the credibility of the general model we present. In the final section, we summarize our perspective and suggest fruitful directions for future research and theorizing. It will be distressingly clear to readers that the available evidence is suggestive at best and totally lacking at worst, so our goal in this chapter is to provide a heuristic synthesis of the available literature in hopes of stimulating further programmatic research.

The Dynamics and Ontogeny of Parent-Infant Interaction

In this chapter, we discuss a number of factors that are likely to affect the quality or compatibility of infant-parent relationships. Before doing so, however, we must first describe the dynamics of compatible infant-parent relationships and then explain *how* the factors discussed later are likely to be influential.

An examination of the interaction that occurs between infants and parents reveals that it is unlike that observed in any other human relationship. When interacting with infants, parents make extensive use of behaviors that are exaggerated variations of the behaviors they employ in other social contexts (Stern, 1974). For example, parents comonly speak to their infants in high-pitched tones and with brief, repetitive utterances, and they employ exaggerated facial expressions, prolonged gazes, and multiple pauses. Stern (1977) suggests that such behaviors are well adapted to the range of stimuli to which infants are most responsive. The exaggerated social behaviors compensate for the infants' limited physical and cognitive abilities and are effective in eliciting and maintaining social responsiveness (e.g., smiles and coos) in infants. Although infants initially have less sophisticated social skills than adults do, they are surprisingly capable partners. They shape social interaction by orienting and responding selectively to social stimulation, actively soliciting stimulation, and withdrawing when overstimulated. As a result, the interaction develops a cyclical nature in which periods of excitement and delight alternate with quiet, less intense periods during which the infants withdraw from stimulation.

Over the first few months, the way in which infant and parent interact becomes individualized and a unique style emerges. The intermeshing of parent and infant behaviors into a characteristic pattern of interaction has been described by Stern (1977) as a joint choreography because both partners play a role in regulating the quality, amount, and timing of behaviors in an attempt to maintain an optimal level of stimulation. As the infant grows older, he or she develops increasingly sophisticated means of monitoring and shaping interaction, and truly reciprocal interchanges result.

After gaining the infant's attention, for example, a father will smile with widened eyes and begin talking in a high-pitched voice to maintain the attention of and elicit a response from the infant. Delightedly, the infant smiles and coos in return, causing the father to pause momentarily before speaking again in animated fashion and moving his face closer to the infant's. She responds by chuckling and bouncing excitedly. Father moves in still closer, his face still exaggeratedly expressive, his speech again repetitive and high-pitched. At this point, the infant may avert her gaze and turn her head slightly away. In response, the father relaxes his posture and withdraws somewhat, waiting until the infant returns her gaze and signals a readiness to play again.

In this example we can see that both parent and infant adjust their behavior in response to the other's cues. The resulting "choreography" is marked by shared pleasure, interest, delight, and surprise—all positive reinforcers that lead the participants to seek out such interactions frequently. These interactions typically end when the stimulation becomes too great for the infant. By varying the stimulation in accordance with the infant's cycles of attention and withdrawal, and by continuing or terminating the interaction when appropriate, the parent can maintain interactions within a narrow, optimal range. Such interactions depend on a system of mutual feedback in which parent and infant provide each other with cues to help regulate the course of the interactions (Brazelton, Koslowski, & Main, 1974; Stern, 1977).

Obviously, there are individual differences in the clarity of these cues and in the partners' abilities to interpret them and respond appropriately. In some dyads, such abated interactions are rare, while in others they become normative. As a result, the degree of intermeshedness varies, with some dyads characterized by discordance and asynchrony. The partners' (and especially the parent's) ability to be flexible when an interaction fails is important since it helps determine whether the pattern will become characteristically asynchronous and discordant.

The defining feature of a compatible infant-parent relationship, we propose, is that the behavior of the two individuals be well meshed, and thus, that the partners be able to communicate efficiently and accurately. This means that each party must be able to "read" the behavior and signals of the other *and* be capable of emitting clear and unambiguous signals to the other. Implicit here is the assumption that compatible relationships are characterized by reciprocity, which is developed and refined as each partner learns to interpret and respond appropriately to the other's behavior.

A key determinant of relationship compatibility appears to be "parental sensitivity." Parental sensitivity refers to the adult's ability to provide contingent, appropriate, and consistent responses to the infant's signals or needs (Lamb & Easterbrooks, 1981). Operationally, this implies that the parent must be able to perceive the infant's signals or needs, interpret them accurately, select appropriate responses, and implement them effectively. Obviously, therefore, the characteristics of both parties affect parental sensitivity, as the clarity of the infant's signals helps determine how easily they can be perceived and interpreted. The *parents'* abilities play a crucial role in the establishment of compatible relationships, however, because although infants can both initiate interaction with and respond to them, maintenance of smooth interaction is initially the responsibility of the parents, who must accurately "read" the infants and respond in a manner that complements their behavior.

By responding sensitively, parents demonstrate to infants that the infants' behaviors have predictable consequences, and these repeated demonstrations foster the development of a sense of perceived personal effectance (Lamb, 1981). In addition, sensitively responsive parents teach infants that they are trustworthy and can be counted on to be available (psychologically and physically) when needed. Infants whose caretakers are nurturant and respond contingently to their needs seem more likely to form secure (compatible) attachment relationships to their caretakers than infants whose parents are insensitive, unresponsive, or unpredictable (Ainsworth, 1973; Ainsworth et al., 1978; Lamb et al., 1984).

Insensitive responding can result from deviations occurring at any point in the perceive-interpret-select-implement sequence of response mediation, and the effects of insensitivity on the enduring quality of the relationship will depend on the extent to which it is characteristic of the dyadic interaction. If, for example, a parent persistently fails to perceive the infant's distress until it has reached high intensity, and then either selects an inappropriate response or implements an appropriate response poorly, incompatibility is likely to result. In such circumstances, the infant learns that the parent's behavior is neither predictable nor responsive to his or her immediate needs, and consequently, that the parent cannot be relied on as a source of comfort or security. The pattern of interaction that develops is asynchronous in that there is poor intermeshing of parent and infant behaviors. Thus, variations in the perceived contingency, quality, and consistency of adult responses significantly influence the degree of compatibility in emergent parent-child relationships.

It is important to recognize that although parent-infant interaction involves reciprocity and mutual participation, the bulk of the responsibility for maintaining and guiding interaction initially falls on the parent, who must sensitively appraise the infant's state and interpose appropriate behaviors in the infant's ongoing behavioral stream. Thus, the parent's sensitivity and flexibility plays a major role in enhancing relationship compatibility. The infant's behavioral repertoire is limited and somewhat haphazardly controlled, whereas adults can make major and minor modifications of facial expressions, postures, and vocal tones in order to accommodate and expand upon the infant's "contributions." For example, several researchers have reported that mothers carry on "proto-conversations" with their young infants, incorporating smiles, coos, and burps into the conversations as though they were intentional communicative responses (Bateson, 1975; Bruner, 1977; Snow, 1977). Parents use exaggerated vocal tones and facial expressions to maintain the infants' attention, and often take on the roles of both participants until the infants are able to participate more fully in interaction. Presumably, infants learn about the give-and-take nature of reciprocal social interaction by participation in these proto-conversations.

Parents must also adapt to and incorporate new infantile behaviors into the parent-infant dialogue, and modify their own role as infants become more sophisticated. This, too, demands sensitivity on their part. Thus, parents guide infants' participation in task-oriented interaction by interpreting cues from the infant to determine at what pace to proceed, when to change the stimulation or task, and when to terminate the interaction (Kaye, 1982; Rogoff, in press; Rogoff, Gilbride, & Malkin, 1983). As the infant's competence increases, the parent withdraws from total control of the situation and allows the infant to take more responsibility. With a 6-month-old, for example, an adult may take responsibility for winding up a jack-in-the-box, and interpreting the sudden popping up of Jack as a funny surprise ("He popped up! Isn't that funny?!"). With a 12-month-old, however, the adult allows the infant to help turn the crank, and simply laughs at Jack's sudden appearance, as if sharing the surprise (Rogoff et al., 1983).

All of the factors that will be mentioned in this chapter (including characteristics of the family ecology and circumstances) presumably affect the quality of relationships by affecting the interactants' abilities to read each other's communicative exchanges. Thus, for example, socioeconomic or emotional stress is likely to preoccupy parents so that they fail to attend adequately to their infantile "conversational partners." Temperament or personality may affect the clarity of signals emitted by either party, the persistence of the individuals engaged in conversation or interaction, and their ability to process the other's signals accurately. It may also produce a mismatch between very different behavioral styles. Other characteristics, such as the infant's gender, may have effects on the parent's motivation which vary depending on his or her desires and attitudes.

We need to emphasize that the degree to which relationships are compatible or incompatible may change—and often does change—over time (Thompson &

Lamb, 1984; Thompson, Lamb, & Estes, 1982). Social, economic, and emotional circumstances often change, for example, and as they do so, we would expect the adult to become more or less preoccupied by these and thus less or more available to attend to the interaction. Changes in relationship compatibility, both positive and negative, are likely to follow. Any resulting deleterious effects are likely to be especially marked in early infancy, when the child's relative immaturity and/or temperamental characteristics place much of the burden for maintaining smooth interaction on the parent. As the child grows older, the parent's attitudes and values may change, the child's signals surely become clearer, and the child's characteristics or capacities may become more or less attractive to the parent. Thus, familiarity may breed either contempt or facility with each other's signals. In short, relationships are dynamic, not static, entities, and their quality can change as circumstances change. Our goal here is to explain individual differences in the quality of relationships at any time, and the way in which change or stability is mediated. Explanation and under- standing of these individual differences is important because they may have a significant impact on the child's development, affecting such factors as the security of attachment, social cognition, peer relationships, self-esteem, and achievement motivation (Ainsworth et al., 1978; Lamb et al., 1984; Sroufe, 1983).

Influences on the Compatibility of Infant-Parent Relationships

Many factors influence the compatibility of any given parent-infant relationship and these factors are interrelated in a complex fashion. The complexity is illustrated by the degree of variation observed among dyads as well as within dyads across different situations. Clearly, infants do not come into the world programmed to establish compatible relationships with their parents; the compatibility or incompatibility of parent-infant relationships must evolve through interactions in which the characteristics of the parents adapt to and become intermeshed with those of their infants (and vice versa) across various contexts. We propose that the compatibility or incompatibility of parent-infant dyads is determined jointly by characteristics of the parent, characteristics of the infant, and characteristics of their social situation. In order to demonstrate the way in which these factors operate, we examine the influence of each set of factors in turn. This may give the impression that these sources of influence operate independently, which we consider unlikely. We consider them separately only to facilitate discussion and analysis, and later we will attempt to illustrate the ways in which these factors interact dynamically so as to influence the quality of parent-child relationships.

Parental Contributions to Compatibility

Parental influences on the compatibility of parent-infant dyads can be traced to personality characteristics, attitudes, expectations, history, and role models. All of these factors seem to affect the adult's sensitivity to the infant, which, as mentioned above, is a crucial determinant of relationship compatibility.

One factor affecting the parent's sensitivity is the amount of experience or practice he or she has had interacting with infants in general and with the specific infant in particular. Frequent interaction provides the adult with practice interpreting infant signals and perfecting successful intervention strategies. In addition, through practice adults develop sensitivity to developmental stages and thus learn to modify their behavior according to the infants' age-appropriate capabilities and needs. Thus, one aspect of sensitive parenting is the ability to accommodate to changing circumstances and needs, which means that the specific components of compatible interactions are continually changing as parents adjust their responses and demands to their infants' developmental level.

The role of experience in shaping parent-infant interactions can be illustrated by considering the case of traditional fathers (see Lamb & Easterbrooks, 1981). Fathers are certainly capable of responding sensitively and contingently, as has been shown both by studies of participative fathers who are directly involved in caretaking (Lamb & Goldberg, 1982; Lamb, Frodi, Hwang, & Frodi, 1982) and by studies of new fathers asked to demonstrate their skills (Parke & Sawin, 1980). However, traditional fathers generally appear less sensitive to their infants than mothers do (Nash & Feldman, 1981). These fathers have few opportunities to interact with their infants and so do not gain experience interpreting subtle cues or selecting and implementing appropriate interventions. Involved fathers have more opportunity to learn from their experiences, at least in part because infants provide them with discriminating feedback that helps consolidate and shape their skills. Although other factors (e.g., role definition) certainly affect paternal sensitivity and the compatibility of the relationships developed, experience probably plays a major role.

The likelihood of successful interaction increasing with experience (at least up to a point) is important also because as parents become more skillful in play or caretaking, their sense of efficacy increases. Goldberg (1977, p. 166) refers to this as the "enhancement of competence motivation." Perceived effectiveness reinforces parents and motivates them to seek further interaction. This gives them more experience and more enthusiasm, both factors that are likely to enhance dyadic compatibility.

Personality characteristics also affect the parent's sensitivity and thus can enhance or interfere with the compatibility of relationships. The extent to which the adult is unempathic or self-centered, for example, probably influences his or her ability to perceive infant signals, as well as the contingency and quality of his or her responses, by producing a mismatch between adult desires and infant needs (Lamb & Easterbrooks, 1981). Repeated attempts to play with a sleepy, fussy baby would be an example of insensitive and noncontingent responding by an unempathic adult. Likewise, the parent's stylistic flexibility may also be important, in that it allows them to accommodate the temperament and changing needs of their infant partners. Parental flexibility also enables adults to adapt to new infantile behaviors, incorporating them into the parent-infant dialogue.

As suggested earlier, the adults' attitudes and expectations regarding the parental role may also affect the nature of parent-infant relationships (Goldberg, 1982; Lamb & Easterbrooks, 1981). Parents who value the parental role highly will judge their self-esteem in accordance with their perceived success at meeting the demands of their chosen role. Thus, mothers who view themselves as primary caretakers, responsible for meeting the infant's needs, will invest their attention and energy in caretaking and nurturance; they will accordingly assess their competence as parents depending on their success in these interactions. By contrast, traditional fathers may believe that caretaking is a maternal responsibility, and that their own responsibility is limited essentially to the financial support of the family. As long as these fathers adequately provide for their families, therefore, their sense of efficacy and self-esteem may remain high, even though their relationships with their children may be of poor quality and their interactions limited. In other words, the effects of perceived success or failure in social interaction are likely to vary depending on the parents' role definitions.

Parents have expectations concerning not only their roles but the infants' roles as well (Goldberg, 1977, 1982). Depending on how closely reality accords with these expectations, the parents' sense of effectance may be enhanced or diminished. Consider, for example, mothers who intend to combine motherhood and employment. They may expect their infants to make few demands of their time, making it easy for them to be part-time caretakers and full-time employees. These expectations may be violated, however, either because they were hopelessly unrealistic, or because the infants' health or temperament makes them unusually demanding. Similarly, parents of infants with specific difficulties (e.g., prematurity, blindness, or Down's Syndrome) have to adjust their expectations before effective interactions and compatible relationships can develop (Goldberg, 1979). Incompatibility is likely to result in such situations unless or until the parents' expectations are redefined.

The attitudes and expectations that adults bring to parent-child relationships are often determined by the adults' personal history and prior exposure to significant role models. The role models provided for mothers and fathers clearly differ substantially in most societies, and it is the culturally approved roles that are likely to be learned. Modes of interaction previously learned in the context of other social relationships may also be generalized to the parent-infant relationship. The social and personal characteristics developed by the individual, as well as the amount of child-care experience acquired earlier in life, should thus affect the adult's ability to establish compatible relationships with his or her own children. Belsky and his colleagues (Belsky, Robins, & Gamble, 1984; Belsky, 1980, 1981) emphasize with particular eloquence the need to view parenting in the context of life-span development, with parenting skills being influenced by characteristics of the parent's developmental history. Consistent with this notion, for example, Gamble and Belsky (1982) found that mothers who perceived their parents as warm and affectionate were themselves characterized by positive self-esteem and emotional responsiveness. Belsky also suggests that earlier experiences can influence personal characteristics such as patience, endurance, and commitment to parenting. Likewise, we would expect characteristics such as egocentrism, flexibility, and sensitivity to be influenced by previous social experiences.

Infant Contributions to Compatibility

In the preceding section, we deliberately ignored the effects of infant characteristics on relationship compatibility in order to explore the influence of adult characteristics. As indicated earlier, however, the characteristics of both parties must play a role in shaping the quality of their relationship. We now examine the effects of infant characteristics on individual differences in the compatibility of parent-infant dyads.

Recently, much attention has been given to infant effects on their caretakers, as it is now commonly recognized that infants can and do influence their parents' behavior in a variety of ways (Bell, 1968, 1971; Bell & Harper, 1977; Lewis & Rosenblum, 1974). Infants are able to affect parental behavior from the moment of birth, thanks to innate behavioral capabilities such as crying and smiling that evoke adult attention and intervention (Frodi, Lamb, Leavitt, & Donovan, 1978a; Korner & Thoman, 1972). Crying makes adults approach and pick up distressed infants (Bell & Ainsworth 1972; Frodi et al., 1978a; Murray, 1979), whereas smiling encourages adults to "stay around," continuing the interaction which the infant evidently enjoys so much (Frodi et al., 1978a; Jones & Moss, 1971). Ethological attachment theorists argue that smiling and crying evolved because they promote survival by encouraging protective adults to approach and/or remain near otherwise helpless infants (Ainsworth, 1969, 1973; Bowlby, 1969). In addition to ensuring survival, however, these behavioral predispositions ensure the frequent social interactions that are formatively important for infants.

In addition to initiating interactions and responding to social bids by their parents, infants can effectively modulate the course of interaction by smiling, babbling, changing their facial expressions, and withdrawing attention (Stern, 1977). Smiles and vocalizations serve to elicit increased social stimulation, whereas crying and falling asleep effectively terminate play. Bell (1974) and Stern (1974, 1977) eloquently describe the way in which infants control the level of stimulation they receive by signaling when play has gone on too long or when the adults' bids are too intense.

When they are able to elicit reliable responses from their parents, infants develop a sense of personal effectance comparable to that developed by their parents (Lamb, 1981). Just as parents gain competence in reading and responding to infants through experience, infants gain competence by effectively eliciting specific types of responses from adults.

Although all infants influence social interactions, there are large individual differences among infants that affect the nature of specific parent-infant relationships. Much research has focused on individual differences in behavioral style or temperament (Goldsmith & Campos, 1982; Rothbart, 1981; Thomas, Chess, & Birch, 1968). In the New York Longitudinal Study, for example, Thomas et al. (1968) defined four common temperament styles: difficult, slow to warm up, average, and easy. The difficult infants—defined as those who reacted intensely to stimuli, were frequently negative in mood, irregular in sleeping and eating patterns, and reacted with aversion and slow adaptation to changes in the environment—were considered to be at risk for developing behavioral problems because of their intrinsic characteristics. In fact, however, such problems developed only when the parents were unable to adapt to the children's characteristics; thus, the "goodness of fit" between child and parental characteristics appeared critical.

Nevertheless, children's temperamental characteristics may influence the behavior and expectations of parents, and thus set the tone of parent-child relationships. Consistent with this reasoning, studies suggest that babies who are sluggish and unresponsive following delivery (perhaps due to perinatal anesthesia and analgesia) are later less involved in social interaction with their mothers (Richards, 1975), and have mothers who are less responsive, affectionate, and report more difficulty in caretaking than mothers in comparison groups (Murray, Dolby, Nation, & Thomas, 1981). Murray et al. suggested that the mother's expectations and behaviors were shaped by the initial unresponsiveness of their newborn infants so that when the infants' behavior returned to normal, their mothers continued to behave as if their infants were unresponsive. Innate temperamental differences may affect the compatibility of parent-infant relationships in the same way, making harmonious relationships more difficult to achieve.

Although a number of researchers have suggested that infant temperament helps determine the quality of interaction, and thus affects the security of infant-parent attachment, there is little agreement about the processes involved (Campos, Caplovitz-Barrett, Lamb, Goldsmith, & Stenberg, 1983). One possibility is that difficult infants require greater effort on the part of parents than do easy infants, who are predictable and easy to read. Consequently, in many cases the parents of difficult infants would appear less sensitive, and poor relationships might develop (Lamb, Chase-Lansdale, & Owen, 1979; Lamb & Easterbrooks, 1981). In at least one study this did not seem to be the case, however: Insecurely attached infants were rated as easy more often than difficult, whereas securely attached infants were rated as difficult more often than easy (Owen & Chase-Lansdale, 1982). The authors suggested that difficult infants may demand and receive more time and attention from busy parents than do easy infants, and thus difficult infants have more opportunity to develop secure attachments. Similar associations were not found by Lamb, Hwang, Frodi, and Frodi (1982) or by Thompson and Lamb (1982), however, suggesting that this counter-intuitive association needs further verification before it can be considered reliable.

Another possibility is that some parents are able to compensate for their infants' difficult temperament, whereas others are unable to do so. If this is the case, it would mean that temperament *per se* does not directly affect the attachment relationship, but that it interacts with characteristics of the adult to shape the compatibility or incompatibility of the relationship. This interpretation would be consistent with the findings obtained in the New York Longitudinal Study by Thomas et al. (1968).

Rothbart and Derryberry (1981) and Kagan (1982) also suggest that infant temperament plays an important role in the development of attachment, and that behavior in the "Strange Situation" (the procedure traditionally used to assess the security of infant-adult attachments) reflects temperament more than it reflects security. They propose that temperamental differences in level of reactivity and self-regulatory processes lead infants to respond with varying degrees of distress to apparently similar situations, thus manifesting varying needs for parental intervention. Using the traditional assessment procedure, these differences in infant behavior would be interpreted as differences in the "security of attachment" (i.e., the compatibility of relationships), whereas they may simply reflect differences in infant temperament. For example, some infants may have a low level of reactivity and so may not experience distress when separated and thus not require much maternal intervention. Other infants may have very effective self-regulatory processes that allow them to calm themselves even in stressful situations. These infants would not be less secure, even though they would be classified as such on conventional measures. Likewise, infants who are highly reactive to stress and soothe very slowly because of their high reactivity and poor self-regulatory processes may erroneously be deemed insecure.

Although temperamental differences probably do affect Strange Situation behavior, the argument that security of attachment is simply and entirely an epiphenomena of temperamental differences is contradicted by the repeated demonstration that infants form relationships of different quality to their mothers and fathers (Grossmann, Grossmann, Huber, & Wartner, 1981; Lamb, 1978; Lamb, Hwang, Frodi, & Frodi, 1982; Main & Weston, 1981; Sagi, Lamb, Lewkowicz, Shoham, Dvir, & Estes, in press). Evidently, the effects of infant temperament on parent-infant relationships and on subsequent social development remain unclear. The matter is complicated further because most studies rely on correlational analyses and parental perceptions rather than on "objective" measures of infant temperament. For our purposes, suffice it to say that temperament is one way in which infants help shape relationships with their parents. The specific effects probably vary depending on how the infants' and parents' temperaments intermesh, as well as on the social context in which the parents and infants are embedded. Current research is designed to explore the temporal and cross-situational stability of temperament and the role of temperamental differences in infant development (e.g., Goldsmith & Campos, in press; Rothbart, 1983).

In addition to individual differences in temperament, infants differ in their degree of social competence and in their ability to affect parental competence.

Goldberg (1977) suggests that individual differences in infant social competence can be traced to individual differences along three dimensions: readability, predictability, and responsiveness. Readability refers to the clarity of infant signals and cues. "Easily readable" infants signal their needs, desires, and states of arousal clearly; this facilitates the adults' decisions about how to intervene. Predictability refers to the extent to which the infants' behavior can be anticipated reliably based on an appraisal of the context and of preceding behaviors. Responsiveness refers to the promptness and contingency of reactions to stimulation.

Socially competent infants, who provide parents with clear signals, behave in a predictable fashion, and respond promptly to adult stimulation, foster smooth reciprocal interactions in which both parents and infants develop feelings of efficacy. In addition, predictable, readable, responsive infants may draw unresponsive parents into interaction by instilling feelings of efficacy in them. The greater the infants' social competence, the more effective and competent are adult partners likely to become, and the more compatible is the relationship likely to be.

By contrast, when infants are unpredictable, unreadable, and unresponsive, parents may be "trapped" in cycles of ineffective interaction because their feelings of failure predominate. Such "incompetent dyads" constitute incompatible relationships in the absence of attempts to compensate for the infants' limited skills. Possible compensations will be discussed when we focus on the "fit" between parents and infants in the next section.

Interactions Between Parental and Infantile Influences

Thus far, we have described the separate contributions of parents and infants to dyadic compatibility or incompatibility, but we know that these influences do not operate independently. Each partner's behavior is shaped by feedback from the other. In the best of relationships, responses are contingent upon the other's behavior and are clearly communicated. Of course, the specific behavioral sequences change as infants mature and gain greater control over their own behavior and a greater understanding of the social environment. Parents also become more skilled at reading and predicting their infants as a result of the infants' maturation. As infants become more socially skillful, parents come to expect more sophisticated responses, and so social games become more complex as the parents vary the contingencies required for success (Bruner, 1977). In compatible relationships, therefore, interaction sequences do not become unchanging rituals; they are constantly changing over time.

To the extent that there is predictability in interaction, a sense of mutual efficacy develops that enhances compatibility. The competence that parents and infants produce in each other also constitutes a useful resource in times of stress (Goldberg, 1977). By corollary, a lack of competence within parent-infant dyads generates internal stress and reduces the dyads' ability to cope with external stress. Goldberg predicts that in such situations, parents and infants benefit from interventions aimed at enhancing both the infants' readability, responsiveness, and predictability and the parents' sensitivity.

Even without such interventions, Goldberg (1979, 1982) reports, parents themselves are often able to compensate for the limited skills of their infants. For example, several researchers have shown that mothers of unresponsive, preterm infants work harder to maintain their infants' attention and alertness than mothers of responsive, full-term infants do (Beckwith & Cohen, 1978; Brown & Bakeman, 1979; DiVitto & Goldberg, 1979; Field, 1977). This is an effective strategy for eliciting some interaction with unresponsive infants and thus gaining some degree of perceived effectance, and it may help explain why, when preterm and full-term infants are followed longitudinally, few enduring differences between two groups are found (Brachfeld & Goldberg, 1978; Leiderman & Seashore, 1975; Sameroff & Chandler, 1975).

Goldberg (1979) discusses other examples of the ways in which parents develop strategies to facilitate social interaction with infants whose capacities are limited. For example, parents of blind infants rely on tactile and kinesthetic stimulation to elicit smiles and vocalizations (Fraiberg, 1977). Mothers of Down's syndrome infants come to expect more muted emotional expressions, and to structure and support the interaction more in order to compensate for their infants' low levels of responsivity (Jones, 1980; Sorce & Emde, 1982). Thus, parent-infant compatibility is possible even within "at risk" dyads, provided that parents adjust their behavior, expectations, and attitudes in accordance with the infants' competence and temperament.

Variations in parental and infantile temperament also affect dyadic compatibility (Rothbart & Derryberry, 1981; Thomas, Chess, & Birch, 1970). In some cases, the parents' temperamental characteristics may intermesh well with those of their infants; in others, parents may have to work at achieving a balance between the infants' temperament and their own. Certainly, the resulting degree of "fit" is jointly determined by parental and infant characteristics. Bell (1974) points out that there are probably upper and lower limits of tolerance for the intensity, frequency, and appropriateness of the partners' behavior, with deviations from these limits making incompatibility likely.

Contributions of the Social Environment

That parent-infant relationships do not exist in isolation from the surrounding social context has been increasingly emphasized by developmental researchers (Belsky, 1981; Bronfenbrenner, 1979; Parke & Tinsley, 1982; Sameroff & Chandler, 1975). Sameroff and Chandler (1975) have proposed that child development must be viewed as a "transactional" process in which children and parents not only influence each other but are also responsive to socioecological factors such as socioeconomic status, social support systems, and environmental stresses. Likewise, Bronfenbrenner (1977) has called for a more broadly based approach to the study of development with a focus on the interaction between children, parents, and the changing environments in which they develop.

In response to these appeals for new approaches to the study of child development and parent-child relationships, attempts have been made to consider simultaneously the characteristics of children, parents, and the social environment. Thus, researchers such as Parke (Parke, Power, & Gottman, 1979; Parke & Tinsley, 1982), Pedersen (1980, 1981), Lamb (Lamb & Easterbrooks, 1981; Lamb et al., 1979), and Belsky (1981) have begun to look at child development from a family perspective. In their view, each parent-child dyad must be considered as elements within mother-father-child triads, or even mother-father-firstborn-secondborn tetrads. Influence patterns are multidirectional in that parents affect children, who themselves affect each of the parents as well as the marital relationship, which in turn affects both parents and children.

Building upon this assumption, Belsky (in press; Belsky et al., 1984) has developed a "contextual theory" of parental competence, in which parental functioning is viewed as the product of a multiply determined system. The major components of this system resemble the factors we have considered to be the major determinants of parent-infant compatibility—namely, personal resources and characteristics of the parent, characteristics of the child, and socio-ecological sources of stress and support. Belsky agrees that these three types of influence are interrelated, such that strengths in any area help buffer the parent-infant relationship when any one component is "at risk." Thus, for example, parents with extensive personal resources and skills are better equipped to deal with difficult children, whereas easy-going children may compensate for parents with few personal resources. Similarly, extensive social support can reduce the negative effects of limited parental resources, difficult child behavior, or high social stress, whereas ill effects due to a lack of social support may be reduced or avoided when the parents' resources are ample or when children have easygoing temperaments and thus make minimal demands of their parents.

According to Belsky, dyadic compatibility is at greatest risk when two or more of the three components are in suboptimal states. In such situations, he suggests, it is crucial that the parents' personal resources be adequate; by contrast, the greatest likelihood of dyadic failure exists when the infants' characteristics provide the only functional buffer. This prediction speaks to the relative importance of the three sources of influence. The effects of socio-ecological factors such as life stress, social support, and marital satisfaction can be especially important in mediating the "fit" between parents and infants, however, when the parents' resources are deficient or the child's characteristics nonoptimal.

Life stress, commonly defined by the incidence of multiple or major negative life changes, is significantly related to the frequency of health problems and psychiatric symptoms (e.g., anxiety, depression) in several populations (Crnic, Greenberg, Ragozin, Robinson, & Basham, 1981; Nuckolls, Cassel, & Kaplan, 1972; Sarason, Johnson, & Siegel, 1978). It therefore seems reasonable to predict that parents who encounter marital, social, or financial stress will be less available and/or responsive to their children because of their irritability or their preoccupation with competing demands for their attention (Cochran & Brassard, 1979; Lamb & Easterbrooks, 1981). This should in turn impair dyadic compatibility, unless the child is unusually resilient and easy-tempered to the point even of reducing the perceived stress by their own cheerful dispositions. By contrast, irritable infants may be sources of additional stress and may thus increase dyadic incompatibility. As Goldberg has suggested, socially competent infants are able to instill feelings of efficacy in their parents. Stressed parents who feel effective with their infants are likely to have more compatible relationships than are stressed parents who feel ineffective.

The effects of stress may also vary as a function of the infants' reactivity and self-regulatory processes, to the extent that reactivity influences the infants' perceptions and interpretations of the stressed parents' behavior, while their self-regulatory abilities influence their response to parental stress. Unreactive children with well-developed self-regulatory capacities may not be as seriously affected by stressed, unsupported parents as are children who are highly reactive and unable to regulate their own states.

Other factors must also modulate the effects of stress, because the statistically significant correlations between life-stress indices and dependent measures of well-being tend to be of low magnitude (Sarason et al., 1978). Sarason et al. suggested that the effects of life stress probably differ from person to person, depending on their individual characteristics and the levels of social support available to them. As a result, some individuals will be greatly affected by moderate levels of stress, whereas others may be relatively unaffected even by high levels.

A relationship between stress and moderating variables such as social support has indeed been found in studies of parent-infant relationships, wherein social support refers to the instrumental assistance and emotional support provided by close relations, friends, and community organizations (Cochran & Brassard, 1979; Crnic, Greenberg, Ragozin, Robinson, & Basham, 1983; Gottlieb, 1981; Henderson, Duncan-Jones, Byrne, & Scott, 1980). In a longitudinal study of mothers and their 3- to 12-month-old infants, for example, Crockenberg (1981) found that mothers who reported low social support were significantly more likely to have insecurely attached infants than were mothers with high social support. However, low social support was associated with anxious attachment *only* when the infants were highly irritable, confirming that characteristics of the social context interact with maternal and infant characteristics in affecting dyadic compatibility. Even more intriguing, the majority of the infants who were not irritable were securely attached even when their mothers reported low social support or were behaviorally unresponsive. Crockenberg suggested that placid and easy-going temperaments allowed these infants to remain unaffected by their mothers' unresponsive behavior, and enabled them to quickly become interactive when their mothers were more responsive.

In a study of premature and full-term infants, Crnic et al. (1981, 1983) similarly found that the amount and quality of social support available to mothers significantly buffered them against the effects of stress. Mothers who reported high levels of stress and high levels of intimate support (that is, support provided by a spouse or partner) reported much greater life satisfaction than did mothers who reported high life stress and low intimate support; in fact, the latter mothers reported the least satisfaction of all groups surveyed. Social support was significantly associated with the mothers' attitudes toward parenting, but, somewhat contrary to Crockenberg's findings, social support did not significantly moderate the effects of stress. Perhaps this was because Crockenberg measured stress in terms of infant irritability, whereas Crnic et al. measured stress in terms of reported stressful life events.

Intimate support is often obtained from a spouse, and thus marital satisfaction may have an important impact on parent-infant dyads. This prediction is supported by the finding that marital satisfaction during pregnancy predicts both adaptation to parenthood and emotional well-being during the first year postpartum (Belsky, 1981; Grossmann, Eichler, & Winickoff, 1980). Research with adolescent mothers, who are especially at risk for parenting failure (Elster, McAnarney, & Lamb, 1983), indicates that social support from relatives or partners often predicts individual differences in the quality of maternal behavior (Colletta, 1981; Montemayor, Gilbride, & Elster, 1983).

Besides families, friends, and partners, the larger community can often be an important source of support for parents. Here a distinction is often made between informal (unstructured) and formal (structured or institutional) support systems (Cochran & Brassard, 1979; Parke & Tinsley, 1982). When informal support systems are unavailable, formal support systems may provide the assistance needed. Community agencies can provide services that are not otherwise available, such as parent education, information about child development, medical care, follow-up programs, parent support groups, and crisis shelters. In most cases, the effects of such support on dyadic compatibility have not been evaluated, but several studies have shown that hospital-based programs during the early postpartum period significantly enhance parental behavior and attitudes (Badger, Burns, & Vietze, 1981; Parke, Hymel, Power, & Tinsley, 1980; Whitt & Casey, 1982; Zelazo, Kotelchuck, Barber, & David, 1977). Moreover, research in settings such as well-baby clinics demonstrates that positive effects accrue when health-care providers applaud the parents' efforts to learn about their infants' needs and idiosyncrasies (Casey & Whitt, 1980; Chamberlin, 1979). By supporting parents' efforts to increase their competence and sense of efficacy, and by attending to behavioral development and providing anticipatory guidance, institutions such as hospitals and pediatric clinics can affect the compatibility of parent-child relationships (American Academy of Pediatrics, 1972; Casey & Whitt, 1980; Chamberlin, 1976). Crnic et al. (1981) even suggest that pediatric assessments should include inquiries about the availability and adequacy of social support networks, so as to identify and intervene with families who may be at risk for parenting problems.

Summary

Individual differences in the compatibility of infant-parent relationships appear to be determined jointly by parental characteristics, child characteristics, and the characteristics of their social ecology. Available evidence regarding the importance of each of these factors has been reviewed above. While few would argue that any of these factors is unimportant, disagreement remains about the complex manner in which these factors interact to shape the quality of individual relationships. In large part, the disagreement here reflects the absence of a compelling body of empirical research; as this becomes available, we anticipate greater clarity and consensus. Some of the most promising speculations about these interactions were discussed above; these ideas and others like them will surely be the focus of intense research in the next few years.

Extreme Incompatibility: A Case Study of Child Maltreatment

We have argued in the preceding section that the compatibility or incompatibility of individual relationships must be viewed as the consequence of a complex interaction among a diverse array of factors that span parental characteristics (including personality, attitudes, and values), infant characteristics (such as temperament, health status, and gender), and the social, emotional, and economic ecology in which the dyad is embedded. Although we believe that this perspective is consistent with the available evidence, it has certainly not been proven, because the "available evidence" is limited indeed. In fact, perhaps the best documentation of the processes we have described comes not from studies concerned with variations within the normal range, but from the literature on child abuse and neglect. Here we find a growing consensus regarding the antecedents of child maltreatment that is entirely in accord with our view regarding qualitative aspects of relationships (Parke, 1977; Parke & Collmer, 1975; Parke & Lewis, 1981). In the present section, therefore, we will review the evidence concerning child maltreatment in an effort to illustrate and support empirically some of the claims and speculations offered above.

As one might expect, theorizing about the determinants of child maltreatment has evolved over time in a pattern of progression mirroring changes in our conception of parent-child compatibility and its determinants. Immediately following the publication of Kempe, Silverman, and Steele's (1962) seminal article on the battered-child syndrome, child abuse was largely viewed as the product of parental psychopathology. Even today, most laypersons and a substantial number of professionals cling to the belief that parents behave abusively because they are "crazy," sadistic, or emotionally disturbed. The accumulated evidence, however, shows no clear or significant relationships between any psychiatric diagnoses or characteristics and the incidence of child abuse. Most abusers, in fact, seem to be depressingly normal. The only parental characteristic consistently associated with abuse is a report by the abusive adult that he or she was maltreated by his or her parents as a child (Oliver & Taylor, 1971; Steele & Pollock, 1968). This may well be a self-serving claim, but it gains some validity from the evidence that female monkeys raised in isolation or by incompetent mothers grow up to be incompetent and abusive mothers themselves (Suomi, 1978). There is also a demonstrated relationship between the amount of punishment a child receives and his or her tendency to later rely upon similarly punitive disciplinary techniques (Erlanger, 1974; Gelfand, Hartmann, Lamb, Smith, Mahan, & Paul, 1974). These findings strengthen the plausibility of a causal relationship between victimization and later abusive behavior. However, no other aspects of parental personality, viewed in isolation, appear to be antecedents of abusive behavior.

Initial enthusiasm about the etiological significance of parental pathology waned in the face of overwhelming empirical disconfirmation. Next to achieve prominence was the sociological perspective, in terms of which child abuse was viewed as the consequence of parental subjection to extraordinary degrees of stress, both economic and socioemotional. Several studies confirm that the incidence of abuse is significantly higher in families characterized by poverty, single parenthood, paternal unemployment, and social isolation—factors that surely make both life in general and parenting in particular stressful experiences (Garbarino, 1976; Garbarino & Crouter, 1978; Garbarino & Stocking, 1979). Stress generates tension and lowers the individual's tolerance for frustration, whereas social isolation robs the individual of social networks and support systems that would otherwise help alleviate the stress. However, *most* poor, single, isolated parents do not behave abusively, so some other factors must play a role in determining when abuse will occur.

In addition, both the psychiatric and sociological models have difficulty explaining why it is that abusive treatment is often (though certainly not always) meted out to one child in the family while others escape unscathed (Milow & Lourie, 1964; Parke & Collmer, 1975). The selective identification of a victim presumably would not occur if either parental pathology or socioeconomic stress alone determined when abuse would occur. Instead, there must be some reason why the parents discriminate against particular children; presumably the characteristics of the child are involved. Empirical evidence that children in fact play a role in determining whether or not they will be abused is slowly becoming available. Studies suggest that preterm, handicapped, difficult, and otherwise "unusual" children are more likely to be abused than are their more "normal" counterparts (see Parke & Collmer, 1975, for a review). Perhaps best established is the relationship between abuse and prematurity (Baldwin & Oliver, 1975; Elmer & Gregg, 1967; Fontana, 1971; Klein & Stern, 1971; Simons, Downs, Hurster, & Archer, 1966; Smith, 1975), though not all studies support this finding (Egeland & Brunnquell, 1979). Moreover, unattractive children are more likely to elicit punishment for transgressions than are physically attractive children (Berkowitz & Frodi, 1978; Dion, 1974), and this finding may help explain why children with "deviant" characteristics are "at risk" for child abuse.

Only a small minority of children who have specific deviant or unattractive characteristics, however, are actually abused or maltreated by their parents. Clearly, therefore, this factor alone, like parental psychopathology and socioecological circumstances, cannot explain the incidence of child mal-treatment. Instead, it seems most likely that all three types of factors *together* determine who will abuse whom and in what circumstances. Thus, we would expect abuse to occur when the demands made by the child (which presumably vary in noxiousness depending on his or her age and characteristics), coupled with the stress occasioned by the social, economic, and emotional circum-stances of the parent, reach a point that exceeds the individual's level of tolerance (itself an aspect of the parent's personality), resulting in an abusive outburst. Abuse also may be potentiated by cultural standards regarding the appropriateness of physical punishment: Abuse appears to be much less common in countries or communities (e.g., China, Singapore, Sweden) that disapprove of physical punishment (Freedman & Freedman, 1969; Garbarino & Stocking, 1979; Goode, 1971; Hwang, 1982; Niem & Collard, 1971; Sidel, 1972; Wong, 1983). In addition, parents' reactions may vary depending on their demands of the child. One factor frequently noted in the child abuse literature is the unrealistic nature of the parents' expectations (Parke & Collmer, 1975). Typically, these involve age-inappropriate demands or expectations that the child is unable to satisfy. The child's failure to comply then provokes punishment when the adult interprets the child's behavior as deliberate disobedience. Again, the intensity of the punishment is assumed to be affected by the stressfulness of the parents' current circumstances.

Some insight into the processes relating parental personality, socioecological circumstances, child characteristics, and the incidence of child abuse can be garnered by considering Berkowitz's theory concerning the determinants of aggressive behavior, and Patterson's description of the vicious cycles that sometimes come to characterize parent-child relationships. Berkowitz (1974) has shown that people are more likely to behave aggressively when they are aroused or stressed. In such psychological states, aggression is not randomly emitted but is more likely to occur in the presence of aggression-eliciting stimuli. Such stimuli are likely to be things or events that are either aversive to the individual or have previously been associated with aggression. Drawing upon these notions, Frodi and colleagues (Frodi & Lamb, 1980; Frodi, Lamb, Leavitt, Donovan, Neff, & Sherry, 1978b) have argued that certain children become aversive in their parents' eyes by virtue of noxious characteristics such as the high-pitched, irritating cry of preterm infants (Lester & Zeskind, 1982), or the added, perhaps unrewarding, effort involved in caring for preterm or handicapped children. As a result, children who have these characteristics are more likely to become targets for their parents' aggression in times of stress. Such stress can be occasioned not only by the demands of parenting (especially when the child has special needs), but also by social, economic, and emotional circumstances, such as unemployment, poverty, social isolation, poor marital relationships, etc. The individual's personality is also important, of course, inasmuch as it determines the parent's tolerance for stress and his or her coping style.

Consistent with these speculations, Frodi et al. (1978b) showed that parents responded more negatively (on both psychophysiological and self-report measures) to the facial features and cry of a premature infant than to that of a full-term infant. Further, they found that abusive mothers responded negatively to both smiles and cries, whereas nonabusive mothers responded differentially—negatively to cries and positively to smiles (Frodi & Lamb, 1980). Similar findings were reported by Disbrow, Doerr, and Caulfield (1977). These findings suggest that abusive parents may come to see all child bids as negative, presumably as a result of prior, unrewarding experiences. Such tendencies on the parents' part surely place children at risk for abuse.

Drawing upon observations of interaction between out-of-control or aggressive boys and their parents, Patterson (1974; Patterson & Cobb, 1971, 1973) has described "vicious spirals" that appear to teach both children and parents the usefulness of aggressive or noxious behavior. Instead of terminating noxious behavior when punished by their parents, these children increase the level of noxiousness, eliciting an even stronger rebuke from their parents. The process continues until one of the interactants gives in. If the parents withdraw first, the children learn that if they persist long enough in their obnoxious behavior, they will get their own way. Parents locked into these cycles may not always give in, however. Instead, they may be pushed so far that their response to the child's escalating provocation amounts to physical maltreatment. As Patterson and Cobb (1971) have written, "There are many grown women with no past history of hitting, who are shaped by interactions with infants and children to initiate physical assaults. . . . The mother learns that hits terminate child behavior" (p. 124). This interpretation of the dynamics leading to abuse is consistent with evidence that abuse often occurs when the child fails to comply with an initially reasonable request from the abuser (Gil, 1970; Patterson & Cobb, 1971).

Summary

An examination of the child abuse literature reveals that child maltreatment, once viewed simply as the product of serious parental pathology, is now viewed as the consequence of a complex interaction among three types of factors: parental characteristics, child characteristics, and characteristics of their social ecology. The relationship among these factors appears to be multiplicative, such that in most cases all three must be involved if abuse is to occur. Our discussion illustrates the way in which compatibility or (in this case) incompatibility is influenced by a variety of factors interacting in a complex fashion.

Conclusion

Although there were some noteworthy exceptions, the majority of studies conducted prior to the late 1960s assumed that patterns of influence within parent-child relationships were unidirectional. Psychologists scorned the existence of constitutionally based temperamental characteristics and instead portrayed children as plastic, malleable organisms entirely shaped by their experiences, especially those involving interactions with their parents.

This tidy interpretive framework was sharply criticized in the late 1960s by Bell (Bell, 1968; Bell & Harper, 1977), who pointed out that statistical associations between child and parental characteristics could plausibly be interpreted as consequences of child-to-parent influences rather than parent-to-child influences. Thus stimulated, researchers came to realize that social influences were typically bidirectional. The characteristics of each partner in any interaction were recognized as determinants not only of how the other would be influenced but also of how he or she would subsequently be affected by the other's behavior. Exploring the processes of interactional influence thus became much more difficult.

By the late 1970s, however, it became clear that a further level of difficulty had to be acknowledged. Parents and children did not constitute dyads existing in vacuums: They were embedded in networks of social relationships and were dependent on others for things like employment, companionship, love, social support, etc. The functioning of each individual, and thus of the dyad, seemed likely to depend in part on the quality of their social ecology.

Today, therefore, researchers and theorists are attempting to develop and test empirically complex models for explaining individual differences in the quality of relationships in order to understand developmental processes. Most would agree that the compatibility or incompatibility of parent-child relationships depends on the interaction among three classes of influence: child characteristics, parental characteristics, and characteristics of the social ecology. The effects of each type of influence have been demonstrated, but developmentalists have only begun to consider the complex interactions among them. Considerable excitement has been generated, however, and we can expect to witness dramatic progress in the next decade. Many would agree that we are at the brink of the most exciting advances in a century of concern with social and personality development.

References

Ainsworth, M. (1969). Object relations, dependency, and attachment: A theoretical review of the infant-mother relationship. *Child Development*, *40*, 969–1025.

Ainsworth, M. (1973). The development of mother-infant attachment. In B. M. Caldwell & H. N. Ricciuti (Eds.), *Review of Child Development Research* (Vol. 3). Chicago: University of Chicago Press.

Ainsworth, M., Blehar, M., Waters, E., & Wall, S. (1978). *Patterns of attachment*. Hillsdale, NJ: Lawrence Erlbaum Associates.

American Academy of Pediatrics. (1972). Statement of Child Health Supervision. *Bulletin of Pediatric Practice, 6,* 3.

Badger, E., Burns, D., & Vietze, P. (1981). Maternal risk factors as predictors of developmental outcome in early childhood. *Infant Mental Health Journal, 2,* 33–43.

Baldwin, J. A., & Oliver, J. E. (1975). Epidemiology and family characteristics of severely abused children. *British Journal of Preventive Social Medicine, 29,* 205–221.

Bateson, M. (1975). Mother-infant exchanges: The epigenesis of conversational interaction. In D. Aaronson & R. Rieber (Eds.), *Developmental psycholinguistics and communication disorders.* New York: New York Academy of Science.

Beckwith, L., & Cohen, S. (1978). Preterm birth: Hazardous obstetric and postnatal events as related to caregiver-infant behavior. *Infant Behavior and Development, 1,* 403–412.

Bell, R. (1968). A reinterpretation of the direction of effects in studies of socialization. *Psychological Review, 75,* 81–95.

Bell, R. (1971). Stimulus control of parent or caretaker behavior by offspring. *Developmental Psychology, 4,* 63–72.

Bell, R. Q. (1974). Contributions of human infants to caregiving and social interaction. In M. Lewis & L. A. Rosenblum (Eds.), *The effect of the infant on its caregiver.* New York: Wiley.

Bell, R., & Ainsworth, M. (1972). Infant crying and maternal repsonsiveness. *Child Development, 43,* 1171–1190.

Bell, R., & Harper, L. (1977). *Child effects on adults.* Hillsdale, NJ: Lawrence Erlbaum Associates.

Belsky, J. (1980). Child maltreatment: An ecological integration. *American Psychologist, 35,* 320–335.

Belsky, J. (1981). Early human experience: A family perspective. *Developmental Psychology, 17,* 3–23.

Belsky, J. (1984). The determinants of parenting: A process model. *Child Development, 55,* 83–96.

Belsky, J., Robins, E., & Gamble, W. (1984). Characteristics, consequences and determinants of parental competence: Toward a contextual theory. In M. Lewis & L. A. Rosenblum (Eds.), *Beyond the dyad.* New York: Plenum.

Berkowitz, L. (1974). Some determinants of impulsive aggression: Role of mediated associations with reinforcements for aggression. *Psychological Review, 81,* 165–176.

Berkowitz, L., & Frodi, A. (1978). Reactions to a child's mistakes as affected by her/his looks and speech. Unpublished paper, University of Wisconsin.

Bowlby, J. (1969). *Attachment and loss* (Vol. 1). *Attachment.* New York: Basic Books.

Brachfeld, S., & Goldberg, S. (1978, April). Parent-infant interaction: Effects of newborn medical status on free play at 8 and 12 months. Paper presented to the Southeastern Conference on Human Development, Atlanta.

Brazelton, T. B., Koslowski, B., & Main, M. (1974). The origins of reciprocity: The early mother-infant interaction. In M. Lewis & L. A. Rosenblum (Eds.), *The effect of the infant on its caregiver.* New York: Wiley.

Bronfenbrenner, U. (1977). Toward an experimental ecology of human development. *American Psychologist, 32,* 513–531.

Bronfenbrenner, U. (1979). *The ecology of human development.* Cambridge, MA: Harvard University Press.

Brown, J. V., & Bakeman, R. (1979). Relationships of human mothers with their infants during the first year of life. In R. Bell & W. Smotherman (Eds.), *Maternal influences and early behavior*. Jamaica, NY: Spectrum.

Bruner, J. (1977). Early social interaction and language acquisition. In H. R. Schaffer (Ed.), *Studies in mother-infant interaction*. New York: Academic Press.

Campos, J., Caplovitz-Barrett, K., Lamb, M., Goldsmith, H., & Stenberg, C. (1983). Socioemotional development. In P. Mussen (Ed.), *Handbook of Child Psychology* (Vol. 2). New York: Wiley.

Casey, P., & Whitt, J. (1980). Effect of the pediatrician on the mother-infant relationship. *Pediatrics, 65*, 815–820.

Chamberlin, R. (1976). What is "adequate well baby care"? *Pediatrics, 58*, 772.

Chamberlin, R. (1979, August). Effects of educating mothers about child development in physicians' offices on mother and child functioning over time. Paper presented to the American Psychological Association, New York City.

Chess, S., & Thomas, A. (1977). Temperamental individuality from childhood to adolescence. *Journal of Child Psychiatry, 16*, 218–226.

Cochran, M., & Brassard, J. (1979). Child development and personal social networks. *Child Development, 50*, 601–616.

Colletta, N. D. (1981). Social support and the risk of maternal rejection by adolescent mothers. *Journal of Psychology, 109*, 191–197.

Crnic, K., Greenberg, M., Ragozin, A., Robinson, N., & Basham, R. (1981, April). The effects of stress and social support on maternal attitudes and the mother-infant relationship. Paper presented to the Society for Research in Child Development, Boston.

Crnic, K. A., Greenberg, M. T., Ragozin, A. S., Robinson, N. M., & Basham, R. B. (1983). Effects of stress and social support on mothers and premature and full-term infants. *Child Development, 54*, 209–217.

Crockenberg, S. B. (1981). Infant irritability, mother responsiveness, and social support influences on the security of infant-mother attachment. *Child Development, 52*, 857–865.

Dion, K. K. (1974). Children's physical attractiveness and sex as determinants of adult punitiveness. *Developmental Psychology, 10*, 772–778.

Disbrow, M. A., Doerr, H., & Caulfield, C. (1977). Measuring the components of parents' potential for child abuse and neglect. *Child Abuse and Neglect, 1*, 279–296.

DiVitto, B., & Goldberg, S. (1979). The development of early parent-infant interaction as a function of newborn medical status. In T. Field, A. Sostek, S. Goldberg, & H. Shuman (Eds.), *Infants born at risk*. Jamaica, NY: Spectrum.

Egeland, B., & Brunnquell, D. (1979). An at-risk approach to the study of child abuse. *Journal of the American Academy of Child Psychiatry, 18*, 219–235.

Elmer, E., & Gregg, G. S. (1967). Developmental characteristics of abused children. *Pediatrics, 40*, 596–602.

Elster, A. B., McAnarney, E. R., & Lamb, M. E. (1983). Parental behavior of adolescent mothers. *Pediatrics, 71*, 494–503.

Erlanger, H. S. (1974). Social class differences in parents' use of physical punishment. In S. K. Steinmetz & M. S. Straus (Eds.), *Violence in the family*. New York: Dodd, Mead.

Field, T. (1977). Effects of early separation, interactive deficits, and experimental manipulations on infant-mother face-to-face interaction. *Child Development, 48*, 763–771.

Fontana, V. J. (1971). *The maltreated child* (2nd ed.). Springfield, IL.: Charles C. Thomas.

Fraiberg, S. (1977). *Insights from the blind*. New York: Basic Books.

Freedman, D. A., & Freedman, N. (1969). Behavioral differences between Chinese-American and European-American newborns. *Nature, 224,* 1227.

Freud, S. (1940). *An outline of psychoanalysis.* New York: Norton.

Frodi, A., & Lamb, M. E. (1980). Child abusers' responses to infant smiles and cries. *Child Development, 51,* 238–241.

Frodi, A. M., Lamb, M. E., Leavitt, L. A., & Donovan, W. L. (1978a). Fathers' and mothers' responses to infant smiles and cries. *Infant Behavior and Development, 1,* 187–198.

Frodi, A. M., Lamb, M. E., Leavitt, L. A., Donovan, W. L., Neff, C., & Sherry, D. (1978b). Fathers' and mothers' responses to the faces and cries of normal and premature infants. *Developmental Psychology, 14,* 490–498.

Gamble, W., & Belsky, J. (1982, March). The determinants of parenting within a family context: A preliminary analysis. Paper presented to the International Conference on Infant Studies, Austin, TX.

Garbarino, J. (1976). Some ecological correlates of child abuse: The impact of socioeconomic stress on mothers. *Child Development, 47,* 178–185.

Garbarino, J., & Crouter, A. (1978). Defining the community context for parent-child relations: The correlates of child maltreatment. *Child Development, 49,* 604–616.

Garbarino, J., & Stocking, S. H. (Eds.), (1979). *Supporting families and protecting children.* Boys Town, NE: Boys Town Center for the Study of Youth Development.

Gelfand, D. M., Hartmann, D. P., Lamb, A. K., Smith, C. L., Mahan, M. A., & Paul, S. C. (1974). The effects of adult models and described alternatives on children's choice of behavior management techniques. *Child Development, 45,* 585–593.

Gil, D. G. (1970). *Violence against children: Physical child abuse in the United States.* Cambridge, MA: Harvard University Press.

Goldberg, S. (1977). Social competence in infancy: A model of parent-infant interaction. *Merrill-Palmer Quarterly, 23,* 164–177.

Goldberg, S. (1979, August). Adaptation to stress in the parent-infant dyad. Paper presented to the Keystone Conference on Parenting, Keystone, CO.

Goldberg, S. (1982). Prematurity. In J. Belsky (Ed.), *In the beginning.* New York: Columbia University Press.

Goldsmith, H., & Campos, J. (1982). Toward a theory of infant temperament. In R. N. Emde & R. J. Harmon (Eds.), *The development of attachment and affiliative systems.* New York: Plenum.

Goldsmith, H., & Campos, J. (in press). The development of temperament: A biobehavioral study. In M. E. Lamb, A. L. Brown, & B. Rogoff (Eds.), *Advances in developmental psychology* (Vol. 4). Hillsdale, NJ: Lawrence Erlbaum Associates.

Goode, W. J. (1971). Force and violence in the family. *Journal of Marriage and the Family, 33,* 624–636.

Gottlieb, B. H. (1981). Social networks and social support in community mental health. In B. H. Gottlieb (Ed.), *Social networks and social support.* Beverly Hills, CA: Sage.

Grossman, F., Eichler, L., & Winickoff, S. (1980). *Pregnancy, birth, and parenthood.* San Francisco: Jossey-Bass.

Grossmann, K. E., Grossmann, K., Huber, F., & Wartner, U. (1981). German children's behavior towards their mothers at 12 months and their fathers at 18 months in Ainsworth's Strange Situation. *International Journal of Behavioral Development, 4,* 157–181.

Henderson, S., Duncan-Jones, P., Byrne, D. G., & Scott, R. (1980). Measuring social relationships: The Interview Schedule for Social Interaction. *Psychological Medicine, 10,* 723–734.

Hwang, C-P. (1982, April). Personal communication.

Jones, O. (1980). Prelinguistic communication skills in Down's syndrome and normal infants. In T. Field, S. Goldberg, D. Stern, & A. M. Sostek (Eds.), *High risk infants and children: Interactions with adults and peers*. New York: Academic.

Jones, S., & Moss, H. (1971). Age, state, and maternal behavior associated with infant vocalizations. *Child Development, 42*, 1039–1051.

Kagan, J. (1982). *Psychological research on the human infant: An evaluative summary*. New York: William T. Grant Foundation.

Kaye, K. (1982). *The mental and social life of babies*. Chicago: University of Chicago Press.

Kempe, C. H., Silverman, F. N., Steele, B. B., Droegemueller, W., & Silver, H. K. (1962). The battered-child syndrome. *Journal of the American Medical Association, 181*, 17–24.

Klein, M., & Stern, L. (1971). Low birth weight and the battered-child syndrome. *American Journal of Diseases of Childhood, 122*, 15–18.

Korner, A., & Thoman, E. (1972). The relative efficacy of contact and vestibular proprioceptive stimulation in soothing neonates. *Child Development, 43*, 443–454.

Lamb, M. E. (1978). Qualitative aspects of mother and father infant attachments. *Infant Behavior and Development, 1*, 265–275.

Lamb, M. E. (1981). The development of social expectations in the first year of life. In M. E. Lamb & L. R. Sherrod (Eds.), *Infant social cognition: Empirical and theoretical considerations*. Hillsdale, NJ: Lawrence Erlbaum Associates.

Lamb, M. E., Chase-Lansdale, L., & Owen, M. (1979). The changing American family and its implications for infant social development: The sample case of maternal employment. In M. Lewis & L. Rosenblum (Eds.), *The child and its family*. New York: Plenum.

Lamb, M. E., & Easterbrooks, M. A. (1981). Individual differences in parental sensitivity: Origins, components, and consequences. In M. E. Lamb & L. R. Sherrod (Eds.), *Infant social cognition: Empirical and theoretical considerations*. Hillsdale, NJ: Lawrence Erlbaum Associates.

Lamb, M. E., Frodi, A., Hwang, C-P., & Frodi, M. (1982). Varying degrees of paternal involvement in infant care: Attitudinal and behavioral correlates. In M. Lamb (Ed.), *Nontraditional families: Parenting and child development*. Hillsdale, NJ: Lawrence Erlbaum Associates.

Lamb, M. E., & Goldberg, W. A. (1982). The father-child relationship: A synthesis of biological, evolutionary, and social perspectives. In L. Hoffman, R. Gandelman, & H. R. Schiffman (Eds.), *Parenting: Its causes and consequences*. Hillsdale, NJ: Lawrence Erlbaum Associates.

Lamb, M. E., Hwang, C-P., Frodi, A., & Frodi, M. (1982). Security of mother- and father-infant attachment and its relation to sociability with strangers in traditional and non-traditional Swedish families. *Infant Behavior and Development, 5*, 355–367.

Lamb, M. E., Thompson, R., Gardner, W., Charnov, E., & Estes, D. (1984). Security of infantile attachment as assessed in the "Strange Situation." *Behavioral and Brain Sciences, 7*, 127–171.

Leiderman, P. H., & Seashore, M. J. (1975). Mother-infant separation: Some delayed consequences. In *Parent-infant interaction*. CIBA Foundation Symposium No. 33. New York: Elsevier.

Lester, B. M., & Zeskind, P. S. (1982). A biobehavioral perspective on crying in early infancy. In H. E. Fitzgerald, B. M. Lester, & M. W. Yogman (Eds.), *Theory and research in behavioral pediatrics*. New York: Plenum.

Lewis, M. & Rosenblum, L. (Eds.). (1974). *The effect of the infant on its caregiver*. New York: Wiley.

Maccoby, E., & Masters, J. (1970). Attachment and dependency. In P. H. Mussen (Ed.), *Carmichael's Manual of Child Psychology* (Vol. 2). New York: Wiley.

Main, M., & Weston, D. (1981). The quality of the toddler's relationship to mother and to father: Related to conflict behavior and the readiness to establish new relationships. *Child Development, 52,* 932–940.

Milow, I., & Lourie, R. (1964). The child's role in the battered-child syndrome. *Society for Pediatric Research, 65,* 1079–1081.

Montemayor, R., Gilbride, K., & Elster, A. (1983, April). Predicting maternal sensitivity in a group of teenage mothers. Paper presented to the Society for Research in Child Development, Detroit.

Murray, A. (1979). Infant crying as an elicitor of parental behavior: An examination of two models. *Psychological Bulletin, 86,* 191–215.

Murray, A., Dolby, R., Nation, R., & Thomas, D. (1981). The effects of epidural anesthesia on newborns and their mothers. *Child Development, 52,* 71–82.

Nash, S., & Feldman, S. (1981). Sex-role and sex-related attributions: Constancy and change across the family life cycle. In M. Lamb & A. Brown (Eds.), *Advances in developmental psychology* (Vol. 1). Hillsdale, NJ: Lawrence Erlbaum Associates.

Niem, T. C., & Collard, R. (1971, August). Parental discipline of aggressive behaviors in four-year-old Chinese and American children. Paper presented at the annual meeting of the American Psychological Association, Washington, D.C.

Nuckolls, K. B., Cassel, J., & Kaplan, B. H. (1972). Psychosocial assets, life crisis and the prognosis of pregnancy. *American Journal of Epidemiology, 95,* 431–441.

Oliver, J. E., & Taylor, A. (1971). Five generations of ill-treated children in one family pedigree. *British Journal of Psychiatry, 119,* 473–480.

Owen, M. T., & Chase-Lansdale, L. (1982, April). The "difficult" baby: Parental perceptions and infant attachments. Paper presented to the International Conference on Infant Studies, Austin, TX.

Parke, R. D. (1977). Socialization into child abuse: A social interactional perspective. In J. L. Tapp & F. J. Levine (Eds.), *Law, justice and the individual in society: Psychological and legal issues.* New York: Holt, Rinehart & Winston.

Parke, R. D., & Collmer, C. W. (1975). Child abuse: An interdisciplinary analysis. In E. M. Hetherington (Ed.), *Review of child development research* (Vol. 5). Chicago: University of Chicago Press.

Parke, R. D., Hymel, S., Power, T., & Tinsley, B. (1980). Fathers and risk: A hospital based model of intervention. In D. Sawin, R. Hawkins, L. Walker, & J. Penticuff (Eds.), *Psychosocial risks in infant-environment transactions.* New York: Brunner/ Mazel.

Parke, R. D., & Lewis, N. G. (1981). The family in context: A multilevel interactional analysis of child abuse. In *Parent-child interaction.* New York: Academic.

Parke, R. D., Power, T. G., & Gottman, J. M. (1979). Conceptualizing and quantifying influence patterns in the family triad. In M. E. Lamb, S. J. Suomi, & G. R. Stephenson (Eds.), *Social interaction analysis: Methodological issues.* Madison, WI: University of Wisconsin Press.

Parke, R. D., & Sawin, D. (1980). The family in early infancy: Social interactional and attitudinal analyses. In F. A. Pedersen (Ed.), *The father-infant relationship: Observational studies in the family setting.* New York: Praeger Special Studies.

Parke, R. D., & Tinsley, B. R. (1982). The early environment of the at-risk infant: Expanding the social context. In D. Bricker (Ed.), *Intervention with at-risk and handicapped infants: From research to application.* Baltimore: University Park Press.

Patterson, G. R. (1974). Interventions for boys with conduct problems: Multiple settings, treatments and criteria. *Journal of Consulting and Clinical Psychology, 42,* 471–481.

Patterson, G. R., & Cobb, J. A. (1971). A dyadic analysis of "aggressive" behavior. In

J. P. Hill (Ed.), *Minnesota Symposia on Child Psychology* (Vol. 5). Minneapolis: University of Minnesota Press.

Patterson, G. R., & Cobb, J. A. (1973). Stimulus control for classes of noxious behavior. In J. F. Knutson (Ed.), *The control of aggression: Implications from basic research*. Chicago: Aldine.

Pedersen, F. (Ed.), (1980). *The father-infant relationship: Observational studies in the family setting*. New York: Praeger Special Studies.

Pedersen, F. (1981). Father influences viewed in a family context. In M. E. Lamb (Ed.), *The role of the father in child development* (2nd ed.). New York: Wiley.

Rajecki, D., Lamb, M., & Obmascher, P. (1978). Toward a general theory of infantile attachment: A comparative review of aspects of the social bond. *Behavioral and Brain Sciences, 1,* 417–464.

Richards, M. (1975). Early separation. In R. Lewin (Ed.), *Child Alive!* Garden City, NY: Anchor Press/Doubleday.

Rogoff, B. (in press). Social guidance of cognitive development. In E. Gollin (Ed.), *Colorado symposium on human socialization: Social context and human development*. New York: Academic Press.

Rogoff, B., Gilbride, K., & Malkin, C. (1983, April). Interaction with babies as guidance in development. Paper presented to the Society for Research in Child Development, Detroit.

Rothbart, M. K. (1981). Measurement of temperament in infancy. *Child Development, 52,* 569–578.

Rothbart, M. K. (1983, April). Development of inhibitory control during infancy. Paper presented to the Society for Research in Child Development, Detroit.

Rothbart, M. K., & Derryberry, D. (1981). Development of individual differences in temperament. In M. E. Lamb & A. L. Brown (Eds.), *Advances in developmental psychology* (Vol. 1). Hillsdale, NJ: Lawrence Erlbaum Associates.

Sagi, A., Lamb, M., Lewkowicz, K., Shoham, R., Dvir, R., & Estes, D. (in press). Security of infant-mother, -father, and -metapelet attachments among kibbutz-reared Israeli children. In. I. Bretherton & E. Waters (Eds.), *The Strange situation: New directions for research. Monographs of the Society for Research in Child Development.*

Sameroff, A. J., & Chandler, M. J. (1975). Reproductive risk and the continuum of caretaking casualty. In F. D. Horowitz (Ed.), *Review of child development research* (Vol. 4). Chicago: The University of Chicago Press.

Sarason, I. G., Johnson, J. H., & Siegel, J. M. (1978). Assessing the impact of life changes: Development of the life experiences survey. *Journal of Consulting and Clinical Psychology, 46,* 932–946.

Sidel, R. (1972). *Women and child care in China*. New York: Hill & Wang.

Simons, B., Downs, E. F., Hurster, M. M., & Archer, M. (1966). Child abuse: Epidemiological study of medically reported cases. *New York State Journal of Medicine, 66.*

Smith, S. M. (1975). *The battered child syndrome*. London: Butterworths.

Snow, C. (1977). The development of conversations between mothers and babies. *Journal of Child Language, 4,* 1–22.

Sorce, J., & Emde, R. (1982). The meaning of infant emotional expressions: Regularities in caregiving responses in normal and Down's Syndrome infants. *Journal of Child Psychology and Psychiatry, 23,* 145–158.

Sroufe, L. (1983). Infant-caregiver attachment and patterns of adaptation in preschool: The roots of maladaptation and competence. In M. Perlmutter (Ed.), *Minnesota Symposia in Child Psychology* (Vol. 16). Hillsdale, NJ: Lawrence Erlbaum Associates.

Steele, B. F., & Pollock, D. A. (1968). A psychiatric study of parents who abuse infants and small children. In R. E. Helfer & C. H. Kempe (Eds.), *The battered child* (2nd ed.). Chicago: University of Chicago Press.

Stern, D. (1974). Mother and infant at play: The dyadic interaction involving facial, vocal, and gaze behaviors. In M. Lewis & L. Rosenblum (Eds.), *The effect of the infant of its caregiver*. New York: Wiley.

Stern, D. (1977). *The first relationship*. Cambridge, MA: Harvard University Press.

Suomi, S. J. (1978). Maternal behavior by socially incompetent monkeys: Neglect and abuse of offspring. *Journal of Pediatric Psychology, 3*, 28–34.

Thomas, A., Chess, S., & Birch, H. (1970). The origin of personality. *Scientific American, 223*, 102–109.

Thomas, A., Chess, S., & Birch, H. (1968). *Temperament and behavior disorders in children*. New York: New York University Press.

Thompson, R., & Lamb, M. E. (1982). Stranger sociability and its relationships to temperament and social experience during the second year. *Infant Behavior and Development, 5*, 277–287.

Thompson, R., & Lamb, M. E. (1984). Infants, mothers, families, and strangers. In M. Lewis & L. Rosenblum (Eds.), *Beyond the Dyad*. New York: Plenum.

Thompson, R., Lamb, M. E., & Estes, D. (1982). Stability of infant-mother attachment and its relationship to changing life circumstances in an unselected middle class sample. *Child Development, 53*, 144–148.

Whitt, J. K., & Casey, P. H. (1982). The mother-infant relationship and infant development: The effect of pediatric intervention. *Child Development, 53*, 948–956.

Wong, S. T. (1983, February). Personal communication.

Zelazo, P., Kotelchuck, M., Barber, L., & David, J. (1977, March). Fathers and sons: An experimental facilitation of attachment behaviors. Paper presented to the Society for Research in Child Development, New Orleans.

Chapter 3

Compatibility and Incompatibility in Children's Peer and Sibling Relationships

Wyndol Furman

Peers and siblings are central figures in children's social worlds. They are not just playmates, but have fundamental roles in shaping a child's course of development. For example, positive peer relations have been found to contribute to the acquisition of appropriate social behaviors, the control of agressive impulses, the development of norms and values, and other aspects of moral and cognitive development (Hartup, 1976). Although research on sibling relationships is not very extensive, siblings too have been found to be important caretakers and socialization agents (Furman & Buhrmester, 1982).

Some children have satisfying relationships with peers and siblings, whereas for others such relationships are problematic. Even children who have satisfying relationships are likely to have more fulfilling relationships with some peers or siblings than with others. An important question is: What factors contribute to compatibility or incompatibility in these relationships? The present chapter is a review of the literature pertaining to this question.

The concept of compatibility is a new one in the literature, and little agreement exists concerning the specific nature of the construct. In his introduction to this volume, Ickes suggested that compatibility might be defined in terms of: (1) the perceived quality of and satisfaction with the relationship, (2) the integrative functioning of the relationship, and (3) the stability of the relationship. His basic ideas are adopted in the present chapter, but some changes are needed because of differences in the construct systems and terminology used in various literatures. In particular, I consider literature pertaining to six potential indices of compatibility: (1) satisfaction with the relationship, (2) feelings of affection or interpersonal attraction, (3) an absence of feelings of dislike or antipathy, (4) frequent rewarding or positive interactions, (5) infrequent punishing or negative interactions, and (6) long-lasting or stable relationships. The first three do appear to be indices of perceptions of quality and satisfaction, and the last is the same as Ickes' concept of stability. However, the category of rewarding or positive interactions incorporates behaviors that do not coincide with Ickes' concept of integrative functioning.

Ickes was referring principally to synchronous or mutual behaviors such as the ability to set shared goals, work together toward them, and resolve conflicts in a mutually acceptable way; he did not intend to incorporate all forms of positive interchange. Developmental psychologists usually do not draw a distinction between synchronous behaviors and other positive behaviors, and thus it is not possible to focus solely on synchronous behaviors. One might, however, expect synchronous behaviors and other positive behaviors to be positively associated with each other. In any event, the pattern of relations among the six indices will be examined throughout this chapter, and the implications for conceptualizing compatibility will be discussed in the concluding section.

Sociometric Status

One approach to studying compatibility in peer relations is to identify the factors associated with popularity. Popular children are well-liked by their peers and, thus, appear to have the personal attributes or interactional styles that foster successful or compatible relations. Literally hundreds of investigators have examined the correlates of sociometric status (see Hartup, 1970, 1983). Although it is not possible to review this literature in detail, some of the principal findings are highlighted in the following sections.

First, however, a few words must be said about the measurement of sociometric status (see Asher & Hymel, 1981). Many investigators have asked children how much they like each of their peers. Popular or accepted peers are those who receive high ratings of likeability, whereas unpopular or rejected peers are those who receive low ratings. This approach assumes that peer acceptance and peer rejection are at opposite ends of the same continuum. However, when children have been asked to name the peers they like the most and those they like the least, investigators have found that those who are not named as most liked are not necessarily named as least liked. In fact, Coie, Dodge, and Coppotelli (1982) proposed that children can be catergorized into five sociometric status groups: (1) the popular—those who are frequently named as most liked and infrequently named as least liked, (2) the rejected—those who are frequently named as least liked and seldom named as most liked, (3) the neglected—those who receive few nominations of either type, (4) the controversial—those who are frequently named as both most liked and least liked, and (5) the average—those whose scores are not extreme on either dimension. The significance of these distinctions will become apparent subsequently. In the literature reviewed here, however, the distinctions are often not made, and we need to be aware of the fact that a variable could be associated with either peer acceptance or peer rejection.

Physical Attractiveness

Like adults, children have clear and definite stereotypes associated with physical attractiveness (see Langlois & Stephan, 1981; Sorrell & Nowak, 1981). When shown photographs of unfamiliar peers, they rate attractive peers as better prospects for friends and expect them to be more likely than unattractive peers to engage in positive behaviors; by the same token, they think that attractive peers are less likely than unattractive peers to engage in negative behaviors (Dion, 1973; Langlois & Stephan, 1977). Moreover, attractive children actually are more popular with their peers than unattractive ones (Cavior & Dokecki, 1973; Kleck, Richardson, & Ronald, 1974).

The basis for the relation between attractiveness and popularity is not very clear. Perhaps children's stereotypes lead them to respond differently to attractive and unattractive peers. Like adults, children may believe that they are more similar to attractive peers than to unattractive ones and, thus, prefer their company (Marks, Miller, & Maruyama, 1981). Alternatively, because unattractive children have been found to be more aggressive and active than attractive children (Langlois & Downs, 1979), behavioral differences may account for the differences in popularity. In fact, Dodge (1983) found that when behavioral differences were controlled for statistically, the relation between sociometric status and attractiveness was no longer significant. Still, issues concerning the mechanisms responsible for this relation between attractiveness and status have not been studied sufficiently (see Langlois & Stephan, 1981). It is clear, however, that children find physically attractive peers to be more appealing than unattractive ones.

Social Behaviors

Although the overall rate of social behavior is not strongly related to sociometric status (Asher, Markell, & Hymel, 1981), the frequency of positive or nonnegative social behavior is. For example, in observational studies of preschool children, popularity has been found to be related to rates of friendly approach and associative behavior (Marshall & McCandless, 1957), giving positive reinforcement (Hartup, Glazer, & Charlesworth, 1967), and dispensing and receiving reinforcing and neutral social behaviors (Masters & Furman, 1981). Similarly, peer acceptance in the elementary-school years has been found to be associated with cooperative and outgoing behaviors (Bonney & Powell, 1953), rates of distributing and receiving positive reinforcement (Gottman, Gonso, & Rasmussen, 1975), and expressing kindness to children (Smith, 1950). Popular adolescents tend to be perceived as friendly and enthusiastic (Gronlund & Anderson, 1957), helpful, good-natured, and the "life of the party" (Elkins, 1958).

What is the relation between sociometric status and negative social behaviors, such as aggression? Usually, the frequency of aggressive or inappropriate behavior has been found to be unrelated to measures of peer acceptance (i.e., frequency of being named as most-liked) (Gottman, 1977; Hartup et al., 1967; Masters & Furman, 1981). In these same studies, however, the frequency of such negative behaviors has been found to be related to measures of peer rejection (i.e., frequency of being named as least-liked). Coie et al. (1982) provide a nice illustration of the relations between sociometric status and different social behaviors in their comparisons of peers' descriptions of popular, rejected, controversial, neglected, and average children. Popular children were described as being cooperative and being leaders, and as not being disruptive, fighting, or seeking help. Rejected children were described in the opposite manner (i.e., disruptive, fighting, and seeking help, and not being cooperative or leaders). Controversial children had some characteristics of popular children and some characteristics of rejected children. On the one hand, they were described as being leaders and average in cooperativeness; on the other hand, they were characterized as being disruptive, fighting, and seeking help. Neglected children were relatively low in visibility and stood out only as being shy. Other researchers have also found neglected children to be quiet and not very talkative (Gronlund & Anderson, 1957). In subsequent studies, investigators have found that children of different sociometric status are not only perceived differently by their peers but also interact differently with them. For example, Dodge, Coie, and Brakke (1982) found that rejected children frequently engaged in aggressive and inappropriate behaviors, whereas neglected children approached their peers only infrequently.

Thus, children who frequently engage in positive social behaviors tend to be liked by their peers. Those who do not are not necessarily disliked. They may simply be ignored, or they may be actively rejected if they behave aggressively or inappropriately. Although relatively few children fall in the controversial category, children of this type should be studied further. They appear to be compatible partners for some peers and incompatible ones for others. Perhaps their behavior differs depending upon the characteristics of their interaction partners, a point that will be returned to subsequently.

Intelligence and Social Cognitive Abilities

In a number of early studies, intelligence and academic achievement were found to be positively related to popularity (see Gronlund, 1959; Hartup, 1970). More recently, investigators have tried to identify specific social-cognitive abilities associated with successful relationships with peers. One social-cognitive skill that has been studied extensively is perspective-taking ability, or the ability to take the other person's point of view. A number of investigators have found perspective-taking ability to be correlated with popularity, although other investigators have not (Shantz, 1983). Another topic of interest has been problem-solving skills, such as the ability to generate alternative solutions to a problem, anticipate the consequences of behaviors, or accurately link means and ends (see Spivack, Platt, & Shure, 1976). Some investigators have found problem-solving skills to be associated with sociometric status, but again, other investigators have failed to replicate these findings (see Krasnor & Rubin, 1981). Finally, some research has focused on children's knowledge about social behaviors or social relationships. For example, compared to unpopular children, popular ones have been found to have greater knowledge about conventional means of helping (Ladd & Oden, 1979) and more mature conceptions of the nature of friendship (Wood, 1976). Intuitively, one would expect perspective-taking ability and problem-solving skills to foster compatible relationships with peers. Some support for this intuition can be found in the empirical literature, but the literature is strikingly inconsistent. Many conceptual and methodological problems exist (see Furman, 1984b), and perhaps the links between social cognition and behavior will be more apparent in future research than they are now.

Physical and Social Skills

The interest in social-cognitive ability has been paralleled by an interest in children's abilities in physical and social activities. Early investigators demonstrated that popular children were more skilled in sports and in social activities such as dancing or playing cards (see Gronlund, 1959). Recent investigators have attempted to identify the specific behavioral components required for effective interactions. In particular, investigators have focused on the behaviors that distinguish the social interactions of popular and unpopular children. For example, popular children have been shown to be more adept than unpopular children in becoming acquainted with a stranger (Gottman et al., 1975). Similarly, Putallaz and Gottman (1981) found that popular and unpopular children use different strategies for entering an ongoing group activity. Popular children tended to use indirect, low-risk strategies in which they tried to integrate themselves into the ongoing activity. In contrast, unpopular children tended to attract attention to themselves and were likely to be rebuffed. Popular children also are more able than unpopular ones to break a cycle of negative exchanges (Asarnow, 1983).

Although the results of these studies are suggestive, it is not yet clear whether these differences reflect differences in ability or simply differences in social performance. Moreover, like the literature on social-cognitive skills, the research on social skills is rather piecemeal in nature, and we do not have a comprehensive theoretical framework for understanding the contribution of different social skills (see Furman, 1984b). The existing research is promising, however, and in the near future we should be able to make considerable progress in identifying the specific skills or behaviors that foster compatibility.

Self-Perceptions

In a number of studies (see Hartup, 1983), children with high self-esteem have been found to be more popular than those with low self-esteem, although extremely high self-esteem may be associated with low popularity as well (Reese, 1961). The difference in popular and unpopular children's self-esteem may be part of a larger cluster of differences in self-perceptions. Hymel (1983) found that unpopular children not only perceived themselves to be less competent in social activities than popular children, but also reported that they were more lonely and less liked by their peers. Compared to popular children, they expected fewer positive outcomes in peer interactions and took less personal credit for social successes. Unpopular children's negative perceptions of their own abilities and the likely responses of their peers could lead them to act in ways that fulfill their expectations. At the very least, such negative perceptions could make it unappealing to interact with them.

Summary

Which children are likely to be popular with their peers? Based on the literature, children who are physically attractive, friendly, cooperative, intelligent, socially skilled, and self-confident are more likely to be popular than those who are not. Intuitively, these findings make sense. Such children seem to be attractive or interesting partners, and they appear to be sensitive to others' needs and desires; for these reasons, interactions with them are likely to be rewarding.

To put these findings in perspective, it should be noted that the literature on sociometric status consists almost exclusively of correlational studies. Differences between popular and unpopular children may be the results of being popular rather than the causes of such. For example, it is easy to imagine that being popular would enhance one's self-esteem. The problem of inferring causality from correlational studies is particularly serious in the case of studies of social behavior. Being popular might well lead to increases in positive social behavior, and research has shown that peers respond differently to popular and unpopular children's social behavior. For example, rejected children's social overtures are more likely to be rebuffed than are other children's overtures (Dodge et al., 1982). Frequent rebuffs may foster a vicious cycle in which the rejected child responds aggressively and in turn is rebuffed again.

Although caution should be used in inferring causality from correlational studies, intuitively it seems likely that most of the variables that have been discussed are antecedents of popularity. Empirical evidence of the causal impact of social behavior on social status can be found in clinical research demonstrating that children who are taught social skills improve in popularity (see reviews by Furman, 1984a; Hops, 1982). Further evidence can be found in the results of several studies that have examined the emergence of sociometric status in peer groups over time (Coie & Kupersmidt, 1983; Dodge, 1983). For example, Dodge (1983) observed groups of boys playing together for a series of eight sessions; following the last session, sociometric interviews were conducted. Children who became popular tended to engage in more cooperative play than children of average status. Children who were subsequently rejected often engaged in inappropriate behaviors, such as hitting peers, whereas children who were later classified as neglected often played alone. Coie and Kupersmidt (1983) report relatively similar results; in addition, they found that after only three sessions of interaction, children's social status in a group of unfamiliar peers was very similar to their sociometric status in their classroom. In effect, the children's typical patterns of interactions seemed to have led them to be accepted or rejected again.

Thus, despite the fact that most studies in this area are correlational, we have some evidence of causal links—at least between social behaviors and socio-metric status. Still, little is known about which variables are most important in determining popularity or how different configurations of variables are related to sociometric status. For example, can children compensate for being unattractive by being socially skilled? A particularly glaring omission in the literature is research on developmental changes in the variables associated with sociometric status. It seems likely that the causes or consequences of popularity change developmentally, but the specific nature of such changes have not been delineated (see Coie et al., 1982, for an exception).

It is also important to recognize that the factors associated with popularity and friendship are not necessarily isomorphic. Certainly, popular children have more friends than unpopular ones, and thus seem to possess personality or social characteristics that foster compatible peer relations. Yet even neglected or rejected children can have a few close friends. Moreover, some personal attributes and interactional styles may contribute to popularity without being particularly relevant to success in forming or maintaining friendships. For example, being a star on a sports team may make one generally liked by peers, but it may not contribute to the development of specific friendships. For adolescents in particular, peer-group status is likely to involve more than the number of close friends one has.

Masters and Furman (1981) found that the variables associated with popularity and friendship selections are distinctly different. In an observational study of preschool children, *overall* rates of reinforcing and neutral social behaviors with peers were found to be predictive of sociometric status, but they were not related to children's specific selection of friends. Instead, peers whom children named as friends were those who engaged in frequent reinforcing and neutral interactions with them *in particular*. Apparently, friendship selections of at least preschool children are based primarily on children's personal experiences with, or impressions of, peers. Perhaps this may explain why there are "controversial" children who are liked the most by some peers and liked the least by others. And, although we found little evidence of such, it also seems possible that children's observations of a target child's behavior with *others* may affect the observers' friendship selections; for example, children may avoid becoming friends with children who do not interact appropriately with other peers.

More generally, then, the factors associated with sociometric status may affect the development and maintenance of specific friendships if they are representative of children's *personal* experiences with or impressions of peers. That is, children's specific impressions of other children's physical attractive-ness, social behaviors, or intelligence may affect the likelihood that they will become friends with them. The influence of peer groups can also be taken into account in this conceptualization. In particular, the group's impression of or experience with a peer may affect a particular child's impression of that peer, which in turn may affect the likelihood that the peer will be selected as a friend. Although these hypotheses are somewhat speculative, some support for them can be found in research on children's friendships.

Friendships

Perhaps more than any other relationship, friendships are described in almost exclusively positive terms. Our friends like and respect us; they are regular companions with whom we share activities; they can be sources of intimate support when times are difficult. If there is a prototype of a compatible relationship, friendship seems like the obvious candidate. After all, if the relationship were not a compatible one, it could and probably would be terminated. By examining the characteristics of these successful relationships, we may be able to identify variables that foster compatibility in peer relations. Investigators studying children's friendships have examined four issues of interest: (1) similarity between friends, (2) interactions with friends, (3) the formation of friendships, and (4) the dissolution of friendships.

Similarity of Friends

Sex, race, and age. One of the most influential factors in friendship choices is sex. Approximately 90% of children's friends are same-sexed peers (Asher, Oden, & Gottman, 1977; Asher, Singleton, & Taylor, 1982). The preference for same-sex peers is apparent both in terms of stated preferences and actual patterns of behavior. It emerges in the early preschool years and persists throughout childhood (see Hartup, 1983). Even in adolescence, when romantic relationships emerge, the vast majority of friends are still same-sex peers (Kandel, 1978b). Moreover, the few cross-sex friendships that occur are much less stable than same-sex ones (Tuma & Hallinan, 1979).

A number of factors seem to be responsible for the sex schism in peer relations. In his review of the literature, Hartup (1983) suggested that parents may foster the sex cleavage by providing different toys for boys and girls and by seeking out same-sex peers to be potential playmates for their young children. Similarly, teachers respond positively to sex-appropriate activities by groups of same-sex peers (Fagot, 1977). Because the play activities of boys and girls differ in many respects (Maccoby & Jacklin, 1974), similarity of interests could foster attraction to same-sex peers, whereas dissimilarities could lead to the avoidance of opposite-sex peers. Children are also likely to acquire the stereotypic belief that boys play with boys and girls with girls. Finally, in the preadolescent and adolescent years, the development of cross-sex friendships may be stymied by the possibility of romantic involvement (Schofield, 1981).

Sadly, race is also an important factor in the selection of friends. Children's ratings of the "likeability" of same- and cross-race peers are not very different, but relatively few peers of a different race are named as best friends (Asher et al., 1982; Schofield & Whitley, 1983). The preference for same-race peers is already apparent by kindergarten (Finkelstein & Haskins, 1983) and increases as children grow older (Asher et al., 1982). In the elementary-school years, the sex cleavage in friendship nominations is greater than the racial cleavage, but by high school the two are comparable in size. Racial hostility, discrimination, and the limited amount of contact between children of different races all make it difficult for cross-race friendships to develop. Moreover, children may attach different social identities to blacks and whites (Schofield, 1981). For example, whites may be perceived as conceited and prejudiced because of their achievement in the classroom, whereas blacks may be perceived as tough and disobedient. The basis of these perceptions could actually be differences in social class, but children may erroneously perceive them to be racial differences. In any event, such conflicting social identities are not conducive to the development of friendships. Thus, while progress is being made in terms of establishing contacts between races, it seems that we still have a way to go before cross-race friendships become commonplace.

In addition to being of the same sex and race, most friends are about the same age (Hartup, 1983). Several factors may contribute to the age concordance in friendships. In our educational system and elsewhere, children have much more contact with peers of the same age than with peers of different ages. Even if children had equal contact with peers of all ages, however, it seems likely that they would develop friendships primarily with those who are close in age to them. Friendships are, by nature, egalitarian relationships, and establishing and maintaining such egalitarianism would seem to be easier when two children are similar in age than when they are different. Children of the same age are also likely to have more similar interests and attitudes than those of different ages. As shall be seen in the next section, such similarities foster the development of compatible relationships.

Attitudes and behavior. Not only do friends tend to be of the same sex, race, and age, but they tend to have other things in common as well. For example, friends have similar interests and activity preferences (Ball, 1981). The educational aspirations and achievement levels of friends are similar also (Ball, 1981; Tuma & Hallinan, 1979). On the other hand, little evidence exists that friends are particularly similar in terms of intelligence or personality characteristics such as extroversion or neuroticism (see Hartup, 1970).

In one of the most comprehensive studies of this topic, Kandel (1978b) examined the degree of similarity in adolescent friendship pairs on a variety of attributes, including sociodemographic characteristics, attitudes, and behaviors. The highest degree of similarity was found on the sociodemographic characteristics of sex, ethnicity, age, and grade in school. In addition, friends were likely to engage in the same behavioral activities, particularly drug-related activities. The degree of similarity in personality characteristics, attitudes, and quality of relationships with parents was negatively low and often nonsignificant. Kandel's findings are consistent with results of other studies that have examined subsets of these variables. Similarity in sociodemographic characteristics and specific behavioral activities seems more important to friendships than similarity in personality characteristics or abstract attitudes.

Of course, these cross-sectional studies cannot address the issue of causation. It is possible not only that children become friends with those who are similar to them, but that they may become similar to their friends as a result of their interactions together. Kandel (1978a) examined the issue of causal direction in a longitudinal study of adolescent friendships. She compared the degree of behavioral and attitudinal similarity in three types of dyads: (1) pairs of adolescents who were friends at both the beginning and the end of the school year (i.e., stable friends), (2) pairs who were friends at the beginning of the year but not the end (i.e., unstable friends), and (3) dyads who became friends by the end of the year (i.e., subsequent friends). At the beginning of the year, stable friends and subsequent friends were found to be more similar than unstable friends, suggesting that similarity played a role in the selection and development of friends. Moreover, stable friends and subsequent friends were even more similar at the end of the year than at the beginning, suggesting that the friendships fostered similarity. Thus, the relation between similarity and friendship formation appears to be a bidirectional one.

Although these findings indicate that similarity is an important factor in fostering compatible peer relations, many questions have not been adequately addressed. Similarity has generally been treated as a unitary, static construct. The results of Kandel's (1978b) research, however, indicate that some kinds of similarity (e.g., sociodemographic characteristics) may be more important than other kinds (e.g., personality characteristics). Moreover, the kind of similarity that is important may vary from child to child. For example, Ball (1981) found that many friends had similar general attitudes toward school and peer activities, but that some friends had one specific primary interest in common (e.g., horseback riding, scouts). One might also expect developmental changes in the types of similarity that are central; however, this issue has received little attention (but see Duck, 1975). In addition, we know relatively little about how the role of similarity changes during the development of a relationship. Some data suggest that similarity plays a role both in selecting potential friends and in maintaining relationships with friends (Kandel, 1978b; Tuma & Hallinan, 1979), but further research is required. In effect, each of these limitations reflects the fact that the principal concern of investigators has been to demonstrate that friends are similar in terms of some attribute. Now that this point has been demonstrated, we need to conceptualize the role of similarity in dynamic terms. That is, we need to see how individuals go about discovering similarities and how such discoveries foster compatible interchanges.

Interactions With Friends

Information about factors associated with compatibility can also be obtained by comparing children's interactions with friends with their interactions with other peers. Not surprisingly, children interact much more with friends than with other peers (Foot, Chapman, & Smith, 1977; Hartup et al., 1967; Masters & Furman, 1981). More importantly, their interactions with friends and non-friends differ qualitatively as well as quantitatively. Reinforcing and neutral interactions occur more often with friends than with other peers, but punishing interactions occur equally often (Masters & Furman, 1981). Smiling, laughing, and other manifestations of positive affect are more common in interactions of friends than in interactions of acquaintances or strangers (Foot et al., 1977; Newcomb & Brady, 1982; Newcomb, Brady, & Hartup, 1979; Schwartz, 1972); in addition, the affective expression of friends, as compared to nonfriends, is more likely to be matched or synchronized (Foot et al., 1977; Newcomb & Brady, 1982). Similar differences in synchrony or mutuality may also occur in task-oriented behavior. For example, during a problem-solving task, friends were more likely to engage in mutual activities and give mutual credit for their accomplishments than acquaintances were (Newcomb & Brady, 1981).

Children expect more help and prosocial behavior from friends than from acquaintances (Furman & Bierman, 1984), and, in fact, they perceive their friends to be more helpful than other peers (Furman & Childs, 1981). On the other hand, observational studies of prosocial behavior have yielded inconsistent results (see Berndt, in press-b). In some cases, children have been found to share more with friends than with others, but in other instances either no differences have been found or else children have been found to share *less* with friends than with others. Berndt (in press-b) suggested that children may be more likely to help or share with friends than with nonfriends when such behaviors result in equitable outcomes. However, when their assistance results in others outperforming them on tasks, children may be less likely to assist friends than nonfriends because their self-esteem is affected more by the results of contests with friends than with nonfriends. Thus, both cooperation and competition may be more likely to occur with friends than with other peers.

Reinforcing social interchanges, positive affect, synchrony, and prosocial behaviors are probably characteristic of friendships of all ages. Developmental changes occur, however, in other characteristics of friendships. For preschool and young elementary-school children, friendships are centered around play activities. In preadolescence and adolescence, friendships become more personal in nature than before. In particular, marked increases occur in the amount of intimacy and self-disclosure in friendships, particularly in girls' friendships. As they grow older, children report both greater self-disclosure (Buhrmester & Furman, 1984; Hunter & Youniss, 1982) and greater knowledge of information about their friends (Diaz & Berndt, 1982). Youniss (1980) proposed that the differentiation of peers into friends and nonfriends is no longer based on the qualities of actions, but instead on the qualities of persons. In particular, emphasis is placed on the similarity of "personalities." One important implication of these developmental changes is that the factors associated with compatibility and incompatibility should change as well. As children grow older, intimacy skills and similarity of underlying values may become more important, whereas play behaviors and similarity in activity interests may become less important.

Relatively little is known about patterns of conflict and negative behavior in friendships. Children report less conflict with friends than with other peers (Furman & Childs, 1981), although such differences were not found in one observational study of children's interactions (Furman, 1983). On the one hand, one might expect less conflict with friends than with other peers because of the affective bond and shared interests of friends; on the other hand, one might expect more conflict because it may be acceptable for friends to disagree openly. In the studies just cited, only the frequency of conflict was examined. Perhaps ability to resolve disagreements successfully is more predictive of compatibility than the sheer frequency of disagreements.

Studies of friends' interactions suggest that positive peer relations are associated with mutual activities, positive affect, prosocial behaviors, and—for preadolescents or adolescents—intimate self-disclosure. As was the case for research on similarity, one must be cautious in making causal inferences on the basis of these cross-sectional comparisons of different types of relationships. For example, under certain circumstances children compete more with their friends than with other peers, but it is doubtful that one would want to conclude that competition fosters friendships. It seems more likely that such competition results from being friends rather than the reverse. Although examples such as this one underscore the importance of caution, most of the behaviors that characterize interactions with friends seem to be ones that would promote compatible relationships.

The Formation of Friendships

The problems in inferring causality in studies of relationships that have already been established have led some investigators to study how peer relationships develop. For example, Gottman (1983) analyzed conversations of dyads of unacquainted children playing together in a home setting. Children who "hit it off" in their first encounter were found to share information successfully, establish common-ground activities, and manage conflicts amiably. Communication clarity, the exploration of similarities and differences, and self-disclosure were also found to be important predictors of success during children's second and third encounters. In a similar study, Furman (1983) observed dyads of unacquainted third-graders interacting in a laboratory setting. Rates of prosocial behavior and mutual activity were found to be associated with interpersonal attraction and concordant social interactions. In addition, children's perceptions of the amount of information sharing that occurred were also predictive of successful interactions, although the *actual amounts* of information sharing that occurred were not. The results of these two studies are certainly consistent with the literature on interactions of friends. However, because these studies only examined the early development of peer relationships, the possibility remains that the factors associated with compatibility may change over the course of the development of a relationship. In fact, in the Furman (1983) study, dyads of acquainted children were also observed and the correlates of successful interaction (mutual fantasy play and statements of similarity) were different from those for unacquainted children.

Furman and Childs (1981) studied the development of peer relationships over the course of a week-long summer camp. On the second, fifth, and seventh day of camp, children rated six facets of their relationships with each of their cabinmates: (1) prosocial support, (2) intimacy, (3) companionship, (4) similarity, (5) affection, and (6) quarreling. On the seventh day, children also rated the degree of friendship with each cabinmate. At all three points in time, children differentiated among their relationships that received high, medium, or low ratings of friendship. Even as early as the second day of camp, relationships that subsequently received high ratings of friendship were characterized by the highest ratings on all five positive characteristics and the lowest ratings on quarreling; the reverse was true for those that subsequently received low ratings of friendship. Moreover, the degree of differentiation among the three levels of friendship increased over the week. For the five positive characteristics, ratings of "high" and "medium" friendships increased, whereas ratings of "low" friendships decreased. On the other hand, ratings of quarreling in "low" and "medium" friendships increased over time, whereas ratings for "high" friendships remained stable. Apparently, positive social behaviors and the absence of conflict foster friendships in childhood.

Relatively few investigators have examined the development of friendships beyond the initial stages of acquaintanceship. Youniss (1980) asked children what things might happen that would lead children to become "friends" or "best friends." Six- to ten-year-old children emphasized the importance of mutual activities and prosocial behavior. Becoming best friends, they said, required spending an increased amount of time together and doing special things together (e.g., sleeping over at the other's house). Twelve- and thirteen-year-old children also reported such behaviors, but unlike younger children, they were more likely to emphasize the importance of self-disclosure and similarity. A comparable pattern of results was obtained in Bigelow and LaGaipa's (1980) study of the experiences children thought had led them to feel closer to friends. The developmental differences found in these studies are consistent with previously described research on developmental changes in intimacy and self-disclosure.

The Dissolution of Friendships

In addition to studying the development of friendships, one can also study the dissolution of such relationships to determine what factors are associated with incompatibility. For example, some investigators have tried to determine which friendships are likely to be stable and which are likely to be unstable. Opposite-sex friendships have been found to be much less stable than same-sex friendships (Tuma & Hallinan, 1979). Perhaps this is so simply because the children are likely to be less similar. This explanation is consistent with Kandel's (1978a) finding that dissimilarity was associated with instability in children's friendships. Alternatively, opposite-sex friendships may be unstable because peers and perhaps adults often disapprove of them.

Another variable associated with stability is age. In particular, young elementary-school children's friendships are less stable than older elementary-school children's or adolescents' friendships, which do not differ in stability (Berndt, 1982). It is not clear, however, why friendships increase in stability with age. Perhaps older children are more careful or thoughtful than younger children in choosing the children with whom they become friends. As children grow older, they also are more likely to have the social skills necessary for maintaining friendships. Young children may outgrow their friendships as they outgrow the childhood games or childhood activities on which their friendships were based. On the other hand, the friendships of older children, which are based on underlying values and attitudes, may be relatively stable because the shared values and attitudes are slow to change. Finally, the intimate nature of older children's friendships may make them more valuable to participants and/ or more resistant to the pressures that lead to dissolution.

Mutual or reciprocated friendships are more stable than unreciprocated ones; in fact, over time, one-way friendships are more likely to dissolve than to become mutual friendships (Gershman & Hayes, 1983; Hallinan, 1979). Mutual feelings of attraction seem essential if friendships are to develop.

Some investigators have examined the reasons given for the dissolution or decay of friendships. Although situational factors, such as a child moving, are certainly responsible for many dissolutions, children's behavior and the characteristics of their relationship often seem to be responsible as well. For example, Berndt (in press-a) found that kindergarten and elementary-school children commonly referred to aggressive behavior or an absence of play in explaining why friendships had broken up. By contrast, third- and sixth-grade children also referred to disloyalty, faithlessness, or the lack of trust and intimacy as well as to aggression and an absence of play. Bigelow and LaGaipa (1980) reported a similar pattern of results, and made the important observation that the factors that lead to decay are not the flip side of those that lead to the development of relationships.

Summary

What can be concluded about the factors associated with compatibility in children's peer relations? Investigators of sociometric status have emphasized the role of personal characteristics such as physical attractiveness, self-esteem, or intelligence, but these variables have not received much attention in research on children's friendships. For example, we do not know if physically attractive children's friendships develop quicker, are more intimate in nature, or are more stable than unattractive children's friendships. Personal characteristics have, however, received considerable attention in research on the impact of similarity. It seems clear that similarity—at least in terms of sociodemographic characteristics or behaviors—fosters compatible relationships.

Like the research on sociometric status, studies of children's friendships underscore the importance of positive social interactions. Mutual activities, positive affect, and prosocial behavior all seem to foster positive peer relationships. For older children and adolescents, self-disclosure and intimacy skills also appear to be important contributors to successful relationships. Much less is known about the role of conflict and negative behaviors. It appears that negative behaviors can lead one to be disliked and, in effect, excluded from becoming a friend. It is not as clear what impact conflict has once relationships have been established, although there are some indications that the presence of an undue amount of conflict or difficulties in resolving conflicts may lead to problems in peer relationships.

Sibling Relationships

Compared to the amount of research on friendships and peer relations, relatively little study has been made of sibling relationships. Certainly, many investigators have examined the effects of birth order, sex of sibling, age spacing, or other family constellation variables on children's personalities and on their social or cognitive characteristics (see Sutton-Smith & Rosenberg, 1970); however, these studies are not investigations of the sibling relationship per se. Observed effects could be a function of the impact of family constellation variables on parent-child or marital relationships rather than on sibling relationships. Most traditional studies of birth order or other family constellation variables do not provide much information about the processes involved because they do not examine empirically the effects that constellation variables have on sibling relationships or other family relationships. Instead, investigators have simply proposed that various effects occur.

Fortunately, some exceptions can be found. In a classic study, Koch (1960) interviewed preschool children about their relationships with their siblings. Children reported greater association with younger siblings or those close in age than with older siblings or those much different in age. In addition, same-sex siblings were more likely to be preferred play partners than opposite-sex siblings were. Not surprisingly, children were more likely to take care of younger siblings than older siblings. Older siblings were seen as more bossy than younger ones, particularly when the age spacing was great. Brothers were perceived as more likely to take or abuse children's property than sisters were. When the age difference was great, children were more likely to quarrel with older siblings than with younger ones. For siblings close in age, boys often seemed to quarrel with older sisters. Children with younger siblings were more likely than those with older siblings to think that their siblings were favored by their mother and more boys than girls thought that their siblings were favored by their mothers.

Although specific findings have varied somewhat, subsequent investigators have also found that children's perceptions of sibling relationships vary as a function of family constellation variables (see Bryant, 1982). In our own research (Furman & Buhrmester, in press), approximately 200 fifth- and sixth-grade children completed questionnaires that assessed 15 characteristics of sibling relationships, such as the degree of companionship, nurturance, dominance, quarreling, and partiality by parents. A principal-components analysis revealed four underlying factors: (1) Warmth/Closeness, (2) Relative Status/Power, (3) Conflict, and (4) Rivalry. These four factors were relatively independent of one another except for Conflict and Rivalry, which were moderately correlated. Analyses revealed that family constellation variables were related to each of the four factors. For example, children with same-sex siblings had higher scores on the Warmth/Closeness factor than those with opposite-sex siblings, and the difference between children with same-sex and opposite-sex siblings was particularly marked when the children were close in age. Older members of dyads were perceived as having more power and status than younger members, particularly when the age difference was wide. Conflict scores were greater when the difference in age was small than when it was large. Finally, children reported that parents gave preferential treatment to their younger siblings, particularly when these siblings were much younger.

In the preceding studies, investigators examined children's perceptions about sibling relationships. Other investigators have examined patterns of interactions between young siblings (see Dunn, 1983). These researchers have consistently found that older and younger members of dyads differ in their behavior. For example, older siblings initiate most of the prosocial and the agonistic interchanges, whereas younger siblings engage in more imitation than older siblings (Dunn & Kendrick, 1982). Prosocial behavior and imitation also occur more frequently in same-sex dyads than in opposite-sex ones, whereas agonistic interactions occur more commonly in opposite-sex dyads than in same-sex ones (Dunn & Kendrick, 1982). Age-spacing effects have not been found very often in observational studies, although Minnett, Vandell, and Santrock (1983) found greater aggression in narrow-spaced dyads of young school-aged children than in wide-spaced dyads.

Although family constellation variables may be associated with compatibility or other aspects of sibling relationships, the size of these relations should not be overstated. In the Furman and Buhrmester (in press) study, we examined the correlations among the four qualitative factors and the family constellation variables (e.g., sex, sibling's sex, relative age, age difference, family size, and the interactions of the five). Not surprisingly, Relative Status/Power was strongly related to relative age ($r = .81$); older children had more status and power than younger children. On the other hand, the correlations between the other three factors and the constellation variables were relatively modest (all r's $< .30$). Similarly, we were very successful in predicting Relative Power/Status factor scores from a regression equation comprised of the family constellation variables and the interactions among them ($R = .84$), but similar regression equations accounted for less than 20% of the variance on the other three qualitative factors (R's $< .45$). Clearly, family constellation variables and qualitative features of the relationship are not interchangeable.

We also found that relationship satisfaction ratings could not be predicted very well from family constellation variables ($R = .32$), but they could when the four qualitative factors were added to the equation ($R = .67$). Moreover, when the qualitative factors were put in the equation first, the family constellation variables did not provide a significant increment in prediction. These results are not particularly surprising; one would expect satisfaction to be related to the qualitative features of relationships. The important point is that the major focus of research should be the qualitative features of sibling relationships and not family constellation variables. In some respects, recent investigators have begun to shift their attention to qualitative features by studying patterns of interaction between siblings. Unfortunately, such studies have principally examined how patterns of interaction are related to family constellation variables.

What other variables may affect the qualitative features of sibling relationships? Parents may play an important role. For example, Bryant and Crockenberg (1980) observed mothers and their children interacting and found that maternal responsiveness to children's needs was positively related to prosocial sibling interactions and negatively related to agonistic sibling interactions. Dunn and Kendrick (1982) observed family interactions after the birth of a second child. Friendly interactions between siblings were much more common if the mother and first-born had had discussions about the new baby's needs and feelings than if they had not had such conversations. It was also found that if the mother had particularly warm and playful interactions with the second-born, agonistic interactions between the siblings were likely to occur. Apparently, siblings' sex, age spacing, and the characteristics of other family relationships affect the degree of compatibility in sibling relationships. Apart from this type of influence, however, little is known about the factors associated with compatibility in sibling relationships. One would expect that important roles would be played by variables such as the social and personality characteristics of each sibling, but the necessary empirical studies have yet to be conducted.

Friendships and Sibling Relationships

To date, no one has attempted to compare and contrast directly the factors associated with compatibility in children's relationships with their friends and with their siblings. Because investigators have generally focused on different aspects of the two types of relationships, the two literatures have remained almost completely isolated from each other. Still, it is possible to generate some reasonable hypotheses about how the nature of compatibility may be similar or different in these two types of relationships.

One obvious similarity is that positive social interactions are associated with compatibility in both. Companionship, prosocial acts, and intimacy seem to be important determinants of attraction in both. In fact, the specific kinds of positive social interactions that occur in the two probably bear some resemblance to each other because both friendships and sibling relationships—in the context discussed here—are relationships between children. The social and cognitive skills required for effective social interactions can also be expected to be similar in the two.

Negative social behaviors and conflict appear to be negatively associated with compatibility in both friendships and sibling relationships. Conflicts and disagreement between children (or adults!) seem inevitable, and, thus, it is essential that children be able to resolve their disagreements amicably if relationships are to be satisfying or, in the case of friendships, even to continue.

Despite these major similarities, the two types of relationships clearly differ. Friends tend to be of the same age, whereas siblings are not, except in the case of twins. As a consequence, friendships are egalitarian in nature, whereas sibling relationships are characterized by some asymmetry in status or power. The role expectations for children and their friends are very similar, but the role expectations for siblings tend to be different, particularly when the siblings differ substantially in age. Older siblings are responsible for nurturing, guiding, and directing younger ones, whereas younger ones are expected to follow and imitate. Accordingly, compatibility in friendships involves maintaining similar roles and an even balance of power, whereas in sibling relationships it involves coordinating two roles that ideally should complement each other.

Inequality between friends needs to be corrected or the relationship can be jeopardized (Youniss, 1980). Siblings expect some inequality and differentiation in roles, although disagreement about the degree of asymmetry can lead to conflict and incompatibility. That is, younger children may expect older ones to have more power and status than they do, but they may still believe that their siblings have too much power or too many privileges. On the other hand, older siblings may be dissatisfied if the differentiation in power is not sufficiently great. Needless to say, older and younger siblings are likely to have different perceptions about the degree of differentiation that is appropriate. Such disagreements may be especially likely to occur when the two are close in age, because the appropriate balance of power is particularly ambiguous in those cases. Such an explanation could account for the fact that children with siblings who are slightly older than themselves are less satisfied with their relationships than those whose siblings are much older (Furman & Buhrmester, in press).

Friendships are also voluntary relationships, whereas sibling relationships are not. Children can always dissolve relationships with friends, an option that is not available to siblings—at least not until they become adults. One consequence of this difference is that the rules of conduct may be stricter in friendships than in sibling relationships. Children are aware of the fact that a serious transgression can result in the loss of a friend, and they usually behave accordingly. In contrast, relationships with siblings generally continue regardless of what occurs. One could argue that serious transgressions may be less likely to occur in sibling relationships than in friendships because siblings have to continue living together, but this hypothesis is probably not correct. Children report substantially more conflict and quarreling with siblings than with friends (Furman & Buhrmester, in press), and insults and antagonistic behavior occur often between siblings. Although friends can be competitive, the intensity of the rivalry that can occur in sibling relationships appears to be much greater than that occurring in friendships. (After all, can one think of a friendship, even a fictitious one, that resembles in its competitive intensity the relationship between the Ewing brothers, Bobby and J.R.?)

Another important difference between the two is that sibling relationships are family relationships, whereas friendships are not. In fact, sibling relationships must be conceptualized as part of a larger system of relationships among all of the family members. Parents are likely to try to shape the nature of sibling relationships directly. In some pilot research, we found that parents have definite opinions about how close siblings should be, how much conflict is permissible, and how different the privileges and responsibilities of different siblings should be. Sibling relationships not only are directly affected by parents' attempts to foster the kind of relationship they desire between their children; they also are indirectly affected by parents' relationships with each of them. For example, sibling rivalry is commonly thought to result from competition for parental attention (Adler, 1929). Conflict occurs frequently in sibling dyads when children perceive that one of them is favored by their parents (Furman & Buhrmester, in press).

Whereas sibling relationships are affected by parent-child relationships, children's specific friendships may be affected by relationships with other peers. Children commonly talk about their other friends and express opinions about what those relationships should be like. Although it is likely that there are differences in the degree of parental and peer influence on sibling relationships and friendships, it should be emphasized that these differences are relative ones. Parents clearly affect children's selection of friends (see Hartup, 1983), and peers sometimes talk about their siblings and share opinions about how those relationships should be.

In conclusion, both similarities and differences exist in the factors associated with compatibility in the two types of relationships, although further research is needed to delineate the specific similarities and differences. We also need to recognize that neither sibling relationships nor friendships are homogeneous categories of relationships. The factors associated with compatibility in sibling relationships may vary depending upon factors such as the relative age and sex of the children. Similarly, best friendships and other friendships need to be distinguished (see LaGaipa, 1979), and perhaps even finer distinctions are required. Obviously, such differentiations complicate the research task. The important point is that empirical work is needed to directly compare different kinds of relationships, be they different kinds of sibling relationships, different kinds of friendships, or friendships versus sibling relationships.

The Concept of Compatibility

In the beginning of this chapter, six indices of compatibility were listed: (1) feelings of affection or interpersonal attraction, (2) an absence of feelings of dislike or antipathy, (3) frequent rewarding or positive interactions, (4)

infrequent punishing or negative interactions, (5) satisfaction with the relationship, and (6) stability of the relationship. Information about the pattern of
relations among these six can be obtained from the literature reviewed here.

Interpersonal attraction and positive social interactions were consistently
found to be linked in research on sociometric status and friendship selections.
Similarly, in our study of sibling relationships (Furman & Buhrmester, in
press), affection and various positive social behaviors such as companionship,
prosocial acts, and intimacy loaded on the same factor of Warmth/Close-
ness.

On the other hand, frequency of conflict or negative interactions has usually
been found to be unrelated to interpersonal attraction or frequency of positive
social interactions. For example, aggressive behavior is not strongly related
to peer acceptance, although it is associated with peer rejection. Similarly, rates
of giving positive and negative reinforcement to peers have been found to be
uncorrelated (Hartup et al., 1967). Studies of sibling relationships present a
similar picture. For example, perceptions of conflict were found to be
independent of perceptions of warmth or closeness (Furman & Buhrmester,
in press). In other research, rates of positive and negative interactions between
siblings have been found to be relatively independent of each other (Bryant &
Crockenberg, 1980; Minnett et al., 1983). Apparently, conflict is not necessarily indicative of a lack of affection. Some siblings or friends who are close
may find conflict to be an appropriate means of resolving differences, whereas
others may believe that it could jeopardize the closeness of their relationships.
Similarly, some siblings who are not close may regularly quarrel with each
other, whereas others may simply try to avoid each other.

Little is known about the pattern of relations between satisfaction and the
other variables. Although the satisfaction variable has commonly been
incorporated in studies of adult relationships, it has not received much attention
in the developmental literature. I suspect that satisfaction is related to both
positive and negative behaviors and sentiments in relationships. It is possible,
however, that it may be related only to the positive ones, if satisfaction and
dissatisfaction are not bipolar opposites in our judgments.

Similarly, few investigators have directly examined relations between
stability and other indices of compatibility. Investigators examining stability in
friendships have focused on characteristics of the persons involved (e.g., sex
and age), but it is not clear how these variables are related to the sentiments or
behaviors of those involved in the relationships. Friendships in which the
feelings of attraction are mutual are more stable than those in which the feelings
are held by one person, suggesting that stability and attraction are related. In
their descriptions of the dissolution of friendships, children commonly refer to
negative acts and conflict, and sometimes refer to the absence of positive social
acts (Berndt, in press-a; Bigelow & LaGaipa, 1980). It appears that stability
may be a function of both positive and negative aspects of the relationships,
although the relevant data are not very extensive. Incidentally, other authors in

this volume argue that stability may not be strongly associated with compatibility. Unsatisfying relationships may persist because the costs of dissolution are too high or because the alternatives are not appealing. This point is well-taken, although stable, unsatisfying relationships are probably more common in adult relationships, particularly romantic ones, than in children's relationships.

In any event, it is clear that compatibility is not a unitary construct. At a minimum, we need a two-factor model that distinguishes between positive sentiments and acts on the one hand and negative sentiments and acts on the other. Positive sentiments and acts are closely linked, and negative sentiments and acts are closely linked, but the two sets can be distinguished. Overall, stability and satisfaction appear to be composite variables that reflect both the positive and the negative elements. Perhaps compatibility and incompatibility should be viewed as separate constructs rather than as bipolar opposites.

The present distinction bears some resemblance to Rodin's (1982) distinction between liking and disliking criteria. According to Rodin, decisions regarding liking and disliking are based on different criteria. Some individuals are excluded as potential friends because they have some quality that leads them to be disliked. Rodin argues that such individuals will never be liked regardless of what likeable characteristics they have. Among those who are not disliked, others are disregarded because they do not meet the liking criteria. In effect, individuals must both *not meet* the disliking criteria and *meet* the liking criteria for a friendship to develop. Disengagement or dissolution can occur because either the criteria for disliking are subsequently met or because the criteria for liking are no longer met. Perhaps the former kind of relationship would terminate more quickly than the latter kind would.

Although Rodin's distinction is consistent with the present one, I am not certain that meeting the disliked criteria fully excludes the possibility of a close relationship. To use the present terminology, I believe it is possible for a relationship to be simultaneously compatible and incompatible. Two individuals who can't live with each other and can't live without each other may be an example of such a relationship. Similarly, isn't it possible to love and hate someone simultaneously?

It is interesting to note that similar distinctions have recently appeared in other related fields. Positive and negative emotions are no longer thought to be opposites (Russell, 1979; Zevon & Tellegan, 1982). Reich and Zantra (1983) distinguished between positive and negative components of well-being, and proposed that life desires were related to the positive components and life demands to the negative components. Perhaps the positive compatibility factor in relationships is linked to the fulfillment of desires and the positive element of well-being, whereas the negative incompatibility factor is associated with the presence of demands and the negative element of well-being. Certainly, it would be valuable to study the links among well-being, life events, and compatibility and incompatibility in relationships.

Sources of Compatibility

In the empirical research, a number of variables have been identified that may contribute to compatibility or incompatibility. Still, the literature is rather piecemeal in nature. Some variables have been studied extensively, whereas other, seemingly promising ones have received little attention. Particularly absent is a framework to guide the search for the factors associated with compatibility or incompatibility. In a recent paper, I described a model of the types of variables that affected patterns of social interactions in relationships (Furman, 1984-b). Particularly relevant to the study of compatibility are four such types: (1) general characteristics of the target child, (2) general characteristics of the partner, (3) interactions between general characteristics of the two, and (4) relationship-specific factors.

General characteristics of the target child. This category refers to person variables such as social competence, personality or social traits, cognitive abilities, or other general attributes of the target child. Studies of sociometric status have examined some such variables, particularly physical attractiveness, self-esteem, and intelligence or other abilities. Although the results of these studies have been encouraging, the variables they examined have received almost no attention in studies of friendships or sibling relationships. As noted earlier, such variables could be important determinants of attraction and compatibility if they are manifested in the context of a specific relationship.

General characteristics of the partner. This category is identical to the previous one except that it refers to the characteristics of the other sibling or peer in the relationship. Of course, the distinction between target child and partner is completely arbitrary in the case of friendships. This category warrants mentioning, however, because greater progress is likely to occur by examining the characteristics of both children in dyads than by examining the characteristics of only one. To the best of my knowledge, such studies have not been conducted yet. In effect, we are ignoring at least half the variance by examining the characteristics of only one child in a relationship. In fact, as will be seen in the next section, we are probably ignoring more than half because the interaction between the general characteristics of the two can contribute as well.

Interaction of the general characteristics of the two individuals. The third category of the model refers to the multiplicative product of the first two categories. Not only can the general characteristics of each child affect their compatibility, but the degree to which these charcteristics mesh well can also affect compatibility. The literature on the role of similarity in friendships illustrates the importance of the interaction of general characteristics. For example, the sex of either child is not predictive of compatibility, but the interaction of the sexes of the two (e.g., same or opposite) is.

As yet, investigators studying children's relationships have not examined other types of potential interaction. Although research on complementary needs in marital relationships has not been very fruitful (Tharp, 1963), perhaps a more sophisticated examination of complementarity would be. More generally, the study of interactions of characteristics would permit us to go beyond simple additive models of the factors involved in compatibility. For example, Jourard and Resnick (1970) found that the degree of self-disclosure was a function of the interaction of both individuals' tendencies to disclose. If either person tended to be self-disclosing, high rates of disclosure occurred. Low rates of disclosure occurred only when both were low self-disclosers. In other words, properties of dyads cannot be predicted by examining the characteristics of the individuals separately; it is necessary to look at their characteristics in conjunction with each other.

Relationship-specific factors. The preceeding category referred to the interaction of the *general* characteristics of the two individuals, but it is also important to consider patterns of interaction or attitudes that are specific to a certain relationship. Such relationship-specific factors would include the impact of the participants' previous interaction (i.e., the history of the relationship), the participants' specific attitudes and feelings toward each other, their pattern of interaction with each other, and their expectations for the future of the relationship. Based on the present review of the literature, it appears that this category contains some of the most important factors associated with compatibility. For example, Masters and Furman (1981) found that children's selections of friends could not be predicted from peers' *general* social behavior, but they could be predicted from peers' social behavior with particular children. Similarly, children commonly refer to dyad-specific incidents in their descriptions of the bases for the strengthening or dissolution of a friendship. Finally, qualitative features of siblings' interactions with each other were found to be strongly associated with their satisfaction with the relationship. In fact, many of these relationship-specific variables can be thought of as either determinants or indices of compatibility. The important point, however, is that they are centrally related to compatibility. In recent years investigators have become increasingly interested in these relationship-specific variables, although as yet few have examined the effects of the history of the relationship. This research should lead to a better understanding of compatibility.

Significance. Each of these four domains of variables are likely to contain important facets or determinants of compatibility. Although not discussed here, environmental factors and the interaction among the different domains (e.g., person by environment interactions) also warrant consideration (see Furman, 1984-b). No attempt has been made to specify the central variables within each domain. This chapter and other chapters in this volume can serve as a guide for that important task. The present model can, however, serve as an organizing framework for research by identifying aspects of compatibility that have not been studied extensively. Research on these aspects could in turn lead us to a better understanding of the nature of compatibility in children's relationships with their peers and siblings.

Acknowledgment. Preparation of this manuscript was supported by grants from the National Institute of Child Health and Human Development (1R01HD 16142) and from the National Science Foundation (BSN 8014668).

References

Adler, A. (1929). *Understanding human nature.* New York: Premier.

Asarnow, J. R. (1983). Children with peer adjustment problems: Sequential and nonsequential analyses of school behaviors. *Journal of Consulting and Clinical Psychology, 51,* 709–717.

Asher, S. R., & Hymel, S. (1981). Children's social competence in peer relations: sociometric and behavioral assessment. In J. D. Wine & M. D. Smye (Eds.) *Social Competence.* New York: Guilford.

Asher, S. R., Markell, R. A., & Hymel, S. (1981). Identifying children at risk in peer relations: A critique of the rate of interaction approach to assessment. *Child Development, 52,* 1239–1245.

Asher, S. R., Oden, S. L., & Gottman, J. M. (1977). Children's friendships in school settings. In L. G. Katz (Ed.), *Current topics in early childhood education* (Vol. 1). Norwood, NJ: Ablex.

Asher, S. R., Singleton, L. C., & Taylor, A. R. (1982). *Acceptance versus friendship: A longitudinal study of racial integration.* Paper presented at the American Educational Research Association, New York.

Ball, S. J. (1981). *Beachside comprehensive.* Cambridge, England: Cambridge University Press.

Berndt, T. J. (1982). The features and effects of friendship in early adolescence. *Child Development, 53,* 1447–1460.

Berndt, T. J. (in press-a). Children's reports of their friends. In M. Perlmutter (Ed.), *Minnesota Symposium on Child Psychology.* Hillsdale, NJ: Erlbaum.

Berndt, T. J. (in press-b). Sharing between friends: Contexts and consequences. In E. Mueller & C. Cooper (Eds.), *Peer relations: Process and outcome.*

Bigelow, B. J., & LaGaipa, J. J. (1980). The development of friendship values and choice. In H. C. Foot, A. J. Chapman, & J. R. Smith (Eds.), *Friendship and social relations in children.* New York: Wiley.

Bonney, M. E., & Powell, J. (1953). Differences in social behavior between sociometrically high and sociometrically low children. *Journal of Educational Research, 46,* 481–495.

Bryant, B. K., & Crockenberg, S. B. (1980). Correlates and dimensions of prosocial behavior: A study of female siblings with their mothers. *Child Development, 51,* 529–544.

Bryant, B. K. (1982). Sibling relationships in middle childhood. In M. E. Lamb & B. Sutton-Smith (Eds.), *Sibling relationships: Their nature and significance across the lifespan.* Hillsdale, NJ: Erlbaum.

Buhrmester, D., & Furman, W. (1984). *Developmental changes in intimacy and companionship with significant others.* Unpublished manuscript, UCLA.

Cavior, N., & Dokecki, P. R. (1973). Physical attractiveness, perceived attitude similarity, and academic achievement as contributors to interpersonal attraction among adolescents. *Developmental Psychology, 9,* 44–54.

Coie, J. D. D., & Kupersmidt, J. B. (1983). A behavioral analysis of emerging social status in boys' groups. *Child Development, 54,* 1400–1416.

Coie, J., Dodge, K., & Coppotelli, H. (1982). Dimensions and types of social status: A cross age status: A cross age perspective. *Developmental Psychology, 18,* 557–571.

Diaz, R. M., & Berndt, T. J. (1982). Children's knowledge of a best friend: Fact or fancy? *Developmental Psychology*, *18*, 787–794.

Dion, K. K. (1973).Young children's stereotyping of facial attractiveness. *Developmental Psychology*, *9*, 183–198.

Dodge, K. A. (1983). Behavioral antecedents of peer social status. *Child Development*, *54*, 1386–1399.

Dodge, K. A., Coie, J. D., & Brakke, N. P. (1982). Behavior patterns of social approach and aggression. *Journal of Abnormal Child Psychology*, *10*, 389–409.

Duck, S. W. (1975). Personality similarity and friendship choices by adolescents. *European Journal of Social Psychology*, *5*, 351–365.

Dunn, J. (1983). Sibling relationships in early childhood. *Child Development*, *54*, 787–811.

Dunn, J., & Kendrick, S. (1982). *Siblings: Love, envy and understanding*. Cambridge, MA: Harvard University Press.

Elkins, D. (1958). Some factors related to the choice status on ninety eighth-grade children in a school society. *Genetic Psychology Monograph*, *58*, 207–272.

Fagot, B. I. (1977). Consequences of moderate cross-gender behavior in preschool children. *Child Development*, *48*, 902–907.

Finkelstein, N. W., & Haskins, R. (1983). Kindergarten children prefer same-color peers. *Child Development*, *54*, 502–508.

Foot, H. C., Chapman, A. J., & Smith, J. R. (1977). Friendship and social responsiveness in boys and girls. *Journal of Personality and Social Psychology*, *35*, 401–411.

Furman, W. (1983). *Aquaintanceship in middle childhood*. Unpublished manuscript, University of Denver.

Furman, W. (1984-a). Enhancing peer relations and friendships. In S. Duck (Ed.), *Personal relationships V: Repairing personal relationships*. London: Academic.

Furman, W. (1984-b). Issues in the assessment of the social competency of normal and handicapped children. In T. Field (Ed.), *Friendships of handicapped and nonhandicapped children*. Ablex.

Furman, W., & Bierman, K. L. (1984). Children's conceptions of friendship: A multimethod study of developmental change. *Developmental Psychology*. 1984, *20*, 925–933.

Furman, W., & Buhrmester, D. (1982). The contribution of siblings and peers to the parenting process. In M. Kostelnik, A. I. Rabin, L. A. Phenice, & A. K. Soderman (Eds.), *Child Nurturance: Vol. 2. Patterns of supplementary parenting*. New York: Plenum.

Furman, W., & Buhrmester, D. (in press). Children's perceptions of the qualities of sibling relationships. *Child Development*.

Furman, W., & Childs, M. K. (1981). *A temporal perspective on children's friendships*. Paper presented at meeting of Society for Research in Child Development, Boston.

Gershman, E. S., & Hayes, D. S. (1983). Differential stability of reciprocal friendships and unilateral friendships among preschool children. *Merrill Palmer Quarterly*, *29*, 169–177.

Gottman, J. (1977). Toward a definition of social isolation in children. *Child Development*, *48*, 513–517.

Gottman, J. M. (1983). How children become friends. *Monographs of the Society for Research in Child Development*, *48*, No. 201.

Gottman, J., & Gonso, J., & Rasmussen, B. (1975). Social interaction, social competence, and friendship in children. *Child Development*, *45*, 709–718.

Gronlund, N. E. (1959). *Sociometry in the classroom*. New York: Harper.

Gronlund, N. E., & Anderson, L. (1957). Personality characteristics of socially accepted, socially neglected and socially rejected junior high school pupils. *Educational Administration and Supervision*, *43*, 329–338.

Hallinan, M. T. (1979). The process of friendship formation. *Social Networks*, *1*, 193–210.

Hartup, W. W. (1970). Peer interaction and social organization. In P. H. Mussen (Ed.), *Carmichael's Manual of Child Psychology* (3rd ed., Vol. 2). New York: Wiley.

Hartup, W. W. (1976). Peer interaction and the behavioral development of the individual child. In E. Schopler & R. J. Reichler (Eds.), *Psychopathology and child development*. New York: Plenum.

Hartup, W. W. (1983). The peer system. In P. H. Mussen (Editor-in-chief) & E. M. Hetherington (Ed.), *Carmichael's manual of child psychology* (4th ed., Vol. 4). New York: Wiley.

Hartup, W. W., Glazer, J. A., & Charlesworth, R. (1967). Peer reinforcement and sociometric status. *Child Development*, *38*, 1017–1024.

Hops, H. (1982). Social skills training for socially withdrawn/isolated children. In P. Karoly & J. Steffan (Eds.), *Advances in child behavior analysis & therapy, Vol. 2: Intellectual & social deficiencies*. New York: Gardner Press.

Hunter, F. T., & Youniss, J. (1982). Changes in functions of three relationships during adolescence. *Developmental Psychology*, *18*, 806–811.

Hymel, S. (1983). *Social isolation and rejection in children: The child's perspective*. Paper presented at Society for Research in Child Development, Detroit.

Jourard, S. M., & Resnick, J. L. (1970). Some effects of self-disclosure among college women. *Journal of Humanistic Psychology*, *10*, 84–93.

Kandel, D. (1978a). Homphily, selection, and socialization in adolescent friendships. *American Journal of Sociology*, *84*, 427–436.

Kandel, D. B. (1978b). Similarity in real-life adolescent friendship pairs. *Journal of Personality and Social Psychology*, *36*, 306–312.

Kleck, R. E., Richardson, S. A., & Ronald, C. (1974). Physical appearance cues and interpersonal attraction in children. *Child Development*, *45*, 305–310.

Koch, H. L. (1960). The relation of certain formal attributes of siblings to attitudes held toward each other and toward their parents. *Monographs of the Society for Research in Child Development*, *25*, Whole No. 4.

Krasnor, L. R., & Rubin, K. H. (1981). The assessment of social problem-solving skills in young children. In T. Merluzzi, C. Glass, & M. Genes (Eds.), *Cognitive assessment*. New York: Guilford.

Ladd, G. W., & Oden, S. L. (1979). The relationship between peer acceptance and children's ideas about helpfulness. *Child Development*, *50*, 402–408.

LaGaipa, J. J. (1979). A developmental study of the meaning of friendship in adolescence. *Journal of Adolescence*, *2*, 201–213.

Langlois, J. H., & Downs, A. C. (1979). Peer relations as a function of physical attractiveness: The eye of the beholder or behavioral reality? *Child Development*, *50*, 409–418.

Langlois, J. H., & Stephan, C. (1977). The effects of physical attractiveness and ethnicity on children's behavioral attributions and peer preferences. *Child Development*, *48*, 1694–1698.

Langlois, J. H., & Stephan, C. (1981). Beauty and the beast: The role of physical attractiveness in the development of peer relations and social behavior. In S. S. Brehm, S. H. Kassin, & F. X. Gibbons (Eds.), *Developmental Social Psychology*. New York: Oxford University Press.

Maccoby, E. E., & Jacklin, C. N. (1974). *The psychology of sex differences*. Stanford, CA: Stanford University Press.

Marks, G., Miller, N., & Maruyama, G. (1981). Effect of targets' physical attractiveness on assumptions of similarity. *Journal of Personality and Social Psychology*, *41*, 198–206.

Marshall, H. R., & McCandless, B. R. (1957). A study in prediction of social behavior of preschool children. *Child Development*, *28*, 149–159.

Masters, J. C., & Furman, W. (1981). Popularity, individual friendship selection, and specific peer interactions among children. *Developmental Psychology*, *17*, 344–350.

Minnett, A. M., Vandell, D. L., & Santrock, J. W. (1983). The effects of sibling status on sibling interaction: Influence of sex of child, birth order, and age spacing. *Child Development*, *54*, 1064–1072.

Newcomb, A. F., & Brady, J. E. (1982). Mutuality in boys' friendship relations. *Child Development*, *53*, 392–395.

Newcomb, A. F., Brady, J. E., & Hartup, W. W. (1979). Friendship and incentive condition as determinants of children's task-oriented social behavior. *Child Development*, *50*, 878–881.

Putallaz, M., & Gottman, J. M. (1981). An interactional model of children's entry into peer groups. *Child Development*, *52*, 986–994.

Reese, H. W. (1961). Relationship between self-acceptance and sociometric choice. *Journal of Abnormal & Social Psychology*, *62*, 472–474.

Reich, J. W., & Zantra, A. J. (1983). Demands and desires in daily life: Some influences on well-being. *American Journal of Community Psychology*, *11*, 41–58.

Rodin, M. J. (1982). Non-engagement, failure to engage, and disengagement. In S. Duck (Ed.), *Personal relationships 4: Dissolving personal relationships*. London: Academic.

Russell, J. A. (1979). Affective space is bipolar. *Journal of Personality & Social Psychology*, *37*, 345–356.

Schofield, J. W. (1981). Complementary and conflicting identities: Images and interaction in and interracial school. In S. R. Asher & J. M. Gottman (Eds.), *The development of children's friendship*. Cambridge, England: Cambridge University Press.

Schofield, J. W., & Whitley, B. E. Jr. (1983). Peer nomination versus rating scale measurement of children's peer preferences in desegregated school. *Social Psychology Quarterly*, *46*, 242–251.

Schwartz, J. C. (1972). Effects of peer familiarity on the behavior of preschoolers in a novel situation. *Journal of Personality & Social Psychology*, *24*, 276–284.

Shantz, C. U. (1983). Social cognition. In P. H. Mussen (Editor in chief) & J. H. Flavell & E. M. Markman (Eds.), *Handbook of Child Psychology*: (4th ed., Vol. 4) (pp. 495–555). New York: Wiley.

Smith, G. H. (1950). Sociometric study of best-liked and least-liked children. *Elementary School Journal*, *51*, 77–85.

Sorrell, G. T., & Nowak, C. A. (1981). The role of physical attractiveness as a contributor to individual development. In R. M. Lerner & N. A. Buson-Rossnagel (Eds.), *Individuals as producers of their development: A life-span perspective*. New York: Academic Press.

Spivack, G., Platt, J. J., & Shure, M. B. (1976). *The problem-solving approach to adjustment*. San Francisco: Jossey-Bass.

Sutton-Smith, B., & Rosenberg, B. G. (1970). *The sibling*. New York: Holt, Rinehart & Winston.

Tharp, R. G. (1963). Psychological patterning in marriage. *Psychological Bulletin*, *60*, 97–117.

Tuma, N. B., & Hallinan, M. T. (1979). The effects of sex, race, and achievement on school children's relationships. *Social Forces*, *57*, 1265–1285.

Wood, H. D. (1976). *Predicting behavioral types in preadolescent girls from psychosocial development and friendship values*. Unpublished doctoral dissertation. University of Windsor.

Youniss, J. (1980). *Parents and peers in social development: A Sullivan-Piaget perspective*. Chicago: University of Chicago Press.

Zevon, M. A., & Tellegan, A. (1982). The structure of mood change: An idiographic/nomothetic analysis. *Journal of Personality & Social Psychology*, *43*, 111–122.

Part II

Behavioral Interdependence:
Social Exchange

Chapter 4

Equity and Intimate Relations: Recent Research

Elaine Hatfield, Jane Traupmann, Susan Sprecher,
Mary Utne, and Julia Hay

Equity theory is a social psychological theory concerned with justice in all interpersonal relationships. Until recently, however, equity principles have been examined only in casual role relations (i.e., employer-employee, philanthropist-recipient, and harmer-victim relations) and have not been examined in more personal relations (see Walster (Hatfield), Walster, & Berscheid, 1978). The distinction between role relationships and personal relationships is a long-standing and important one (see Cooley, 1902; Tonnies, 1887). Given the importance of primary, intimate relations, it would be a grave omission to overlook such relations in theory and research on interpersonal behavior.

In this chapter, we will begin by reviewing equity theory and the theoretical debate as to whether or not equity considerations *should* apply to intimate relations. Then we will summarize the recent evidence indicating that equity principles *do* seem critically important in our most significant relations.

Equity Theory: An Overview

The most recent formulation of equity theory, by Walster (Hatfield), Walster, and Berscheid (1978) and Hatfield and Traupmann (1980), evolved from the earlier versions of equity theory by Adams (1965) and Homans (1974). The theory contains four interlocking propositions:

Proposition I: Individuals will try to maximize their outcomes (where outcomes equal rewards minus punishments).

Proposition IIA: Groups (or rather, the individuals comprising these groups) can maximize collective rewards by evolving accepted systems for equity, and will attempt to induce members to accept and adhere to these systems.

Proposition IIB: Groups will generally reward members who treat others equitably, and generally punish members who treat others inequitably.

Proposition III: When individuals find themselves participating in inequitable relationships, they will become distressed. The more inequitable the relationship, the more distress they will feel.

Proposition IV: Individuals who discover that they are in inequitable relationships will attempt to eliminate their distress by restoring equity. The greater the inequity that exists, the more distress they will feel, and the harder they will try to restore equity.

Theoretically, an equitable relationship is said to exist when the person evaluating the relationship concludes that both participants' relative gains are equal. Inequity can arise if one participant's ratio of outcomes to inputs is either larger or smaller than his or her partner's. According to the theory, individuals who find themselves in inequitable relationships will become distressed. The overbenefited will feel guilty about their favorable state of affairs, while their underbenefited partners will feel angry or resentful. These feelings of distress will lead the inequitably treated individuals to initiate steps to restore equity and balance to the relationship. It is assumed here that a state of equity (and its accompanying psychological comfort) is desired.

The Theoretical Debate

Theoretically, equity theory should apply to *all* relationships—from those of the most casual acquaintances to those of the most intimate lovers. A careful scrutiny of research applications of equity theory, however, reveals a bias toward the examination of casual relationships (see Walster (Hatfield), Walster, & Berscheid, 1978). In general, early equity researchers studied relationships between persons who barely knew each other. In study after study, such casual role relationships as philanthropist-recipient, employer-employee, and harmer-victim were observed to determine how participants react when they find themselves either exploiting others or being exploited. So long as researchers examined such casual role relations, equity theory was well received (see Adams & Freedman, 1976).

More recently, however, equity theorists have begun to argue that intimate relations, too, might be dependent on an equitable exchange of rewards. In reaction to this step forward, however, several objections were raised. Holding the traditional Western view of love as involving altruism and selflessness, many theorists have insisted that "true love" transcends equity considerations. In an equally forceful voice, another group of theorists have argued that concerns with fairness are important in love relations. Following are excerpts from both sides of the theoretical controversy.

Equity theory is not applicable to love relationships. Some critics argue that intimate relations are special relations—untainted by crass considerations of social exchange. These critics include those who do not hesitate to apply exchange and equity principles to more casual relations, but object to their application in special relations.

Chadwick-Jones (1976), an exchange theorist, observes:

> On the topic of love, exchange theorists tended to have very little to say for the very good reason that, in love, and in unconditional commitment, there can be no exchange. (p. 2)

Brunner (1945) also states that love is special:

> The sphere in which there are just claims, rights, debits and credits, and in which justice is therefore the supreme principle, and the sphere in which the gift of love is supreme, where there are no deserts, where love, without acknowledging any claim, gives all—these two spheres lie as far apart as heaven from hell. . . . If ever we are to get a clear conception of the nature of justice, we must also get a clear idea of it as differentiated from and contrasted with love. (p. 104)

Other eminent theorists agree with the contention that love relationships should, and do, transcend "selfish" concerns. See for example, Douvan (1974), Fromm (1956), Kennedy (1980), Mills and Clark (1980), Murstein (1980), Rubin (1973), and Wexler (1980).

Equity theory is applicable to love relationships. Other theorists insist that in love relationships, as in less intense relationships, persons are deeply concerned with considerations of fairness. For example, Tedeschi (1974) observes:

> Fromm defined love as primarily giving, not receiving. . . . The nature of true love is contrasted to the behavior of the marketing character . . . the difference between true love and the false love of the marketing character is a matter of timing, illusion, and appearances. . . . The person should believe that he is willing to give without selfish intent, but implicitly his behavior depends upon expected reciprocity at some later, unstated time, and in a form to be decided upon by the other person. (p. 211)

Perhaps the strongest proponents of the equity perspective have been behavioral and family therapists. For example, Sager (1976) observes:

> In work with marital couples and families, the concept of individual marriage contracts has proven extremely useful. . . . The term *individual contract* refers to a person's expressed and unexpressed, conscious and beyond awareness concepts of his obligations within the marital relationship, and to the benefits he expects to derive from marriage in general and from his spouse in particular. But what must be emphasized above all is the reciprocal aspect to the contract: what each partner expects to give and what he expects to receive from his spouse in exchange are crucial. Contracts deal with every conceivable aspect of family life: relationships with friends, achievements, power, sex, leisure time, money, children, etc. . . . It is most important to realize that, while each spouse may be aware of his own needs and wishes on some level of awareness, he does not usually realize that his attempts to fulfill the partner's needs are based on

the covert assumption that his own wishes will thereby be fulfilled. When significant aspects of the contract cannot be fulfilled, as is inevitable, and especially when these lie beyond his own awareness, the disappointed partner may react with rage, injury, depression, or withdrawal, and provoke marital discord by acting as though a real agreement had been broken. (pp. 4–5)

Other theorists from a variety of areas also agree that equity considerations are critically important in intimate relations. See, for example, Bernard (1964), Blau (1964), Lederer and Jackson (1968), McCall (1966), Patterson (1971), Scanzoni (1972), and Storer (1966).

Who is right—the theorists who insist that intimate relationships transcend equity considerations or the theorists who insist that issues of fairness and justice are very relevant to intimate relations? In the past few years, researchers have begun to collect some data designed to address this controversy. For the most part, these data have not been available to the larger audience of researchers in general. The "pro" and "con" advocates in this debate inevitably publish in very different journals—each side insisting that the others' research is based on an inappropriate paradigm, is poorly done, and is poorly written. In addition, much of this research remains unpublished. This chapter was designed to briefly review the existing literature, published or not, so it becomes available to researchers.

Specific Equity Hypotheses for Intimate Relationships

Theorists have derived five specific hypotheses from Equity theory that are applicable to intimate relationships (see Hatfield, Utne, & Traupmann, 1979). In brief, the hypotheses suggest that the more equitable relationships are, the more compatible they will be (i.e., the more satisfying they will be and the longer they will last). (The hypotheses follow, somewhat, the progression of a relationship—from the developing intimacy of the dating stage, to the long-term commitment and accompanying crises of a marriage, to the point of dissolution.) The hypotheses are as follows:

Hypothesis 1: In the casual and steady dating period, couples who feel that their relationships are equitable will be more likely than couples in inequitable relationships to move on to more intimate relationships. (For example, equitable couples will be especially likely to become sexually involved—and to continue to date, live together, or marry.)

Hypothesis 2: Equitable relationships will be compatible relationships. Men and women in equitable relationships should be more content than men and women who are receiving either far more or far less than they feel they deserve. The more inequitable their relationships, the more distress they should feel.

Hypothesis 3: Since inequities are disturbing, couples should continue to try to resolve them over the course of their relationships. Men and women who feel underbenefited should be motivated to demand more from their partners. Men and women who feel overbenefited should find ways to meet the demands of their partners. Thus, all things being equal, relationships should become more and more equitable over time.

Hypothesis 4: In all relationships, there are certain crisis periods (e.g., when a dating couple marries, when the first child arrives, when the children leave home, when someone loses his or her job or retires). At such times of precipitous change, relationships become unbalanced. If couples are contacted before, during, and after such crises, it is likely that couples will find the crisis period very unsettling, and will work to reestablish equity . . . or move in the direction of dissolution of the relationship.

Hypothesis 5: Among the committed relationships, equitable relations will be especially stable. Individuals in equitable relations will be more likely to perceive their relationships as long-term *and* will be more likely to have relationships intact months and years later.

A Review of Existing Research

Let us consider the recent data that have been collected in an effort to support, or to rebut, these equity hypotheses.

Hypothesis 1: In the casual and steady dating period, couples who feel that their relationships are equitable will be more likely than couples in inequitable relationships to move on to more intimate relationships. (For example, equitable couples will be likely to become more sexually involved—and to continue to date, live together, or marry).

In one study, Hatfield, Walster, and Traupmann (1978) interviewed 537 college men and women who were casually or steadily dating someone. Men and women were asked to rate the equity of their current relationship via *The Walster (1977) Global Measure*. (If they were not currently in a relationship, they were asked how equitable their last serious relationship had been before they had split up.) Specifically, the participants were asked: "Considering what you put into your dating relationship, compared to what you get out of it . . . and what your partner puts in compared to what he/she gets out of it, how well does your dating relationship stack up?" Based upon the respondents' estimates of their own inputs and outcomes and their partner's inputs and outcomes, the men and women were classified as overbenefited, equitably treated, or underbenefited in their dating relationships.

The researchers found that equitable relationships were more compatible (i.e., more stable) relationships. Couples in equitable relationships were more likely than couples in inequitable relationships to be moving toward a more intimate relationship. In terms of sexual intimacy, they found that equitable couples were more sexually active. In general, couples in equitable relationships were having sexual intercourse, while those in inequitable relationships tended to stop before "going all the way."

The authors also asked the respondents who were sexually intimate why they had gone that far. The participants in relatively equitable relations were more likely to say that they had intercourse because they *both* wanted to. For example, they were more likely to rate high such reasons as "mutual physical desire" or "enjoyment." Those who felt extremely overbenefited or extremely underbenefited were less likely to say that sex was a mutual decision.

While one aspect of being sexually intimate is engaging in sexually intimate behaviors, another important aspect of sexual intimacy is being *satisfied* with the sexual relationship. Traupmann, Hatfield, and Wexler (1981) interviewed 189 college men and women to investigate whether those who felt equitably treated had more compatible and satisfying sexual relations than those who felt either underbenefited or overbenefited. The authors received some support for their hypothesis. Equitably treated men and women felt more "loving and close" and more physically satisfied after sex with their partner than inequitably treated men and women did.

Another aspect of moving the relationship to greater intimacy is expecting the relationship to evolve into a more permanent one. In the above study of young dating men and women, by Hatfield, Walster, and Traupmann (1978), equitable relationships were found to be generally stable. While equitably treated men and women were confident that they would still be together in 1 year and in 5 years, the overbenefited and underbenefited were less optimistic about the future. If their relationships were not already in disarray, they expected that they soon would be. Furthermore, the equitable couples' confidence and the inequitable couples' pessimism may have been warranted. In a follow-up study 3½ months later, couples in equitable relationships were more likely to still be together than the other couples were.

In another study, Sprecher-Fisher (1980) interviewed a volunteer sample of 50 college dating couples. She also found that equitably treated men and women were more certain than their underbenefited and overbenefited counterparts that they would still be together in the future (equity was measured both via *The Walster 1977 Global Measure* and by a more detailed measure). In addition, 4 years after the initial interview, 48 of the 50 dating couples were interviewed once again to determine if they were still together. Of the 48 couples, 24 had broken up and 24 were still together. Using path analysis, Sprecher-Fisher found that inequities can lead to the termination of the relationship, but only when mediated by psychological distress. In other words, couples have to be distressed by inequities before they consider taking such a drastic step as breaking up.

Conclusion. These studies suggest that dating couples in equitable relations are more likely than other couples to move toward increasing intimacy. Couples in equitable relations are more likely to be sexually involved and sexually satisfied, and are more likely to expect their relations to evolve into more permanent ones.

Hypothesis 2: Men and women in equitable relationships should be more content than men and women who are receiving either far more or far less than they feel they deserve. The more inequitable their relationships, the more distress they should feel.

According to Equity theorists, equitable relationships are compatible (i.e., more satisfying) relationships. Researchers have found this prediction to be an intriguing one, and thus, more research effort has gone into testing it than any other. Most theorists have found it easy to see why men and women who feel that they are getting far less than they deserve from their relationships (who feel that they are being "ripped off" by their partners) should be upset. These men and women may well feel unloved ("If you really loved me, you wouldn't treat me this way") as well as deprived of real benefits. But there is another, more interesting side to this hypothesis. According to Equity theory, men and women who feel that they are getting far *more* than they deserve should also feel distressed. On the one hand they are undoubtedly delighted to be receiving such benefits. However, they know they do not deserve them, and this should make them feel uncomfortable. Berscheid, Hatfield, and Bohrnstedt (1973) provide a graphic description of why an "embarrassment of riches" is often just that:

> Among the *Psychology Today* respondents who are currently in stable relationships, 58 percent say that they are equally matched . . . we wondered what happens to a person who beats the odds, who wins a partner far more desirable than himself. Equity theory predicts that he or she might not be so lucky after all. For one thing, he will worry about losing his mate, who has every reason to leave him; he may feel he could never do so well again.
>
> Waller, citing the epigram that "in every love affair there is one who loves and one who permits himself to be loved," pointed out that such inequitable relationships are costly to both partners. The less dependent person may feel guilty and uncomfortable about exploiting his or her mate while continuing to do so; the more dependent partner suffers exploitation and insecurity. Waller concluded that such lopsided affairs soon come to a sad conclusion. (p. 30)

Figure 4-1 depicts the relationship that Equity theorists *expect* to exist between equity and contentment/distress. (See Austin & Walster, 1974a, 1974b.)

Researchers have collected considerable evidence that couples at all stages of involvement—from dating and newlyweds to couples married for many years—do care deeply about equity. In the study referred to earlier, Hatfield et al. (1978) asked casually and steadily dating students how equitable their relations were and how content they were with them. To measure contentment, daters were given Austin's (1974) *Measure of Contentment/Distress*, which asks couples: "When you think about your relationship as a whole—what you put into it and what you get from it, and what your partner puts into it and what your partner gets out of it—how does that make you feel?" Respondents were asked how "content," "happy," "angry," and "guilty" they felt. An overall index of affect was calculated by summing the respondents' "content" and "happy" scores and subtracting their "anger" and "guilt" scores: Affect = content + happy − angry − guilty. The higher the total score, the more content (and the less distressed) they were.

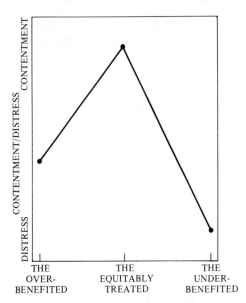

Figure 4-1. The hypothesized relationship between equity and contentment/distress.

These researchers found that men and women who were involved in relatively equitable relationships were far more content and happy than were their greatly overbenefited *or* greatly underbenefited peers. The greatly overbenefited felt extremely guilty about their favored position, while the greatly underbenefited felt extremely angry about the way they were being treated. Identical results were secured by Traupmann, Hatfield, and Wexler (1981) in a replication study. In her survey of 50 dating couples, Sprecher-Fisher (1980), too, replicated the curvilinear relationship between equity and contentment/distress. In addition, she secured some unexpected results. While, in general, equitable couples were more content than inequitable couples, men and women appeared to differ in which type of inequity was more distressing. Women were especially upset when they received too much, whereas men were most upset when they received too little. (This is a finding that has subsequently appeared in several other studies.)

After the dating studies appeared, some critics argued cogently that these data on dating and newlywed couples are not really relevant to the question of whether equity considerations are important in *committed, long-term* intimate relationships. For example, Rubin (1973) stated that only *early* in relationships are people concerned with equity:

> The principles of the interpersonal marketplace are most likely to prevail in encounters between strangers and casual acquaintances and in the early stages of the development of relationships. As an interpersonal bond becomes more firmly established, however, it begins to go beyond exchange. In close relationships one becomes decreasingly concerned with what he can get from

the other person and increasingly concerned with what he can do for the other. (pp. 86–88)

Murstein and MacDonald (1977) agreed with Rubin that although equity considerations shape dating and newlywed relationships, they should not and do not operate in more committed ones. Murstein and MacDonald observe:

An exchange-orientation [was] hypothesized to be quite appropriate for limited or beginning friendships, and exchange-oriented couples were predicted to develop greater friendship intensity than other combinations—perceived exchange equity is almost impossible to obtain in marriage because of greater sensitivity to self than to other. It was hypothesized that exchange-orientation is inimical to marriage adjustment. (p. 1)

At least three studies exist, however, to indicate that equity considerations *are* important in committed and long-term relationships.

Traupmann, Peterson, Utne, and Hatfield (1981) interviewed a random sample of 118 newlywed couples from a variety of occupational backgrounds. Equity was assessed via both a global measure (Walster (1977) Global Measure) and a detailed measure (Traupmann, Utne, & Walster (1977) Scales). These researchers found that newlywed couples are distressed by inequity. Men and women who felt equitably treated were more content than those who felt either overbenefited or underbenefited. Similar to the findings reported above for dating couples (Sprecher-Fisher, 1980), there was a trend for husbands and wives to react differently to advantageous and disadvantageous inequities. Men were more negatively aroused by negative inequities, whereas women were more aroused by positive inequities.

Schafer and Keith (1980) interviewed more than 300 married couples who ranged in age from 19 to 88. The couples were selected in a random area sample designed to include couples who were married for various lengths of time and who were at various stages of the family life cycle. Equity was measured within the context of performance in the family roles of cook, housekeeper, provider, companion, and parent. Husbands and wives evaluated their own and their spouses' levels of effort in the different roles, and equity was determined by taking the difference in the scores of self-evaluation and evaluation of the partner. The prediction that husbands and wives who felt either overbenefited or underbenefited would report higher levels of depression than equitably treated persons received strong support.

In yet another study, Traupmann, Hatfield, and Sprecher (1981) interviewed a random sample of 400 middle-aged and elderly women (ages 50 to 92) living in Madison, Wisconsin. The subjects were asked to think about their lives and say how equitable their relationships had been at various stages in their lives— when they were dating, newlywed, and in their 30s, 40s, 50s, 60s, 70s, and 80s. (They indicated their impressions via *The Hatfield (1978) Global Measure*.) They were then asked to recall, using the *Austin (1974) Measure of Contentment/Distress*, how they had felt about their state of affairs during each of these periods.

As can be seen from Figure 4-2, the results of the Traupmann et al. (1981) study provide additional confirmation for the contention that equity and fairness remain of concern to individuals over the life span.

There is one exception, however, to this clear pattern of results. Traupmann and Hatfield (1983) asked the women in the preceding study how equitable they perceived their current relationships to be and how contented/distressed they were by this *at the present time.* Although the open-ended interview data suggested that elderly women were deeply concerned about equity, the data did not reflect this. Both the overbenefited and the equitably treated women were equally content with the status quo. It was only the underbenefited who expressed any dissatisfaction. This finding raises an interesting possibility. Perhaps late in life, the overbenefited come to feel comfortable about their good fortune. They become confident, finally, that it will last. Of course, the data suggest that one never adapts to underbenefit. Unfortunately, though, the measures of equity used in this study were developed for use with dating and newlywed couples, and perhaps they are simply not appropriate for an older-aged sample. Which of these possibilities is correct will have to be determined by subsequent research.

Conclusion. There is evidence that inequity is distressing for couples at all ages and at all stages of a relationship—dating couples, newlywed couples, couples married an average amount of time, and those married a long time. Equitable relations do appear to be the most compatible relations. Everyone seems to feel

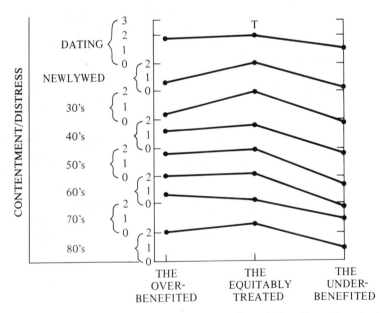

Figure 4-2. The relationship between the equity of a relationship and contentment/distress of each stage in a woman's life.

most content in equitable relations. In general, men and women seem to feel uncomfortable receiving either far more or far less than they think they deserve. It appears that one never gets used to injustice.

Hypothesis 3: Since inequities are disturbing, couples should continue to try to resolve them over the course of their relationship. Men and women who feel underbenefited should be motivated to demand more from their partners. Men and women who feel overbenefited should find ways to meet the demands of their partners. Thus, all things being equal, relationships should become more and more equitable over time.

When couples find themselves experiencing distressful inequities, there are two ways in which they can restore equity to the relationship. Individuals can restore *actual* equity by inaugurating real changes in the relationship; that is, they can alter their own inputs or encourage their partners to alter theirs. Alternatively, individuals can restore *psychological* equity by trying to convince themselves (and their partners) that everything is fair.

Is there any evidence to indicate that inequitable couples do try to restore actual or psychological equity over time? Only one study exists that suggests that relationships may become more equitable over time. Schafer and Keith (1981) interviewed a random sample of more than 300 married couples. They examined how perceptions of equity/inequity change at different developmental stages of the family life cycle. The researchers selected couples that fell into one of four family life cycle stages: (1) early child-raising, (2) children are older and beginning to leave home, (3) children have left home and couple is in middle age, or (4) retirement. They found that perceptions of equity in the family roles of cooking, housekeeping, provider, companion, and parent tended to increase over the life cycle for both husband and wife. The greatest increases in perceived equity tended to occur between Stage 2 and Stage 3—a period when the couple is middle-aged and their children have left home.

Unfortunately, other studies, using slightly more sophisticated measures of equity, have *not* found any evidence that relationships become more equitable over time.

In a study referred to earlier, Hatfield, et al. (1978) interviewed 537 college men and women about their relationships. In a follow-up study, 3½ months later, they interviewed the men and women a second time. The respondents were asked: Were they still going with their partners? How equitable were their relationships at the *present time*? (If they were not currently in a relationship, they were asked how equitable their last serious relationship had been in the few months before they had broken up.) Although Hatfield et al. did not analyze these data of interest to us, their data were available to us. They appear in Table 4-1.

From inspection of Table 4-1, we can see (1) how casual daters, steady daters, and those living together or married differ in their perceptions of how equitable their relationships are, and (2) how people's perceptions change over time. These results provide *no* evidence that relationships become more and

Table 4-1. The Equity of a Couple's Relationship Over Time

	N	*Time 1* How Equitable is Relationship?[a]	*Time 2* How Equitable is Relationship?[a]	Change[b]
Relationship				
All couples who are still together; Daters, Living Together, Married)	181	1.23	1.25	−.02
All couples who are still apart, or who have separated	115	3.67	5.43	−1.75
$F_{Total}(1.294) =$				5.01*
Finer Grained Analyses				
Couples who are still together				
Casual Daters	(20)	2.14	1.84	+.30
Steady Daters	(129)	.98	1.26	−.28
Living Together	(20)	2.23	.59	+1.63
Married	(12)	.78	1.33	−.56
$F_{Linear}{}^{c} (1/176) =$		.72	.69	.02
Couples who are still apart				
Casual Daters	(42)	4.57	4.37	+.20
Steady Daters	(37)	4.46	5.37	−.87
Couples who have separated				
Casual Daters	(14)	3.35	4.57	−1.22
Steady Daters	(20)	.78	8.65	−7.87
$F_{Linear}{}^{d} (1/256) =$		14.81***	1.56	1.82
F_{Linear} B		.10	26.23***	19.79***
$F_{Linear\ A \times Linear\ B}$		.64	3.59*	5.00*

[a]The higher the number, the more inequitable couples perceive their relationships to be.
[b]A + (positive) change indicates that the couple's relationship is becoming more equitable over time; a − (negative) change indicates that it is becoming less equitable.
[c]Analyses for Still-together couples only.
[d]Analyses for all couples—Still-together, Still-apart, and Separated.
  *$p < .05$
  **$p < .01$
***$p < .001$

more equitable over time. Intimates of various statuses (casual daters + steady daters *vs.* couples living together + the married) do not differ from one another in the perceived equity of their relationships. (Linear F [1,176], Time 1 = .72, n.s.)

Nor is there any evidence that intimates' relationships became any more equitable during the 3½ months of the study. For couples who are still together, the change from Time 1 to Time 2 was virtually nonexistant (F[1,176] = .00, n.s.).

What *is* interesting is how men and women's memories of their relationships changed. If a relationship died, men's and women's perception of how equitable it *had been* in its last few months changed precipitously. (The F[1,256] Linear B effect—assessing the difference between the Still Together groups [M = +.02 change], the Still Apart's [M = −.30], and the Separated groups, [M = −5.13]—is 19.79; *p* < .001.) In this case, rather than inequity breeding instability, instability seems to breed a *perception* of inequity.

Additional evidence that the fairness of couples' relationships may not increase over the life span comes from the previously cited interview study of a random sample of 400 elderly women living in Madison, Wisconsin. (Unfortunately, for our purposes, their husbands were not interviewed.) Traupmann et al. (1981) asked the women to indicate via *The Hatfield (1978) Global Measure*, how equitable their marriages had been at various stages in their lives. The women were asked: Did they perceive that their marriages became more and more equitable over time? Stayed about the same? Got less and less fair over time? Varied randomly? As can be seen from Figure 4-3, there is no evidence to support Hypothesis 3. During the early days of dating and marriage, women generally recalled feeling overbenefited. For almost all of the remainder of their lives, however, they felt slightly underbenefited. It was only at the close of their lives that they began to feel fairly treated.

These data raise an intriguing question: If the authors had interviewed men, would they have secured the same pattern of results? Some theorists suggest they would. For example, Lobsenz and Murstein (1976) observe that if men and women "keep score" in their marriages, they both will come out feeling "ripped off." Both men and women, they argue, feel underbenefited most of their lives.

Bernard (1972), on the other hand, argues that men and women should differ markedly in how fair they feel their marriages are. She argues that there is a "His" marriage and a "Her" marriage. In the dating period, women have the advantage. Later on, however, men do. These data support this contention for women, but unfortunately, without data for husbands, we do not know how older men react to the fairness in their relationships.

Conclusion. While one study exists to suggest that perceptions of equity may increase over time, most research provides no support for the contention that relationships become more equitable over time.

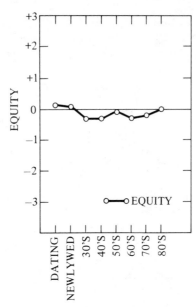

Figure 4-3. Women's perceptions of the equity of their marriages throughout their lives.

Hypothesis 4: In all relationships there are certain crisis periods. At such times of precipitous change, relationships will often become unbalanced. If couples are contacted before, during, and after such crises, it is likely that couples will find the crisis period very unsettling, and will work to reestablish equity . . . or move in the direction of dissolution of the relationships.

The preceding evidence suggests that most couples start off in fairly well-matched relationships (see Hypothesis 1). In time, however, there will be changes in the relationship balance; relationships that were once equitable become inequitable. Change in the balance of equity may occur in a variety of ways. *Getting acquainted*: Regardless of how well dating couples think they know each other, once they begin living together they are likely to make some marked discoveries about themselves and their partners. They may come to realize that the relationship that they thought would be so perfect, so fair, is, in fact, grossly inequitable. *Day-to-day changes*: Over the years, people change. Such mundane changes, too, may produce inequities. Still other changes occur later in life (i.e., during the empty-nest period, retirement or illness). *Dramatic changes*: Sometimes dramatic changes occur in partners' assets and liabilities. Eventually, the impoverished medical student evolves into an affluent doctor. The good provider may be laid off. The overweight wife may join Weight Watchers.

There is a limited amount of survey data that support the contention that any change in the equity of a relationship can send reverberations throughout the entire system. For example, the Depression afforded Komarovsky (1971) an opportunity to study the impact of dramatic changes on the marital balance. Komarovsky reasoned: "In the traditional patriarchal view of the family, the husband is expected to support and protect his wife . . . she, in turn, is expected to take care of his household, to honor and obey him" (p. 2). What happens, Komarovsky asked, when a man loses his job? Does he begin to lose authority?

During the winter of 1935–1936, Komarovsky contacted 58 families who were receiving public assistance. In all of the families, the husband had been the family's sole provider before the Depression. When the Depression hit, this changed: The men lost their jobs and were forced to go on relief. Komarovsky interviewed family members to find out what impact, if any, this change had on the husband and wife's relationship. Komarovsky found that in 13 of the 58 families, when the husband lost his ability to support his family, he began to lose his authority.

Two major types of changes occurred in families: (1) In some families, the couple's relationship evolved into a more egalitarian one. For example, in one family, the man began, for the first time, to take on part of the household duties. In another family, a Protestant father who had formerly forbidden his children to go to a Catholic school now relented. (2) In a very few cases, the husbands' and wives' status was reversed. The dominant husband became subordinate. For example, in one family, so long as the husband was employed, his wife had treated him with careful respect. Once the Depression hit, she no longer bothered to be so polite; she began to blame her husband for unemployment, to ignore his wishes, to complain about his behavior, to argue with him, to nag him constantly, and to criticize him sharply even in front of the children. In another family, the husband admitted: "There certainly was a change in our family, and I can define it in just one word—I relinquished power in the family. . . ." (p. 31).

There is other survey evidence to indicate that crisis periods may change the balance of power in ways that restore equity to the marital relationship. Also studying the effects of unemployment from the Depression, Angell (1936) and Cavan (1959) found that men who became unemployed also lost power in the family, especially if respect and authority were contingent upon earnings. In addition, there is cross-sectional research to suggest that if the status quo (which is usually the husband being the provider) changes, there will also be changes in the relative power of the couple. Scanzoni (1970, 1972) surveyed 900 marriages from all socioeconomic levels and found that the better the husband's performance in the economic system, the more likely it was that the wife believed her husband deserved greater power in the relationship. Those husbands who were not as successful in acquiring status, prestige, and wealth tended to have wives who believed in an equal distribution of power. Aldous (1969) and Gillespie (1971) found that working wives with an independent source of income may have more power than those who stay at home with no independent income. In a sample of 231 dating couples, Peplau (1978) found that the higher the educational and career goals of women, the more power they had in the relationship. Goode (1956), in a study of divorce, commented that "willful failure in the role of breadwinner is often met by willful destruction of the sexual and social unity of the marriage" (p. 63).

Conclusion. There is, then, considerable anecdotal and survey evidence that indicates indirectly that couples *do* try to "fine-tune" the equitableness of their relationships. As yet, however, researchers have collected little compelling survey or experimental data to test directly this intriguing hypothesis.

Hypothesis 5: Equitable relationships will be especially stable relationships. Individuals in equitable relations will be more likely to perceive their relationships as long-term and will be more likely to have relationships intact months and years later.

According to Equity theory, if a couple's relationship becomes grossly inequitable, and if it becomes too costly to restore equity psychologically or actually, they could be tempted to sever the relationship. Dating couples who are unhappy with their relationships may find it relatively easy to end things. As we saw in discussing Hypothesis 1, the most inequitable dating relationships simply end. (See Hill, Rubin, & Peplau [1976] for a further discussion of this point.)

What about couples who have been married? Once couples marry, their lives become more intertwined, and separation becomes much more difficult. In the traditional notion, marriages last forever—they are for "better or worse." In addition to the moral and religious issues, there are very practical costs to divorce. Divorce is very costly in both emotional and financial terms. When a long-married couple separates, parents and friends are stunned, close friends often stop calling, and one of the parents often loses the rights of visitation to his or her children. (See Bohannan, 1971; Hunt & Hunt, 1977; and Napolitane & Pellegrino, 1977.) Thus, when married men and women, after trying to set things right in a marriage, ruefully concede failure, they may first respond by withdrawing *psychologically* from the situation—to bury themselves in their work, or give their all to their children, their friends, or to backgammon. Yet if a marital relationship is unbalanced enough, for long enough, couples do sometimes opt for separation or divorce. In 1973, 913,000 couples opted for an annulment or a divorce. Udry (1971) calculated that 20 to 25% of first marriages end in annulment, desertion, or divorce.

Is there any evidence that equitable marriages are more compatible (i.e., stable) than inequitable ones? In the study referred to earlier of 118 newlyweds who were interviewed immediately after their marriage and a year later, Utne, Hatfield, Traupmann, and Greenberger (1981) found that even a few weeks after their marriages, couples who feel equitably treated in their relationships are more secure about their marriages than are either overbenefited or underbenefited men and women. In the study, the couples were asked how often they had considered moving out, how often they had considered getting a divorce, and whether they thought they would still be together in 1 year and in 5 years. Equitably treated spouses were more certain of the stability of the relationship than were inequitably treated spouses. An interesting difference, however, was found between men and women in how likely they were to consider moving out or getting a divorce. While *underbenefited* men were more likely than other men to report having considered moving out or getting a divorce, *overbenefited* women were more likely than other women to have considered getting out of the relationship.

Another indication of the compatibility (i.e., stability/instability) of the relationship is the willingness of a spouse to become sexually involved with someone outside the marriage. Hatfield, Traupmann, and Walster (1979) predicted that inequitable relationships would be fragile relationships, because men and women who feel that they are not getting their just deserts in their marriage may be especially likely to explore a fleeting, or more permanent, love affair. To test their hypothesis, the authors reanalyzed the data from a survey study conducted by *Psychology Today*. In 1973, *Psychology Today* readers had been asked to express their feelings about dating, living together, or being married. Sixty-two thousand readers returned the 109-item questionnaire, and 2000 questionnaires were sampled for analysis. The researchers stratified the sample on sex and age to approximate the national distributions.

In the original survey, the respondent's willingness to engage in extramarital sex had been assessed in two ways: (1) how soon after they began living with or married their partner they first had sex with someone else, and (2) how many

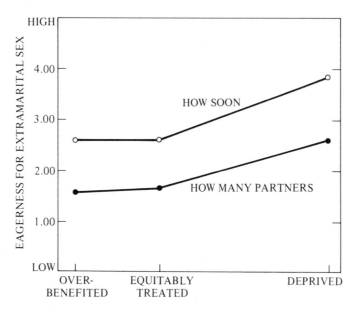

Figure 4-4. The relationship between equity and eagerness for extramarital sex.

people they had had extramarital affairs with. The researchers defined underbenefited respondents as those who had a partner who was less desirable than themselves. Equitably treated respondents were those who had a partner of equal social desirability, and overbenefited respondents were those who had a partner more socially desirable than themselves.

The researchers found some support for their hypothesis. They found that, on the average, equitably treated and overbenefited men and women waited 12 to 15 years before becoming sexually involved outside the relationship. Under-benefited men and women, on the other hand, began extramarital sex 6 to 8 years after marriage. In addition, underbenefited men and women had more extramarital affairs than did their equitably treated and overbenefited counter-parts. See Figure 4-4.

Conclusion. It appears that equitable relations are likely to be more compatible (i.e., stable) than inequitable ones. In equitable relationships, both partners are motivated to be faithful.

Summary and Discussion

We have reviewed a fair amount of research indicating that Equity theory does provide a convenient paradigm for examining romantic and marital relation-ships. Evidence was presented to support the contention that equitable relationships are compatible relationships. Specifically, we found the following:

1. In early stages of a relationship, couples who feel that their relationships are equitable are more likely to move to more intimate relationships than are couples in inequitable relationships (Hypothesis 1).
2. Men and women in equitable relationships are more content than men and women who are receiving either far more or far less than they feel they deserve (Hypothesis 2).
3. Equitable relationships are more stable than inequitable relationships (Hypothesis 5).

However, only one study indicated that relationships may become more equitable over time (Hypothesis 3)—most of the research suggests that relationships do not become more *or* less equitable with time. In addition, only indirect evidence was found to indicate that couples try to "fine tune" their relationship as a result of crises that may occur (Hypothesis 4). It is clear that more research is needed to examine these last two hypotheses.

In the five hypotheses we prepared initially, we assumed that the causal direction was *from* perceptions of inequity *to* psychological distress and/or the desire to terminate the relationship. However, because the research we reported is correlational in nature, a causal direction cannot automatically be assumed. A plausible argument could also be made that general feelings of dissatisfaction and discontent with the relationship could lead to perceptions of inequity. Some intimate relations, for example, arise out of passionate love—the type of love that can be very intense, but also very fleeting. Once the critical spark of passion dissipates, one or both partners may want to terminate the relationship, but may need to seek a more rational explanation for wanting out, other than simply an absence of excitement. The distraught lovers may, for example, search for other ways that the relationship may be imperfect (e.g., they may notice gross inequities that they were able to blindly ignore before).

While in real life there is probably a reciprocal relation between perceptions of inequity and incompatibility (feelings of distress), the causal direction predicted from Equity theory (inequity → incompatibility/distress) seems particularly plausible as an explanation for most of the above data in light of two considerations: First, although it is fairly easy to understand how the individual who becomes dissatisfied with a relationship could suddenly perceive how "cheated" he or she is in the relationship, it is a little more difficult, using such a causal direction, to explain the association between *advantageous* inequity and distress. Second, there is a voluminous amount of experimental evidence examining other types of relationships (i.e., industrial relationships) that indicates that inequities *do* lead to feelings of distress (see Adams & Freedman, 1976).

As we reviewed the research related to the five Equity hypotheses, an unexpected "finding" seemed to emerge. In at least three of the studies reviewed above, men and women were found to react differentially to inequities. In a sample of 50 dating couples (Sprecher-Fisher, 1980), in a sample of 189 casually and steadily dating couples (Traupmann, Hatfield, & Wexler, 1981), and in a sample of 118 newlyweds (Traupmann, Peterson, Utne, & Hatfield, 1981), a consistent difference in men's and women's concern with equity emerged. While women became unusually upset when they were overbenefited, men seemed to be able to take overbenefit more in stride. Conversely, while women seemed to be able to endure underbenefit with more equinimity, men were extremely upset by it. How do we explain the fact that women are more upset by overbenefit than men? Why is the opposite true for men?

Hay and Horton (1981) argue that women may be more sensitive, in general, than men to issues of fairness and justice in interpersonal relations. These authors explain that justice concerns are more salient to those with little power. Because women traditionally have had much less power than men, they should be especially concerned with the equity/exchange aspects of relationships. Although it may not require special sensitivity to fairness issues to recognize and react to being underbenefited, it may require such sensitivity to recognize and react to being overbenefited. Women, who traditionally have had less power, may be socialized to be more sensitive to such issues.

A second possibility to consider is that the types of resources that men offer women (which subsequently lead the women to feel overbenefited) are different from the types of resources women offer men. The differential reaction of males and females to feeling overbenefited/underbenefited may be due more to something inherent about the type of resources controlled by men and women than to any sex difference in reaction to inequity per se. It is likely, for example, that the woman who is receiving too many extravagant gifts from her lover will feel a different kind of distress (and perhaps a more intense type) than the man who feels that his wife is devoting too much time to housework. It would be interesting to examine how men and women react to inequities when controlling for the types of resources exchanged.

A third, less exciting possibility to consider is that these gender "differences" are not differences at all. Although the same pattern of results has been detected in several studies, in none of these studies were the differences statistically significant. More research will help clarify these issues.

While it was found that young dating and newlywed women are uneasy about receiving more than they deserved, elderly women appeared to feel comfortable with overbenefit. In the sample of women aged 50 to 92, both the overbenefited and the equitably treated women were content with the way things were. Only the underbenefited were dissatisfied. In light of the possible explanations we gave above for the sex differences in reactions to inequity among young people, why might women, as they get older, become less distressed about being overbenefited? One possibility is that the older women (who report feeling underbenefited for the bulk of their lives) feel that they finally deserve their just awards—and feel no remorse about accepting them. Another possibility is that they become less concerned with any possible future consequences of being overrewarded. More research is needed on how reactions to inequity change over the life cycle for both men and women.

The Future of Equity Research

The debate we have considered thus far concerns the question: "Do principles of equity operate in love relations?" The evidence we have considered makes it clear that they do. Is this the end of the debate? Hardly. When eminent theorists are so sharply divided on an issue, the ultimate answer to the question "Who is right?" often turns out to be "Both of them are."

We might expect subsequent research to try to find some principles to determine who is especially concerned about equity in love relations, and under what conditions. In fact, research working toward such an understanding already exists. Let us *briefly* review the research, and suggest some areas for further investigation.

1. Who is especially concerned with equity/inequity?

As yet, very little research has been conducted to examine how personality variables may mediate perceptions of inequities and subsequent reactions to such inequities. We do not know what types of individuals are especially concerned with equity and/or especially intolerant of perceived inequities once they are perceived.

Some work, however, has been done by Murstein and his associates (see Murstein & MacDonald, 1977; Murstein, MacDonald, & Cerreto, 1977) to suggest that people may differ in the degree to which they are concerned with equity in their relationships. These researchers developed an *Exchange Orientation Scale*, which measures the degree to which people have an "exchange mentality"—carefully maintaining a balance sheet and insisting that equity be maintained at all times, regardless of circumstances, in their relationships. A person who scores high on the scale tends to be primarily concerned with achieving an "equivalent or itemized exchange" and less concerned with meeting the other's needs. According to these researchers, individuals who are highly exchange-oriented tend to have negative personality traits (see discussion below).

Ways in which other, more traditional personality constructs may be related to concern with equity/inequity are clearly speculative at this point. Utne and Kidd (1980) have suggested that whether the individual has an *internal* or *external* locus of control may affect how distressed he or she becomes over inequities. Because persons with an external locus of control believe that reinforcements are not contingent on their own behavior, they may be less likely to suffer self-concept distress. They tend to believe that what happens to them has little to do with the self. They tell themselves that the inequities are beyond their control. Conversely, internals may be more likely to experience self-concept distress as a result of inequities because they do believe that what happens in their lives has a great deal to do with the self . . . and little to do with the environment.

Self-esteem may also be related to concern with inequities in ways that have yet to be explored. Similar to the hypothesized difference predicted between internals and externals, it is possible that individuals with high self-esteem may be more likely than those with low self-esteem to experience self-concept distress. The higher the self-esteem, the more likely it is that the individual will become distressed over possible violations of self-expectations and moral standards (see Glass, 1964).

It is clear that much research could be conducted in the future to examine how people differ in their degree of concern about equity in their relationships.

2. In what types of relationships are people especially concerned with equity?

In some types of relationships, equity and exchange may be especially salient issues; in other types of relationships, individuals may be less concerned with such issues. One promising avenue for investigating how relationships may differ in affecting their members' concern for equity/inequity comes from the work of Clark and Mills (1979) and Mills and Clark (1980) (see Chap. 5 of this volume). They argue that there are two distinctly different types of relationships—communal and exchange. In communal relationships, intimates give out of love and concern for the other. They avoid exchanging tit for tat. In exchange relationships, on the other hand, people give to get. They carefully keep mental score of what is being exchanged—and who is ahead and who is behind.

Mills and his associates have conducted a series of laboratory experiments designed to illustrate this distinction. Men and women are brought together and asked to work on a task. If the newly acquainted couple is eager to begin a "communal" romantic relationship, they are found to "signal" this by carefully *not* exchanging "tit for tat." If they are motivated to avoid establishing a romantic relationship, they keep things on an exchange basis; after receiving aid, they pay the other back, in kind, immediately.[1]

Some theorists have even argued that people may set up inequities in their intimate relations for special purposes. Adams (1976), for example, points out that intimates may purposely generate inequities in order to increase their overall return. Men may shower beautiful women with presents in order to buy their love. The fabeled "Jewish mother" tries to tie her children to her either with gifts (i.e., by overbenefiting them) or with guilt (by presenting an image of herself as extremely underbenefited). So, sometimes, intimates may seek out inequities in order to demonstrate their affection for others . . . or in order to control them.

What is needed is research designed to explore *how* concern for equity may differ in different types of relationships, and how inequities may be used for different purposes in different types of relationships.

3. Under what conditions and situations are people especially concerned with equity?

It may be that there are certain conditions or certain situations in which people are especially concerned with equity—or especially intolerant of inequities. For example, inequities may be tolerated by the participants as long as they are receiving the rewards they most want—or as long as their costs are not too great. Perhaps it is only when people stop getting what they most want that they become especially concerned with justice and fairness. A husband who feels that he has always been "cheated" by his demanding wife, for example, may not become distressed until she refuses his sexual requests.

Leventhal (1980) has stated that a concern with inequity and injustice may be especially salient under those conditions when there are sudden and obvious changes in what is exchanged. This would suggest that concerns with equity may be especially salient when there are dramatic shifts in the relationship (e.g., when the husband gets a promotion or when the wife suddenly loses 40 lb).

Finally, whether people are especially concerned with equity may vary as a function of what alternatives to the relationship exist. If the individual perceives that there are no viable alternatives to the relationship (that is, has a "low

---

[1] The Mills scenario is one possible way in which aid recipients may signal that they want a special (communal) relationship with another. A second, quite different scenario is possible, however. One can also signal that he or she desires a more communal relationship by "upping the ante." When a person is given a present (and thus, is put in an overbenefited position), he or she may wait (it would be considered peculiar to respond too quickly), and then find just the right present to give in return (perhaps escalating a little). Relationships are often furthered by a series of increasing commitments (Dillon, 1968; Mauss, 1954). (Essentially one is communicating: "I care about you," "You can trust me," "I will be fair.")

comparison level for alternatives"), he or she may not be that concerned with how equitable and just the relationship is. Conversely, if the individual perceives that there are desirable alternatives to the present relationship (has a "high comparison level for alternatives"), he or she may be able to better afford being concerned with the equity in the relationship (Thibaut & Kelley, 1959).

4. What are the consequences of encouraging people to be concerned with equity?

One of the most interesting debates to arise recently is between Murstein (1980) and Hay and Horton (1981). Murstein and his associates (see Murstein, 1977, 1978; Murstein & MacDonald, 1977, Murstein, MacDonald, & Cerreto, 1977) argue that a concern with *short-term* equity can have a disastrous impact on an intimate relationship. Things go best, they argue, when couples do things out of love for each other. A generous spirit sparks generosity in return. A "score-keeping mentality" causes everyone to be dissatisfied.

As described above, these researchers give couples the *Exchange Orientation Scale* (a scale designed to tap an extreme concern with short-term inequities).[2] Their findings have suggested the following associations:

1. Those who tend to be "uneasy much of their lives," "suspicious," "compulsive," "paranoid," "fearful," "defensive," and "insecure" are most concerned with equity (Lobsenz & Murstein, 1976; Murstein, 1978). People who are not "exchange-oriented" tend to be caring, giving, and trusting individuals (Lobsenz & Murstein, 1976; Murstein, 1978).
2. The "spirit and meaning" of marriage as an institution is degraded by an exchange-oriented approach to marriage (Lobsenz & Murstein, 1976). In addition, a concern for balanced exchange in any type of close relationship "leads to trouble." Murstein finds that an "exchange orientation" is related to poor dyadic adjustment for married couples (Murstein, MacDonald, & Cerreto, 1977), for cohabitators (Milardo & Murstein, 1979), and for same-sex friends (Murstein, MacDonald, & Cerreto, 1977).

Hay and Horton (1981), on the other hand, argue that Murstein and his colleagues are actually arguing for the status quo. If men's and women's relations are to change and grow, couples must openly acknowledge their concern with justice and work out fair agreements. In addition, they point out that there are problems with the *Exchange Orientation Scale*. Ideally, in a scale designed to measure concern with equity, there would be an equal number of items measuring concern with giving (overbenefit) *and* taking (underbenefit.) Essentially, the *E Scale* asks only about intimates' concern over being

---

[2]There is some ambiguity as to whether Murstein means to equate concern with exchange with concern with equity. In Murstein, MacDonald, and Cerreto (1977), he argues that the two concepts have nothing to do with each other. In Murstein (1977), he indicates that the *E-Scale* does measure concern with equity. In this chapter, for the sake of discussion, we have assumed that the two are related.

"cheated." Worse yet, the questions are worded so that in order to express a concern with fairness (which could, theoretically, be a positive or a negative trait), one must reveal oneself to be "selfish, rigid, and petty." It is not surprising, then, that persons scoring high on Murstein's *Exchange Orientation Scale* are neurotic and unhappy and have unsuccessful relationships. In the future, researchers may want to create a more value-free scale that measures concern with both advantageous inequity and disadvantageous inequity. Only then can we more clearly delineate what the consequences and correlates are of being especially concerned with equity and exchange.

5. Under what conditions can injustice exist in love relations?

Theorists are sharply divided as to whether or not love relations are ever unfair. Family therapists, such as Napier and Whitaker (1978), argue that families are a perfectly balanced system. Everyone must be getting something out of the status quo if it is to survive. Thus, what may seem at first glance to be an exploitative relationship will turn out to be an exquisitely balanced exchange on further examination. In love, they argue, there are no bullies, no victims. (This observation reminds us of a "sainted" wife we once interviewed. Neighbors agreed that she was shabbily treated by her brutal husband—who happened to be an Episcopal priest. He was a hard-driving cleric who longed to be a bishop. She never spoke of his shabby treatment of her. She told no one . . . except, it turns out, her husband's bishop—the very man in charge of his promotion.) On the other hand, Marxist theorists such as Wexler (1980) and Kennedy (1980) argue that marriages can hardly be equitable if they take place in a context in which men have the economic advantage.

If inequities can exist in a marriage, under what conditions will they be especially disruptive? Under what conditions will they be tolerated? Only further research will provide some answers.

In this chapter, we have traced some promising lines of research which may enable Equity theory and its critics to come up with a synthesis that will tell us more about how love and a concern with justice can coexist and promote each other.

References

Adams, J. S. (1965). Inequity in social exchange. In L. Berkowitz (Ed.), *Advances in experimental social psychology* (Vol. 2, pp. 267–299). New York: Academic Press.
Adams, J. S., & Freedman, S. (1976). Equity theory revisited: Comments and annotated bibliography. In L. Berkowitz & E. Hatfield-Walster (Eds.), *Advances in experimental social psychology* (Vol. 9, pp. 43–90). Boston: Academic Press.
Aldous, J. (1969). Occupational characteristics and males' role performance in the family. *Journal of Marriage and the Family, 31,* 707–712.
Angell, R. C. (1936). *The family encounters the depression.* New York: Charles Scribner's Sons.

Austin's (1974) Measure of Contentment/Distress. Reported in E. Hatfield-Walster, G. W. Walster, & E. Berscheid, *Equity: Theory and research* (p. 243). Boston: Allyn and Bacon, 1978.

Austin, W., & Walster (Hatfield), E. (1974a) Participants' reactions to "Equity with the World," *Journal of Experimental Social Psychology, 10,* 528–548.

Austin, W., & Walster (Hatfield), E. (1974b). Reactions to confirmations and disconfirmations of expectancies of equity and inequity. *Journal of Personality and Social Psychology, 30,* 208–216.

Bernard, J. (1964). The adjustments of married mates. In J. T. Christensen (Ed.), *Handbook of marriage and the family* (pp. 675–739). Chicago: Rand McNally. 675–739.

Bernard, J. (1972). *The future of marriage.* New York: World Publishing.

Berscheid, E., Hatfield, E., & Bohrnstedt, G. (1973). The body image report. *Psychology Today, 7,* 119–131.

Blau, P. M. (1964). *Exchange and power in social life.* New York: Wiley & Sons.

Bohannan, P. (Ed.) (1971). *Divorce and after.* Garden City, NY: Doubleday Anchor.

Brunner, E. (1945). *Justice and the social order.* London: Luderworth Press.

Cavan, R. S. (1959). Unemployment: Crisis of the common man. *Marriage and Family Living, 21,* 139–146.

Chadwick-Jones, J. K. (1976). *Social exchange theory: Its structure and influence in social psychology.* London: Academic Press.

Clark, M. S., & Mills, J. (1979). Interpersonal attraction in exchange and communal relationships. *Journal of Personality and Social Psychology, 37,* 12–24.

Cooley, C. H. (1902). *Human nature and the social order.* New York: Charles Scribner's Sons.

Dillon, W. S. (1968). *Gifts and nations.* The Hague: Mouton.

Douvan, E. (1974). *Interpersonal relationships: Some questions and observations.* Paper presented at the Raush Conference.

Fromm, E. (1956). *The art of loving.* New York: Harper and Row.

Gillespie, D. (1971). Who has the power? The marital struggle. *Journal of Marriage and the Family, 33,* 445–458.

Glass, D. C. (1964). Changes in liking as a means of reducing cognitive discrepancies between self-esteem and aggression. *Journal of Personality, 32,* 520–549.

Goode, W. J. (1956). *After divorce.* Glencoe, IL: Free Press.

The Hatfield (1978) Global Measure. Reported in E. Hatfield, M. K. Utne, & J. Traupmann, Equity theory and intimate relationships. In Robert L. Burgess & Ted L. Huston (Eds.), *Social exchange in developing relationships* (p. 112). NY: Academic Press, 1979.

Hatfield, E., & Traupmann, J. (1980). Intimate relationships: A perspective from Equity theory. In S. Duck & R. Gilmour (Eds.), *Personal relationships I: Studying personal relationships* (pp. 165–178). London: Academic Press.

Hatfield, E., Traupmann, J., & Walster, G. W. (1979). Equity and extramarital sex. In M. Cook & G. Wilson (Eds.), *Love and attraction: An international conference* (pp. 323–334). Oxford: Pergamon Press.

Hatfield, E., Utne, M. K., & Traupmann, J. (1979). Equity theory and intimate relationships. In R. L. Burgess & T. L. Huston (Eds.), *Social exchange in developing relationships* (pp. 99–133). New York: Academic Press.

Hatfield, E., Walster, G. W., & Traupmann, J. (1978). Equity and premarital sex. *Journal of Personality and Social Psychology, 37,* 82–92. Reprinted in M. Cook and G. Wilson (Eds.), *Love and attraction: An international conference* (pp. 309–323). Oxford: Pergamon Press, 1979.

Hay, J., & Horton, T. (1981). An exchange orientation: Is it good for marriage? Unpublished manuscript.

Hill, C. T., Rubin, Z., & Peplau, L. A. (1976). Breakups before marriage: The end of 103 affairs. *Journal of Social Issues, 32*, 147–167.

Homans, G. C. (1974). *Social behavior: Its elementary forms* (rev. ed.). New York: Harcourt, Brace, Jovanovich.

Hunt, M., & Hunt, B. (1977). *The divorce experience*. New York: McGraw-Hill.

Kennedy, R. D. Jr. (1980). A Marxist perspective: The production of cooperative intimate relations. Unpublished manuscript.

Komarovsky, M. (1971). *The unemployed man and his family*. New York: Octagon Books.

Lederer, W. J., & Jackson, D. D. (1968). *The mirages of marriage*. New York: W. W. Norton & Co.

Leventhal, G. S. (1980). What should be done with equity theory? New approaches to the study of fairness in social relationships. In R. Gergen, M. S., Greenberg, & R. Willis (Eds.), *Social exchange: Advances in theory and research*. New York: Picnum.

Lobsenz, N. M., & Murstein, B. I. (1976, September). Keeping score: It's fine for football games but disastrous for a marriage. *Woman's Day*, 146–154.

Mauss, M. (1954). *The gift: Forms and functions of exchange in archaic societies*. Glencoe, IL: Free Press.

McCall, M. M. (1966). Courtship as social exchange: Some historical comparisons. In B. Farber (Ed.), *Kinship and family organization* (pp. 190–200). New York: John Wiley and Sons.

Mills, J., & Clark, M. S. (1980). Exchange in communal relationships. Unpublished manuscript.

Mills, J., & Clark, M. S. (1980). Communal and exchange relationships. Paper presented at the 1980 meetings of the Society of Experimental Social Psychologists, Palo Alto, CA.

Murstein, B. I. (1978). *Exploring intimate lifestyles*. New York: Springer Publishing Company.

Murstein, B. I. (1980). The limit of exchange in equity theories. Unpublished manuscript.

Murstein, B. I., & MacDonald, M. G. (1977). The relationship of "exchange orientation" and "commitment" scales to marriage adjustment. Unpublished manuscript, Connecticut College.

Murstein, B. I., MacDonald, M. G., & Cerreto, M. (1977). A theory of the effect of exchange-orientation on marriage and friendship. *Journal of Marriage and the Family 39*, 543–548.

Napier, A. Y., & Whitaker, C. A. (1978). *The family crucible*. NY: Harper and Row.

Napolitane, C., & Pellegrino, B. (1977). *Living and loving after divorce*. New York: Rawson Associates.

Patterson, G. R. (1971). *Families: Applications of social learning to family life*. Champaign, IL: Research Press Co.

Peplau, L. A. (1978). Power in dating relationships. In J. Freeman (Ed.), *Women: A feminist perspective* (pp. 106–121). Palo Alto, CA: Mayfield.

Rubin, Z. (1973). *Liking and loving: An invitation to social psychology*. New York: Holt, Rinehart, and Winston.

Sager, C. (1976). *Marriage contracts and couple therapy*. New York: Bruner-Mazel.

Scanzoni, J. (1970). *Opportunity and the family*. New York: Free Press.

Scanzoni, J. (1972). *Sexual bargaining: Power politics in the American marriage*. Englewood Cliffs, NJ: Prentice-Hall.

Schafer, R. B., & Keith, P. M. (1980). Equity and depression among married couples. *Social Psychology Quarterly, 43*, 430–435.

Schafer, R. B., & Keith, P. M. (1981). Equity in marital roles across the family life cycle. *Journal of Marriage and the Family*, *43*, 359–367.

Sprecher-Fisher, S. (1980). Men, women, and intimate relationships: A study of dating couples. Unpublished master's thesis, University of Wisconsin-Madison.

Storer, N. W. (1966). The social system of science. New York: Holt, Rinehart, and Winston.

Tedeschi, J. T. (1974) Attributions, liking and power. In R. L. Burgess & T. L. Huston (Eds.), *Foundations of interpersonal attraction* (pp. 193–215). New York: Academic Press.

Thibaut, J. W., & Kelley, H. H. (1959). *The social psychology of groups*. NY: John Wiley and Sons.

Tonnies, F. (1957). *Community and society: gemeinschaft and gesellschaft*. East Lansing, MI: Michigan State University Press. (Original work published 1887)

Traupmann, J., & Hatfield, E. (1983). How important is marital fairness over the lifespan? *International Journal of Aging and Human Development*. 17, 89–101.

Traupmann, J., Hatfield, E., & Sprecher, S. (1981). The importance of "fairness" for the marital satisfaction of older women. Unpublished manuscript.

Traupmann, J., Hatfield, E., & Wexler, P. (1983). Equity and sexual satisfaction in dating couples. 22, 33–40.

Traupmann, J., Peterson, R., Utne, M., & Hatfield, E. (1981). Measuring equity in intimate relations. *Applied Psychological Measurement*. 5, 467–480.

The Traupmann-Utne-Walster (1977) Scales. Available in E. Hatfield-Walster, G. W. Walster, & E. Berscheid, *Equity: Theory and research* (pp. 236–242). Boston: Allyn and Bacon, 1978. For reliability and validity information see Traupmann, J., Peterson, R., Utne, M., & Hatfield, E. Measuring equity in intimate relations. *Applied Psychological Measurement*, 1981, 5, 467–480.

The Traupmann, Utne, Hatfield (1978) Scales: Participants' perceptions of equity/ inequity. In R. L. Burgess & T. L. Huston (Eds.), *Social exchange in developing relationships* (pp. 112–113). New York: Academic Press, 1979.

Udry, J. R. (1971, September). Commentary. *Sexual Behavior, 23*.

Utne, M. K., Hatfield, E., Traupmann, J., & Greenberger, D. (1984). Equity, marital satisfaction, and stability. Journal of Social and Personal Relationships.

Utne, M. K., & Kidd, R. F. (1980). In G. Mikula (Ed.), *Justice in social interaction*. Berne, Switzerland: Hans Huber.

The Walster (1977) Global Measure. Described in E. Hatfield-Walster, G. W. Walster, & E. Berscheid. *Equity: Theory and research* (pp. 234–236). Boston: Allyn and Bacon.

Walster, E., Walster, G. W., & Berscheid, E. (1978). *Equity: Theory and research*. Boston: Allyn and Bacon.

Wexler, P. (1980). Intimacy: A critical social analysis. Unpublished manuscript.

Chapter 5

Implications of Relationship Type for Understanding Compatibility

Margaret S. Clark

Compatibility involves getting along with another in a congenial, harmonious fashion, and it is easy to predict how certain behaviors will affect compatibility. For example, being attentive to what another person says should increase or at least maintain compatibility. In contrast, insulting another should decrease compatibility or keep it at a low level. It is difficult, however, to predict how certain other behaviors will influence compatibility. For example, imagine someone giving you an expensive birthday gift, perfectly suited to your needs. Would it make you feel closer to the giver and solidify the relationship, thereby enhancing compatibility? Or would it seem inappropriate, make you feel awkward and uncomfortable, and therefore decrease compatibility? Alternatively, imagine how you would react if someone whom you just helped immediately paid you for that help. Would it be annoying and decrease feelings of compatibility? Or would it seem entirely appropriate?

In the latter examples you can probably imagine having either reaction— depending upon *who* the other person was. If your spouse gave you the perfect gift, it would probably make you happy. If a mere acquaintance did so, it would probably evoke awkward feelings. If your best friend was the one to pay you back for help, the response might be annoying. If it were a client with whom you regularly did business, repayment would seem desirable.

Although I doubt that many people would argue with these examples, to date social psychologists have almost entirely neglected the variable of relationship type in their research on compatibility. Nonetheless, a small amount of work on this issue recently has been done and it will be reviewed in this chapter. My goal is to convince the reader that if we wish to understand compatibility in relationships, we cannot neglect the variable of relationship type. Specifically, a distinction between two types of relationships, communal and exchange, and the norms that govern when benefits should be given in each, will be described. These different norms suggest that many behaviors ought to have differential effects on compatibility in communal versus exchange relationships. Research supporting the distinction and its implications for compatibility will be reviewed and discussed.

Two Types of Relationships: Communal and Exchange

In earlier papers, Judson Mills and I (Clark & Mills, 1979; Mills & Clark, 1982) have drawn a distinction between two types of relationships based on the rules governing the giving of benefits in those relationships.[1] Some relationships are characterized by members' obligations and, usually, by their desire to be especially responsive to each other's needs. These *communal relationships* are often exemplified by relationships with kin, romantic partners, and friends. In other relationships people do not feel this special responsibility for the other's needs. Although they feel some low level of communal orientation to most people, and will respond to each other's needs in emergencies or when they can give a benefit to the other at little cost to themselves (Mills & Clark, 1982), they do not feel a special responsibility for each other's needs. Rather, they give benefits with the expectation of receiving comparable benefits in return, and when they receive a benefit they feel an obligation to return a comparable benefit.[2] These *exchange relationships* are often exemplified by relationships with strangers, acquaintances, and people with whom we do business.

What Determines Type of Relationship With Another?

The type of relationship we have with another person may be culturally dictated or freely chosen. The culture dictates, for instance, that communal norms are to be followed with family members. Regardless of whether we like or dislike our relatives, we are *supposed* to care about their welfare. The culture also dictates that exchange norms should be followed with people with whom we do business.

There are, in addition, times when we must *decide* what norms to follow in relationships with others. Some determinants of one's desire for a communal relationship include the attractiveness of the other, the availability of the other

---

[1] I assume, as have several others (e.g., Deutsch, 1975; Lerner, Miller & Holmes, 1976; Leventhal, 1980; Mikula, 1981; Reis, 1982), that many different rules for giving and receiving benefits exist. For instance, benefits can be distributed in relationships according to (1) each person's inputs, (2) the equality principle, (3) needs, (4) ability, (5) the effect they will have, and so on (Deutsch, 1975). In addition, I assume that the rule chosen for use at any given time is dependent upon individual differences, situational variables, and the type of relationship one has or expects to have with the person with whom one is interacting. Only relationship type is considered in this chapter, however.

[2] Throughout the chapter the term benefit is used. A benefit is defined as something of value that one person intentionally gives to another (Mills & Clark, 1982). Note that this definition excludes many things of value that a person may derive from a relationship that the other does not *intend* to give to the person. For instance, just by being in a relationship, a person may gain status in outsiders' eyes (Sigall & Landy, 1973) but the status gained would not be considered a benefit.

for a communal relationship, and one's *own* availability for a communal relationship.

Consider one's own availability for a communal relationship first. The more communal relationships one has, the *less* likely one should be to desire additional ones. Having at least some communal relationships with others is valuable for a number of reasons. For instance, having someone else responsible for one's needs should provide a sense of security. On the other hand, participation in such relationships requires that one be responsive to the other's needs as well. As a person has more and more communal relationships, the benefits derived from adding an additional one should diminish while, at the same time, the person's responsibility for others' needs increases. Moreover, as more communal relationships are added, conflicts regarding whose needs one should respond to in the event that different people's needs arise at the same time may increase as well. For these reasons, the more communal relationships a person already has, the *less* likely that person should be to form a communal relationship with a new person.

Everything just said about a person's *own* availability for a communal relationship also applies to the other's availability. Consequently, the more communal relationships the other is perceived to have, the less likely a person may be to desire or anticipate being able to form a new communal relationship with that other.

Finally, the other's attractiveness should influence choosing to form a communal relationship. In communal relationships, members have an implicit agreement to be concerned for each other. This implicit agreement requires some expectation that the relationship will be a long-term one. It requires that one be willing to let the other respond to one's needs as they arise and that one be willing to respond to the other's needs as they arise. In addition, given such a commitment to each other, members of such relationships are often perceived as a "unit" by outsiders, and attributes of one person reflect upon the other (cf. Sigall & Landy, 1973). Consequently, it is understandable why members should be most likely to desire communal relationships with people who are attractive in terms of physical appearance, personality, and/or intelligence. However, this desire may be tempered by the realization that one may not be able to form a relationship with very attractive others if one's own attributes are not terribly attractive (Berscheid, Dion, Walster & Walster, 1971).

Exchange relationships, on the other hand, do not involve special responsibilities for one another's needs and they may be very short term (e.g., one's relationship with a taxi driver) *or* they can be long term. But even long-term exchange relationships may be fairly easily ended at any time simply by "evening" the score and then leaving the relationship. Thus, one tends not to be as closely identified with an exchange partner as with a communal one. Because exchange relationships are less intimate and can be ended relatively easily, attractiveness should be less important (although not entirely unimportant) to forming exchange relationships than to forming communal ones. Exchange relationships should most likely occur when one person needs or desires a benefit from the other and can benefit the other in repayment.

Variation in Certainty About and Strength of Relationships

Both communal and exchange relationships can vary in terms of the participants' feelings of *certainty* that that kind of relationship actually exists (Mills & Clark, 1982). For example, a college freshman assigned to share a dorm room with another person may, on the first day, find the other to be quite friendly and expect a communal relationship. However, the freshman may be uncertain as to whether such a relationship actually does or will exist. Later, after the roommates have actually followed communal norms for awhile, their certainty will be greater. Similarly, exchange relationships can vary in certainty. For example, a store manager may grant credit to a new customer, expecting that that customer will pay the bill. However, the manager may be unsure that the customer will pay. Later, assuming that the customer *has* paid his or her bills, the owner will be more certain of the relationship.

In addition to varying in certainty, communal but not exchange relationships vary in strength (Mills & Clark, 1982). This means that communal relationships can be ordered in terms of the degree of responsibility assumed by one person for the other's needs. A parent, for instance, may feel a greater responsibility for his or her child's needs than for his or her friend's needs. The relationship with the child is stronger than the relationship with the friend. These differences in strength may prevent conflict when a person is responsible for the needs of more than one other at a given time. For example, a person who needs to get to the airport might be upset if her friend turns down her request for a ride. However, if the friend explains that she must stay home to take care of her sick child, the person will probably understand.

Table 5-1. Some Characteristics of Communal and Exchange Relationships

Communal Relationships	Exchange Relationships
1. Characterized by a special responsibility for the other beyond that level of responsibility felt for any other person.	1. *No* special responsibility for the welfare of the other beyond that felt for any other person.
2. Most benefits are given in response to needs or to demonstrate a general concern for the other. Benefits are not given with the expectation of receiving specific repayments nor as repayments for specific benefits received in the past.	2. Most benefits are given with the expectation of receiving specific repayments or *as* repayments for specific benefits received in the past.
3. Certainty about, desire for and strength of these relationships vary.	3. Certainty about and desire for these relationships vary. Strength of these relationships is not assumed to vary.

Variation in Desire for Existing Relationships

Usually people who have communal or exchange relationships with another also *desire* those relationships. However, that may not always be the case. For example, when a person marries, the person may inherit a new set of culturally dictated communal relations known as in-laws. The person may feel compelled to follow communal norms with these people, but may not be very happy about it. Similarly, although people ordinarily freely choose to participate in exchange relationships, they may at times find themselves in an undesired exchange relationship. For example, a person in need of a plumber's assistance may not wish to enter into an exchange relationship with a certain plumber, but if that plumber is the only one available, the person may still do so.

The attributes of communal and exchange relationships just discussed are summarized in Table 5-1. I turn now to a discussion of the importance of these attributes for understanding compatibility.

Implications of the Communal/Exchange Distinction for Compatibility

There are specific classes of behaviors which the communal/exchange distinction implies should have differential impact on compatibility depending upon relationship type. Not every such behavior can be discussed. Only those behaviors are included for which there is research evidence indicating that the behavior really is considered to be more appropriate, desirable, or expected in one type of relationship than in the other. For some of these behaviors, direct evidence will be presented that they do indeed differentially affect indices of compatibility such as attraction or resentment. For other behaviors, the fact that they occur with differential frequency in these two types of relationships will be used to infer that they may differentially affect compatibility within those relationships.

For discussion purposes I have organized these behaviors into two groups: (1) behaviors that follow from exchange norms and (2) behaviors that follow from communal norms. "Exchange behaviors" are discussed first.

Behaviors That Follow From Exchange Norms

Any behavior that allows one to keep track of and to accurately balance what is given and received in a relationship ought to maintain or promote compatibility in exchange relationships. On the other hand, such behaviors may actually be detrimental to compatibility in communal relationships since they may imply that one person does not desire a communal relationship with the other. Several such exchange behaviors are discussed here, including: (1) prompt repayment for benefits received, (2) giving and receiving comparable rather than non-comparable benefits, (3) requesting repayments from others, and (4) keeping track of the individual inputs into joint tasks or activities.

Promptly repaying others for specific benefits received. In exchange relationships, the rule for distributing benefits is that they are given to repay specific past debts or with the expectation of receiving a comparable benefit in return. Therefore, promptly repaying others for benefits received is an appropriate behavior in these relationships, and should promote compatibility. However, prompt repayment should not be important to maintaining compatibility in communal relationships. Indeed, to the extent that this behavior indicates preference for an exchange rather than a communal relationship, it may actually decrease compatibility. Very few studies have examined the impact of repayment for specific benefits in both communal and exchange relationships. Nonetheless, those that have done so support the predictions just described.

In one study (Clark & Mills, 1979, Study 1), undergraduate men were recruited to participate in an experiment with an attractive, friendly, female confederate. Both participants worked simultaneously on individual tasks for which each could win points toward extra credit that would help them complete a course requirement. In all cases the man was induced to help the attractive woman complete her task. Then she either thanked him *or* thanked him *and* repaid him with one of her extra-credit points. At this point the experimenter casually manipulated the type of relationship desired. While the woman was in a different room, the experimenter remarked that she was anxious to go on to the second part of the study, either: (1) because she was new at the university, did not know many people, and had signed up for the study as a good way to meet people (communal conditions) or (2) because she had signed up for the experiment because it would end at a time convenient for her husband to pick her up and go to their home, which was some distance from the campus (exchange conditions).[3]

Finally, supposedly in preparation for a second task, the subject filled out an impressions form describing the woman. From responses on this form, a measure of attraction was derived. The results were clear. Subjects led to desire an exchange relationship liked the woman significantly more if she repaid him than if she did not. In contrast, subjects led to desire a communal relationship liked the woman significantly better if she did *not* repay him than if she did. Thus, the impact of repayment for a specific benefit on compatibility does appear to depend upon relationship type.

A second study (Clark & Vanderlipp, in press) also supports the idea that repayments for specific benefits are important for maintaining compatibility in

---

[3]Note that this manipulation relies on the ideas expressed earlier regarding when a communal relationship will be desired. Specifically, the other person was always attractive and we assumed (1) that most male freshmen would be available for a communal relationship and (2) that if the other was new at the university and consequently also available, a communal relationship would be desired. On the other hand, we assumed (3) that if the other was married and consequently unavailable, an exchange relationship would be preferred. Clear evidence for the effectiveness of these manipulations in producing desires for communal and exchange relationships has been collected and is described in a manuscript available from the author (Clark, 1984b).

exchange but not in communal relationships. In each session of this study, a female subject participated with a female confederate. Shortly after the subject's arrival, the other person was either described as new at the university and as wanting to meet people (communal conditions) or as being in a hurry since her husband would be picking her up (exchange conditions). Furthermore, communal subjects were led to believe that they would have a discussion of common interests with the other, whereas exchange subjects were led to expect a discussion of differences in interests. The experiment supposedly dealt with how people got to know one another and it began with subjects filling out some pretests. During a break in the pretesting, the confederate asked the subject to take and fill out a lengthy questionnaire for a class project. All subjects agreed. Then the other person either paid the subject $4 from "class funds" or offered no repayment, explaining that class funds had run out. Subsequently, the experimenter returned and asked both participants to fill out one more pretest. On this form, subjects rated how exploitative they perceived the confederate to be and answered other questions designed to tap liking.

In the exchange conditions, the results paralleled those of the Clark and Mills (1979) study just described. Subjects who were not repaid felt more exploited by the other and liked the other less than those who were repaid. In contrast, failure to repay had no impact on feelings of exploitation or attraction in communal relationships. Thus, once again evidence was obtained that specific repayments are essential to maintaining compatibility in exchange but not in communal relationships.

The results of the Clark & Vanderlipp (in press) study differed from those of the Clark and Mills (1979) study in that repayment had no negative effects on general attraction in communal relationships. Perhaps this was because in this study, unlike that of Clark and Mills (1979), repayment came from a third source (class funds) and not from the confederate herself. Therefore, it may not have been taken as an indication of the confederate's attitude toward the subject. This, of course, suggests that repayment need not *always* reduce compatibility in a communal relationship. If the other is offering repayment for reasons clearly independent of the relationship, it may not have this effect.

Giving and receiving comparable benefits. The evidence that repayment for specific benefits is appropriate in exchange but not communal relationships suggests that factors that would cause a benefit given to *look* like a repayment for a benefit previously received would be reacted to positively in exchange but not in communal relationships. One such factor is the *comparability* of benefits given to those previously received (Mills & Clark, 1982).

In an exchange relationship, giving a benefit comparable to one previously received should be more desirable than giving a noncomparable benefit. A comparable benefit clearly indicates that the debt incurred by receiving the prior benefit has been eliminated. In contrast, in communal relationships, giving and receiving noncomparable benefits should be preferred. Noncomparable benefits are less likely to be viewed as repayments. They should be more likely to be perceived as having been given out of concern for the recipient's welfare.

A series of three studies (Clark, 1981) supports these ideas. In two of these studies, subjects were presented with descriptions of one person giving something to another, then of that other person giving something to the first. Half the time the two benefits were the same; for example, two lunches (comparable conditions). Half the time they were different; for example, a lunch and a ride home (noncomparable conditions). After reading these descriptions, all subjects rated the degree of friendship they believed existed between the two people. In both studies, perceived friendship was significantly lower when comparable rather than noncomparable benefits were given. The third study revealed that, as expected, comparable benefits were more likely than noncomparable benefits to be seen as repayments. In contrast, noncomparable benefits were more likely than comparable benefits to be perceived as having been given for such communal reasons as "to start a friendship" or "out of appreciation."

Requesting repayments from others. Requesting a repayment is still another behavior that should seem appropriate and desirable in exchange but not in communal relationships, and a second study reported by Clark and Mills (1979) supports this prediction. In this study, female subjects anticipated participating, along with an attractive female confederate, in a task involving forming words with letter tiles. Type of relationship was varied at the start of the study in much the same manner as in the Clark and Mills (1979) and Clark and Vanderlipp (in press) studies described above. As in the first Clark and Mills (1979) study, the participants worked independently on tasks for which they could earn points toward extra credit. This time, however, the confederate finished first, and in the four conditions relevant to the discussion here, the confederate helped the subject.[4] Later in the session the confederate either requested a repayment or explicitly indicated that she wanted no repayment. Finally, the subject's liking for the confederate was assessed.

As predicted, subjects in the exchange condition liked the other significantly more when she requested a repayment than when she did not. In contrast, communal subjects liked the other significantly more when she did *not* request a repayment than when she did. Thus, in exchange relationships, requesting a repayment seems to increase compatibility relative to explicitly indicating that one does not desire such a repayment. On the other hand, the reverse strategy appears to be the best for promoting compatibility in a communal relationship.

Keeping track of inputs into joint tasks. The final behavior to be discussed is keeping track of individual inputs into joint tasks for which there will be a reward. According to exchange norms, people should receive benefits in

---

[4]In half of the conditions, aid was *not* sent. However, these conditions are not described here as they are not relevant to reactions to requesting repayment. They are described later in this chapter.

proportion to their inputs into a task. This calls for keeping track of inputs. In contrast, according to communal norms, benefits should be divided according to needs. The needier person should receive more benefits, or if needs are equal, benefits should be divided equally. It is not necessary to keep track of individual inputs in order to follow this rule.

Three studies provide evidence that members of exchange relationships are more likely than members of communal relationships to keep track of inputs into joint tasks (Clark, 1984a). In all three, subjects were recruited to participate in an experiment in which they would work on a joint task with another person. They were to search a matrix of numbers and circle specified sequences. The task instructions emphasized that the *pair* would receive a reward for each sequence circled.

In the first study, male subjects were recruited to participate along with a female confederate. They were led to expect a communal or an exchange relationship with her in much the same way as used in the studies already discussed. The subject and the confederate were instructed to take turns searching for sequences. The confederate always went first and circled sequences in red or black pen. Then the subject, who had access to both a red and black pen, took a turn circling numbers. If a different color pen was chosen by significantly more than half the subjects in a condition, that was taken as evidence that subjects were making an effort to keep track of inputs. If a different color pen was chosen by significantly *less* than 50% of the subjects, that was taken as an indication that subjects were *avoiding* keeping track of inputs. In the first study, as predicted, subjects expecting exchange relationships seemed to keep track of inputs; 88.2% of them selected a different color pen— significantly more than expected by chance. By contrast, subjects expecting communal relationships seemed to *avoid* keeping track of benefits; only 12.5% selected a different color pen—significantly *fewer* than expected by chance.

Two additional studies reported by Clark (1984a) also support the idea that keeping track of individual inputs into joint tasks is important in exchange but not in communal relationships. These studies further suggest that once a communal relationship is *established*, it may no longer be important to go out of one's way to *avoid* any appearance of following exchange norms. Simply following communal norms may be sufficient. In these two studies, *pairs* of existing friends signed up together. Then they were scheduled to participate in the task just described, paired either with their friend as a partner or with a stranger from a different set of friends. In both studies, when paired with a stranger, subjects showed a significant tendency to pick a different color pen, whereas when paired with a friend they did not. However, in neither of these studies did subjects paired with a friend show any evidence of intentionally *avoiding* picking a different color pen.

From these studies we may infer that keeping track of inputs into joint tasks is important for maintaining compatibility in exchange but not communal relationships. Furthermore, actually *avoiding* keeping track of inputs may be called for in communal relationships prior to the time that those relationships are firmly established.

Cautionary Notes Regarding the Impact of Exchange Behaviors

Several exchange behaviors have now been identified that ought to differentially influence compatibility in exchange and in communal relationships. These are summarized in the top half of Table 5-2. At this point, however, the reader should be cautioned regarding some boundary conditions on these effects.

Compelling needs. First, there are instances in which receiving a benefit, even a comparable benefit, immediately after having given one should *not* appear to be a repayment and consequently should not impede compatibility in communal relationships. Specifically, the benefit should not impede compatibility if the recipient has a compelling *need* for it. Similarly, receiving a request for a benefit after having been given one should not impede compatibility in communal relationships *if* the person requesting the benefit has a compelling *need* for the benefit (Mills & Clark, 1982). In such cases, where the needs of the recipient are very salient, the benefits received or requested are not likely to be thought of as repayments, but rather as responses to needs.

Turn-taking. A second cautionary note has to do with turn-taking, which gives some appearance of involving exchange norms but in fact is not incompatible with communal norms. Turn-taking is appropriate in communal relationships when needs are equal, when there is no clear evidence regarding needs, *or* when there are no clear compelling needs. For instance, a husband and wife who are both busy and who would both like to avoid doing the dishes, might take turns performing this chore.

Table 5-2. Some Behaviors That Should Differentially Affect Compatibility in Exchange and Communal Relationships

Behavior	Type of Relationship	
	Exchange	Communal
1. Prompt repayment for specific benefits	+	−
2. Giving and receiving comparable benefits	+	s
3. Requesting repayment	+	−
4. Keeping track of individual inputs into joint tasks	+	−
5. Helping	s	+
6. Accepting/seeking help	s	+
7. Distributing rewards according to needs	s	+
8. Use of consensus rather than majority rule as a decision strategy	s	+
9. Responsiveness to emotions	s	+
10. Taking the other's perspective	s	+

Note. + indicates that the behavior promotes or maintains compatibility
       − indicates that the behavior detracts from compatibility or keeps compatibility low
       s indicates that the impact of the behavior on compatibility depends upon the situation

Transactions involving money. Finally, it should be noted that one type of benefit—i.e., money—seems to be appropriately given and received according to the exchange rules in *both* communal and exchange relationships (except perhaps in the very strongest of communal relationships).

Certainty. As noted previously, both communal and exchange relationships vary in certainty, and this factor may influence the extent to which exchange behaviors will have the effects on compatibility discussed thus far. First, when one desires but is uncertain about having an *exchange* relationship with another, "exchange behaviors" may be especially welcome because they indicate that the desired relationship actually exists. Second, certainty about *communal* relations may also affect the impact of exchange behaviors in those relationships, albeit in more complex ways. In these relationships, the effect of certainty probably depends upon how easily the exchange behavior may be explained away in communal terms. If an exchange behavior cannot be "explained away" in communal terms, (e.g., a cash repayment for a favor just done), it may be *most* distressing in relations about which one *had* felt certain. People may be quite invested in such relationships, so their possible loss should be especially distressing. If, however, the exchange behavior *can* be "explained away" in communal terms (e.g., an offer of help after one has given the other help), people should be more likely to "explain it away" in communal relationships about which they are certain than in ones about which they are uncertain. Consequently, such behaviors may be *less* detrimental to compatibility in communal relationships about which one feels certain than in those about which one is uncertain.

Strength. Not only do communal relationships vary in certainty, they may also vary in strength, and this too may influence the impact of "exchange" behaviors on compatibility in communal and exchange relationships. For instance, strength may have an impact when it comes to giving and receiving money. As already noted, except in the very strongest communal relationship, money is treated in exchange terms. Thus, repaying money may not produce awkward feelings in communal relationships and indeed should *prevent* such feelings. An exception to this rule, however, may occur in very strong communal relations such as those between spouses and between many parents and children. In such relationships, explicit repayment of money may reduce compatibility.

The strength of communal relations may also have an impact on how people react to the inappropriate presence of exchange behaviors in these relationships. It is likely that the stronger a communal relationship, the more important it is to the participants. Thus, people may be especially distressed when someone with whom they believed they had a strong communal relationship begins displaying exchange behaviors.

Variation in desire for a communal or an exchange relationship. To this point in my discussion of the impact of exchange behaviors in communal and exchange relations the implicit assumption has been made that people *desire* these respective types of relationships. However, as noted earlier, levels of desire can vary. It is probably the case that the greater a person's desire for a communal or exchange relationship, the more distressing violations of the norms appropriate to that relationship will seem.

Behaviors That Follow From Communal Norms

So far this chapter has focused on "exchange" behaviors. The distinction between communal and exchange relationships also implies the existence of "communal behaviors" which ought to have differential effects on compatibility in exchange and communal relationships. These are behaviors that indicate that one feels a special obligation to be responsive to the other's needs and expects the other to be responsive to one's own needs as well. They include: helping, accepting help without attempting repayment, taking needs into account when distributing jointly earned rewards, using decision-making rules that take everyone's needs into account, being responsive to the other's emotional state, and taking the other's perspective when something positive or negative happens to the other. I turn now to evidence for the differential importance of these behaviors in communal and exchange relationships.

Helping. In communal relationships, helping should occur more often and should be more important to maintaining compatibility than in exchange relationships. Evidence for this proposition comes from five studies (Bar-Tal, Bar-Zohar, Greenberg & Herman, 1977; Clark & Mills, 1979, Study 2; Clark & Ouellette, 1983; Daniels & Berkowitz, 1963; Waddell & Clark, 1982).

In the Bar-Tal et al. (1977) study, subjects were asked to imagine themselves as a member of an athletic team who had missed a bus to a very important tournament. The person did not have a car, and knowing that dismissal from the team would result if he or she did not arrive on time, phoned someone to request a ride. The type of relationship with the person called was systematically varied. In three conditions, subjects imagined that the other was either a parent, a sibling, or a close friend. (As noted earlier, these relationships often exemplify communal relationships.) In the remaining two conditions, subjects imagined that they attempted to call their friend, but that the friend was not in. Instead, they reached either an acquaintance or a stranger. (As noted earlier, these relationships often exemplify exchange relationships.) Regardless of the relationship condition, the student always asked the person called for help. At this point, half the subjects imagined that the other gave help whereas half imagined a refusal. Finally, each subject rated how obligated he or she believed the other was to help as well as how grateful or resentful the subject would feel as a result of the other's response.

The results revealed that subjects perceived parents, siblings, and friends to be more obligated to help them than acquaintances or strangers. In addition, if help was given, subjects said that they would feel the most gratitude toward a stranger, acquaintance, and close friend, less toward the sibling, and least toward the parent. On the other hand, in the help-refused situation, the results indicated that subjects would feel more resentment toward parents, siblings, and close friends than toward acquaintances and strangers. These results support the idea that expectations of receiving help are greater in a communal than in an exchange relationship. Furthermore, they indicate that although one may not gain much in terms of gratitude by helping in communal relationships, it is important to help in these relationships in order to *prevent* feelings of resentment.

Next consider a similar study by Waddell and Clark (1982), which also supports the idea that helping is more important to maintaining compatibility in communal than in exchange relationships. In a portion of this study, subjects were asked to imagine themselves in situations in which they had a need (e.g., their car was out of gas). Then they imagined (1) a parent and (2) a romantic partner (communal relationships), as well as (3) a coworker/fellow student they did not know well and (4) a landlord (exchange conditions) helping them *or* failing to help them in each situation. Finally, they indicated what their feelings would be in each situation.

The results fit well with the results of the Bar-Tal et al. study. Helping was perceived to be more likely and appropriate in communal than in exchange relationships. Furthermore, subjects reported that they would feel more hurt and exploited as a result of a communal relation failing to fulfill their need than as a result of an exchange relation failing to fulfill their need. Thus, once again helping seems to be more important for maintaining compatibility in communal than in exchange relationships. If it is not offered, it may result in more resentment (Bar-Tal et al., 1977) and hurt feelings in communal than in exchange relationships.

In these particular studies, there was no evidence of helping actually proving to be detrimental in exchange relationships. Indeed, helping in exchange relationships led to greater reports of gratitude than it did in communal relationships. This is not surprising. Helping is not necessarily inappropriate in exchange relationships. As noted earlier, people seem to feel a low level of communal obligation to almost any other human. Thus, low-cost help or help in an emergency is acceptable in such relationships. Furthermore higher-cost help is also perfectly acceptable *when the recipient can repay the other*. Repayment was not ruled out in the Bar-Tal et al. or in the Clark and Waddell scenarios.

There should be some cases, however, in which helping in an exchange relationship would cause negative reactions. Specifically, when there is no emergency, helping surpasses some minimal level, and the ability for the recipient to pay back is explicitly ruled out or would be aversive to the person who must pay it back, reactions to receiving help should be negative. Research on reactions to receiving such help from a stranger supports the hypothesized role of these boundary conditions (e.g., Gergen, Ellsworth, Maslach, & Seipel, 1975). Moreover, if the other offers help in such a way as to imply a desire for a communal relationship which the recipient does not desire, reactions may be negative. For instance, imagine someone whom you do not particularly want as a friend unexpectedly arriving on your doorstep to help you move into your new apartment. Contrast that with your reactions in the same situation if the person were a friend.

Next, consider two experimental studies by Clark and Ouellette (1983) and Daniels and Berkowitz (1963) in which actual helping was measured in relationships that subjects should have expected to be communal or exchange. These two studies clearly show that helping is greater in communal than exchange relationships. The primary purpose of the Clark and Ouellette (1983) study was to test the idea that the mood of a potential recipient of help would have a greater impact on helping in communal than in exchange relationships, and the results relevant to that hypothesis will be discussed shortly. What is important here is that a manipulation of expectation of a communal or an exchange relationship very similar to that used in the Clark and Mills (1979, Study 1) study produced large differences in the amount of help given within a relationship. Specifically, in this study, subjects were led to expect a communal or an exchange relationship with an attractive other of the opposite gender. Later on, the other person needed help blowing up some balloons, and the subject could help her. As predicted, subjects in the communal conditions spent significantly more time helping the other than did subjects in the exchange conditions, and they blew up significantly more balloons.

Similar results were obtained in the study by Daniels and Berkowitz (1963). Although these authors did not set out to study the impact of relationship type on helping, they included a "liking" manipulation in their study that probably manipulated expected relationship type and they also measured helping. Specifically, they recruited pairs of male subjects, half of whom were told that they had been paired with each other in such a way "that they would probably like their partners and that they were especially well matched" (communal) and half of whom were apologetically told "that conflicting time schedules sometimes prevented the assembly of congenial pairs" (p. 43) (exchange). All subjects were then led to believe that they would be working under the other's supervision. However, half of them were told that their performance would be important in determining an evaluation of their supervisor and consequently his chance at winning a prize (chance to help available), whereas the other half were told that their performance would be unimportant in determining their supervisor's evaluation (no chance of helping). When their performance would not affect their supervisor's outcome, relationship type did not influence how hard the subjects worked. In contrast, when their performance could help their supervisor, subjects worked significantly harder in the "communal" condition than in the "exchange" condition.

Finally, consider one last result from the Clark and Mills (1979, Study 2) experiment described earlier for other purposes. This study included conditions in which subjects who were led to desire a communal or an exchange relationship with another received help from that other. When the helper could not be repaid, receipt of such help increased liking in communal relationships, but actually decreased liking in exchange relationships.

Taken together, these studies demonstrate that helping (with no expectation of repayment) is more *expected* in communal than in exchange relationships

(Bar-Tal et al., 1977; Waddell & Clark, 1982), that it will increase liking in beginning communal relations (Clark & Mills, 1979), and that it is important to maintaining compatibility in established communal relations (Bar-Tal et al., 1977; Waddell & Clark, 1982). It is also a more *common* behavior in communal than in exchange relationships (Clark & Ouellette, 1983; Daniels & Berkowitz, 1963).[5] On the other hand, these studies show that everyday helping is *not* expected in exchange relationships and that while helping in an emergency and/or when an opportunity to repay is available may increase liking in exchange relationships (Bar-Tal et al., 1977; Waddell & Clark, 1982), in nonemergency situations in which repayment is ruled out it may actually decrease liking (Clark & Mills, 1979; Gergen et al., 1975). From this evidence, it seems reasonable to conclude that helping is more important to maintaining compatibility in communal than in exchange relationships.

Accepting help without repayment. Following communal norms, of course, implies not only that one ought to *give* help without expecting repayment, but also that one ought to *accept* help graciously without attempting repayment. Evidence for this hypothesis comes from a study described earlier. In this study (Clark & Mills, 1979, Study 1), the reader will recall, subjects were led to expect a communal or an exchange relationship with an attractive other, and all subjects were then induced to aid the other. Subsequently, the other simply thanked or thanked and repaid the subject. What is now worth emphasizing about this study is that *communal* subjects liked the other who accepted their aid without attempting repayment better than those who repaid, whereas just the opposite was true in the exchange conditions. In other words, graciously accepting help without repayment is important to maintaining compatibility in communal but not exchange relations. A somewhat different finding that nonetheless fits nicely with this one is reported by Shapiro (1980). He observed that whereas people will seek low-cost help from either friends *or* nonfriends, they will seek more help from friends than from nonfriends when the help becomes costly.

Taking needs into account in distributing jointly earned rewards. When one thinks of helping, what usually comes to mind is a situation in which one person has a need and another chooses to draw upon his or her own resources in order to respond to that need. However, another way to help a needy other is to allocate rewards from a jointly performed task according to needs rather than according to an equality or a contribution principle. Thus, people in communal relationships ought to show a greater tendency than people in exchange relationships to distribute jointly earned rewards according to needs (cf. Deutsch, 1975).

---

[5]If one assumes that another's attractiveness creates a desire for a communal relationship, then studies showing that people help attractive others more than less attractive others (Benson, Karabenick, & Lerner, 1976; Kelley & Byrne, 1976; West & Brown, 1975) lend further support to the ideas expressed here.

Few data are available on this point, but what are available support the hypothesis. Lamm and Schwinger (1980) examined how the potential recipients' interpersonal relationships would influence whether allocators would take needs into consideration when distributing between them the proceeds of their joint work. In this study, subjects were asked to read a story about two people who jointly wrote an essay, putting an equal amount of effort into it. Subsequently the essay was sold for 300 German marks. Both people needed to buy books to prepare for some upcoming exams and neither had a source of money. Person A, the needy person, needed 200 marks to buy the books, whereas Person B, the less needy person, needed only 50 marks. Persons A and B were described as being mere acquaintances or as being close friends. The subjects' job was to indicate how he or she would allocate the 300 marks between A and B. The allocations were to be final and no loans were possible. Lamm and Schwinger (1980) found that the needier essay writer was awarded a significantly greater proportion of the marks when the recipients were portrayed as friends than when they were portrayed as casually acquainted. Consistent results were also reported in a follow-up study by Lamm and Schwinger (1983).

Dividing rewards or costs equally in the absence of information about needs. If there is no evidence of differential needs in a communal relationship, then the best way to demonstrate concern for everyone's needs is to divide rewards or costs equally. However, although an equal division of rewards or costs generally should promote compatibility in communal relationships, it may seem inappropriate and detract from compatibility in exchange relationships if inputs have been unequal.

A number of studies support this reasoning. For instance, Austin (1980) had pairs of female friends and pairs of female strangers work together on a puzzle. When they finished, the results were quickly "analyzed" and bogus feedback was prepared showing that one member had done more work than the other. Then the feedback was given to one member of the pair along with $5 and the following instructions from the experimenter: "The guidelines I give decision makers is to divide the money on the basis of the task scores, but the decision maker has discretion to take other factors into account and to make whatever decision she feels is most appropriate" (p. 405). Subjects who worked with a friend, whether they performed better or worse than their partner, tended to divide rewards equally. In contrast, strangers behaved more selfishly. They divided rewards equally if they themselves had performed poorly but according to input if they themselves had excelled. Studies with children also indicate that friends are more likely than strangers to divide rewards equally (Benton, 1971; Lerner, 1974). Finally, Greenberg (1983) found that if two people divide a restaurant check equally, observers are more likely to perceive them as friends than if they divide it according to what each person had ordered.

All of these studies are consistent with the idea that when there is no clear evidence for differential needs, dividing rewards equally will contribute to compatibility in communal relationships but not in exchange relationships, although the impact of allocation procedures in different types of relationships on measures of compatibility per se has yet to be specifically examined.

Choice of decision-making rules in a group. Given the norm to be responsive to needs, members of communal relationships ought to prefer a decision-making rule that takes everyone's needs into account (e.g., consensus) to one that may result in one or more members' needs being neglected (e.g., majority rule). In contrast, members of exchange relationships ought to consider majority rule and consensus to be equally appropriate and desirable. Members of exchange relationships have no special obligation to be responsive to one another's needs, yet it is not clear that they should avoid taking others' needs into account either.

Evidence for these predictions is provided by a recent laboratory experiment (Sholar & Clark, 1982). In this study, subjects were recruited for a study of group problem solving. Upon arrival, they were told they had been assigned to groups on the basis of pretests they had completed at the beginning of the semester. These tests had supposedly indicated that they were likely to become friends with the other members of their group (communal conditions) *or* that they were unlikely to have met the other members of their group before (exchange conditions). Then, five tasks were described. The group was asked to select one of these tasks, and group members were assigned to use either majority rule or consensus to make their choice. Finally, as part of a "premeasure," each subject rated how appropriate he or she perceived the assigned decision-making rule to be.

The results were as expected. Communal subjects rated consensus as being significantly more appropriate than majority rule. Exchange subjects rated these decision procedures as equally appropriate. Furthermore, exchange subjects rated both rules as more appropriate than majority rule was rated as being by communal subjects. This makes sense from our theoretical perspective in that *only* the communal subjects in the majority-rule condition were assigned to use a rule that might lead them to violate communal group norms (by neglecting the needs or ignoring the preferences of some group members). This suggests that the use of group decision rules that take everyone's needs into account is another behavior important to maintaining compatibility in communal, but not exchange, relationships.

Responsiveness to the other's emotional state. One more class of behaviors that ought to be more important to maintaining compatibility in communal than in exchange relationships includes those behaviors indicating responsiveness to the other's emotional state. The norm to be responsive to another's needs in communal relationships clearly implies that one should pay attention to cues indicating another *has* a need, and primary among such possible cues is the other's emotional state.

Are people actually more responsive to the other's emotional state in communal than in exchange relationships? A recent study by Clark and Ouellette (1983) suggests that they are. In this study, described previously in the section on helping, subjects participated in a creativity study with a person with whom they were led to expect either a communal or an exchange relationship. Subjects were given a chance to help the other by blowing up balloons, and it has already been pointed out that they helped more in the communal than in the exchange conditions. What is relevant here is that the mood state the other projected was *also* varied so as to be either sad or neutral. The sad state should have indicated greater need on the other's part, and, as expected, in the communal conditions subjects gave more help when the other was sad than when the other was not. On the other hand, the other's sadness had no impact on subjects' helping in the exchange conditions.

Taking the other's perspective. Finally, consider the implications of the communal norm of responsiveness to others' needs for whether one should take the other's perspective when something positive or negative befalls the other. In communal relationships, this norm implies that members ought to take each other's perspective. Thus, in communal relationships, one should become happier when the other is happy and sadder when the other is sad. In other words, subjects in communal relationships should maintain "equality of affect" (Mills & Clark, 1982). Furthermore, as a result of taking the other's perspective, one should be more likely to attribute the other's success to personal dispositions and to attribute the other's failure to situational factors since this is the tendency people show when making judgments about themselves (Zuckerman, 1979). All of this should not apply to the same extent in exchange relationships.

A study that provides a test of some of these ideas is reported by Finney and Helm (1982). These researchers had subjects watch another person play a Prisoner's Dilemma Game. The other person was either a friend of the subject or a stranger to the subject. During the time the subject was watching, the other person either lost or won the game. After watching the other, the subjects completed some scales which asked them to rate the degree to which the player's outcome was due to the situation and the degree to which it was due to personal factors. It also asked subjects to rate their own emotional reaction to what happened to the player. As predicted, when the players succeeded, observers who were friends of the players attributed significantly more personal responsibility for the players' success and reported feeling significantly better about that outcome than did observers who were not friends of the players. Also as predicted, when the players failed, observers who were friends of the players attributed significantly less personal responsibility for the players' failure and reported feeling significantly worse about the outcome than did observers who were strangers to the players. These results suggest that taking the other's perspective may be called for and may contribute to maintaining compatibility in communal relationships, but is not necessary for maintaining compatibility in exchange relationships.

Cautionary Notes Regarding the Impact of Behaviors Called for in Communal Relationships

Behaviors called for by communal norms which may differentially influence compatibility in exchange and communal relationships have now been identified. They are summarized in the bottom half of Table 5-2. At this point, as with our discussion of exchange behaviors, the reader should be cautioned about boundary conditions regarding reactions to these behaviors.

Impact of these behaviors in exchange relationships depends upon situational factors. Whereas behaviors called for by exchange norms are typically inappropriate in communal relationships, behaviors called for by communal norms are *not* always inappropriate in exchange relationships (see Table 5-2). Rather, their appropriateness appears to depend upon situational factors. For instance, because most people probably feel weak communal obligations with just about anyone else (Mills & Clark, 1982), if behaving in any of the communal ways discussed (e.g., helping, accepting help, taking another's perspective, or whatever) is very low in cost or is required by an emergency, such behaviors are likely to be appropriate in relationships that would otherwise be exchange in nature. Furthermore, even as the costs of the behaviors called for by communal norms rise in nonemergency situations, many of them (e.g., helping, accepting help) are acceptable if mutually agreed-upon arrangements for repayments are made. What is clear, however, is that except in extreme emergency situations in which the subject is the only one available to help, communal behaviors are not *required* in exchange relationships as they are in communal relationships and that some communal behaviors, such as refusing to let another repay, may reduce compatibility in exchange relationships (Clark & Mills, 1979; Gergen et al., 1975).

Certainty. Just as certainty about the existence of a relationship may influence reactions to exchange behaviors, so too may it influence reactions to communal behaviors. First, if one desires but is unsure of having a communal relationship with another, having one's needs taken into account in any of the ways just discussed may be especially welcomed.

Second, uncertainty about *exchange* relationships may also influence reactions to communal behavior. As with the effect of exchange behaviors in communal relations, these effects may depend upon how easy it is to "explain away" the communal behaviors. If such behaviors are easy to "explain away," one may be more likely to discount them in an exchange relationship about which one is certain as opposed to uncertain. In contrast, if the behavior cannot be easily explained away in exchange terms, communal behaviors may be more disruptive in exchange relationships about which one *had* felt certain than in other exchange relationships.

Strength. Variations in the strength of communal relations may be very important in determining just how people in communal relationships will react to adherence to the various communal behaviors discussed thus far. First, such variations have clear implications for understanding when people in communal relations will react negatively to the absence of behaviors such as those described above. For instance, when the reason for the absence is that the other had to meet a conflicting obligation of at least equal magnitude in a stronger communal relationship, then the absence of helping, emotional responsivity, or whatever should not reduce compatibility. By implication, the absence of communal behaviors in strong communal relations may generally produce more distress than their absence in weaker relations.

Desire. Finally, the less the desire for a communal relationship, the less negative should be reactions to the absence of these behaviors in communal relationships. Similarly, the less the desire for an exchange relationship, the less negative may be any reactions to the inappropriate presence of communal behaviors in those relationships.

Conclusion

Considerable evidence has now been reviewed indicating that to understand the impact of many behaviors on compatibility, one must take relationship type into account. The work reviewed here, however, represents just the beginning of possible research on this topic. Further studies likely will reveal many additional behaviors whose impact on compatibility depends upon relationship type. Indeed, further research will probably reveal other relationship types (and subtypes) with their own implications for understanding compatibility.

I believe that research on compatibility which takes relationship type into account will be important not only because it will reveal new findings about compatibility, but also because it will provide a useful framework within which past research on interpersonal relationships can be reviewed. As Berscheid (1982) has pointed out, in the past social psychologists' laboratory studies of attraction have tended to focus on relationships between strangers who have never seen each other before and who never expect to see each other in the future. My guess is that such relationships are almost always viewed in exchange terms and that many findings from such studies will not generalize to communal relationships. As an example, consider a study by Gergen et al. (1975) in which a person who received help from a stranger tended to like that stranger better if the stranger repaid him than if he specifically said he did not want repayment. The study by Clark and Mills (1979) described earlier shows that this finding can be replicated when participants in a study expect an exchange relationship, but that just the opposite effect is obtained when participants expect a communal relationship.

More recently, social psychologists have increasingly focused their attention on actual friendships, romantic relationships, and family relationships. Many have pointed out that these are the relationships that are most important to us and that it is more important to study these relationships than the "artificial" ones that exist in laboratory studies. I agree. However, again, I believe we must be cautious in interpreting the results of such studies. These are probably communal relationships and their results may not generalize to either short-term or long-term exchange relationships.

References

Austin, W. (1980). Friendship and fairness: Effects of type of relationship and task performance on choice of distribution rules. *Personality and Social Psychology Bulletin, 6,* 402–408.

Bar-Tal, D., Bar-Zohar, Y., Greenberg, M. S., & Herman, M. (1977). Reciprocity behavior in the relationship between donor and recipient and between harm-doer and victim. *Sociometry, 40,* 293–298.

Benson, P. L., Karabenick, S. A., & Lerner, R. M. (1976). Pretty pleases: The effect of physical attractiveness, race, and sex on receiving help. *Journal of Experimental Social Psychology, 12,* 409–415.

Benton, A. A. (1971). Productivity, distributive justice, and bargaining among children. *Journal of Personality and Social Psychology, 18,* 68–78.

Berscheid, E. (1982). Attention and emotion in interpersonal relationships. In M. S. Clark & S. T. Fiske (Eds.), *Affect and cognition: The seventeenth annual carnegie symposium on cognition.* Hillsdale, NJ: Erlbaum.

Berscheid, E., Dion, K., Walster, E., & Walster, G. W. (1971). Physical attractiveness and dating choice: A test of the matching hypothesis. *Journal of Experimental Social Psychology, 7,* 173–189.

Clark, M. S. (1981). Noncomparability of benefits given and received: A cue to the existence of friendship. *Social Psychology Quarterly, 44,* 375–381.

Clark, M. S. (1984a). Record keeping in two types of relationships. *Journal of Personality and Social Psychology, 47,* 539–557.

Clark, M. S. (1984b). *Availability and attractiveness of the other as determinants of a desire for a communal or an exchange relationship.* Unpublished manuscript.

Clark, M. S., & Mills, J. (1979). Interpersonal attraction in exchange and communal relationships. *Journal of Personality and Social Psychology, 37,* 12–24.

Clark, M. S., & Ouellette, R. (1983). *The impact of relationship type and the potential recipient's mood on helping.* Unpublished manuscript, Carnegie-Mellon University.

Clark, M. S., & Vanderlipp, B. (in press). Perceptions of exploitation in communal and exchange relationships. *Journal of Social and Personal Relationships.*

Daniels, L. R., & Berkowitz, L. (1963). Liking and response to dependency relationships. *Human Relations, 16,* 141–148.

Deutsch, M. (1975). Equity, equality, and need: What determines which value will be used as the basis of distributive justice? *Journal of Social Issues, 31,* 137–149.

Finney, P. D., & Helm, B. (1982). The actor-observer relationship: The effect on actors' and observers' responsibility and emotion attributions. *The Journal of Social Psychology, 117,* 219–225.

Gergen, K. J., Ellsworth, P., Maslach, C., & Seipel, M. (1975). Obligation, donor resources and reactions to aid in a three nation study. *Journal of Personality and Social Psychology, 31,* 390–400.

Greenberg, J. (1983). Equity and equality as clues to the relationship between exchange participants. *European Journal of Social Psychology, 13,* 195–196.

Kelley, K., & Byrne, D. (1976). Attraction and altruism: With a little help from my friends. *Journal of Research in Personality*, *10*, 59–68.

Lamm, H., & Schwinger, T. (1980). Norms concerning distributive justice: Are needs taken into consideration in allocation decisions? *Social Psychology Quarterly*, *43*, 425–429.

Lamm, H., & Schwinger, T. (1983). Need consideration in allocation decisions: Is it just? *The Journal of Social Psychology*, *119*, 205–209.

Lerner, M. J. (1974). The justice motive: "Equity" and "parity" among children. *Journal of Personality and Social Psychology*, *29*, 539–550.

Lerner, M. J., Miller, D. T., & Holmes, J. G. (1976). Deserving and the emergence of forms of justice. In L. Berkowitz & E. Walster (eds.), *Advances in experimental social psychology*, Vol. 9. New York: Academic Press.

Leventhal, G. S. (1980). What should be done with equity theory? New approaches to the study of fairness in social relationships. In K. J. Gergen, M. S. Greenberg, & R. H. Willis (Eds.), *Social Exchange: Advances in theory and research*. New York: Plenum Press.

Mikula, G. (1981). Concepts in distributive justice in allocation decisions: A review of research in German-speaking countries. *The German Journal of Psychology*, *5*, 222–236.

Mills, J., & Clark, M. S. (1982). Exchange and communal relationships. In L. Wheeler (Ed.) *Review of Personality and Social Psychology*. Beverly Hills: Sage. pp. 121–144.

Reis, H. T. (1982). The multi-dimensionality of justice. In R. Folger (Ed.), *The sense of injustice: Social psychological perspectives*. New York: Plenum Press.

Sholar, W. A., & Clark, M. S. (1982). Deciding in communal and exchange relationships: By consensus or should majority rule? Paper presented at the meetings of the Eastern Psychological Association, Baltimore.

Sigall, H., & Landy, D. (1973). Radiating beauty: The effects of having a physically attractive partner on person perception. *Journal of Personality and Social Psychology*, *28*, 218–224.

Waddell, B., & Clark, M.S. (1982). Feelings of exploitation in communal and exchange relationships. Paper presented at the meetings of the Eastern Psychological Association, Baltimore.

West, S. G., & Brown, T. J. (1975). Physical attractiveness, the severity of the emergency and helping: A field experiment and interpersonal simulation. *Journal of Experimental Social Psychology*, *11*, 531–538.

Zuckerman, M. (1979). Attribution of success and failure revisited, or: The motivational bias is alive and well in attribution theory. *Journal of Personality*, *47*, 245–287.

Part III
Emotional Interdependence

Chapter 6

Compatibility, Interdependence, and Emotion

Ellen Berscheid

Incompatibility is surely the scourge of the realm of interpersonal relationships. It appears with the frequency of the common cold, but unlike that nuisance, incompatibility often proves fatal to many relationships. Furthermore, those who succumb to it often enjoy neither an easy death nor a quick one. As the explanatory epitaph on the death certificates of these doomed relationships, the word "incompatibility" often fails to capture the misery, frustration, and broken dreams that were its agonizing symptoms, as well as the heroic efforts of individual will, and of therapeutic intervention, that sometimes precede the final judgment.

If only because incompatibility is held responsible for the demise of so many relationships, it is not surprising that its mirror image is highly desired. When asked what we are looking for in a marital partner, a coworker, or a friend, "compatibility" usually appears prominently on our list of attributes. If a person were to reply, "Someone with whom I'm incompatible," he or she would likely be regarded as a candidate for the services of the nearest mental-health professional, for the proposition that compatibility is a good property for a relationship to have has the status of a cultural "truism"—a proposition so obviously true that it is not in need of examination.

What *is* perhaps in need of examination, and what is surprising given the value we place on compatibility, is why many of us are not conspicuously successful in contracting compatible relationships for ourselves while avoiding the incompatible ones. It is apparently not so easy for us to determine with whom we shall be compatible—or for how long. Nor is it easy for us to understand why it is sometimes so difficult to transform the incompatible relationship, when it ineluctably appears in our lives, into a more compatible one. Why, for example, when we have tried so hard, and when we have spent every Monday night for the past six months in relationship counseling, are we still stuck in a relationship that is clearly, and seemingly irrevocably, incompatible?

In fact, sometimes it is even not so easy to understand just exactly what compatibility really is. Compatibility seems to be known largely by the company it keeps; that is, it appears to acquire much of its meaning from its assumed cohorts, those *other* properties of relationships that appear to be the traveling companions of compatibility. Compatible relationships, for example, are frequently assumed also to be "enduring" relationships, to be "satisfying" relationships, and to be "healthy" relationships, among other qualities. But when looked at apart from these other, undeniably good properties for a relationship to have, the meaning of compatibility itself often dissolves into a diaphanous mist.

To take just one example of the problem the concept of compatibility presents, consider the following incident. While writing this chapter, the author was interested to hear a man of her acquaintance exclaim that he had found, on his recent vacation to the West and after years of search, the woman with whom he wanted to spend the rest of his life. When asked what it was about this woman and/or their relationship that produced such unprecedented enthusiasm and willingness to (for the second time) contemplate the marital contract, he replied, and not unpredictably, "We're so compatible! It's unbelievable!"

This was a striking statement because this man, having experienced a particularly unhappy and "incompatible" first marriage, had given a great deal of thought to the attributes required of the next (if there were to be a next) marital partner. The prerequisites on his lengthy list were specific and concrete: She must, first and foremost, *not* smoke. In addition, she should not drink. Further, she should be a Protestant and—desirable but not necessary—a faithful church-goer. She should be not older than 30 years of age, and, preferably, never married. She should be well-educated and intelligent, and able to discuss some of the more esoteric intellectual writers of the day, as well as contemporary politics. She should—and this for him was a necessary condition—be interested in art and antiques, and if she had a particular interest in American pottery and American Indian baskets, so much the better (and if she happened to own a rare Gruby vase, she could expect a proposal of marriage on the spot). It was also desirable that she be attractive in appearance and, given his personal taste, fair of hair, eyes, and skin.

Now, given the probability that a person who embodied such a constellation of attributes actually existed somewhere on this planet, multiplied by the probability that this man would ever meet such a person, and that probability estimate multiplied in turn by the probability that such a woman would return his overtures, even a beginning student of interpersonal attraction would have to predict that this man was destined for a life of singledom. Thus, his announcement that his search had ended was greeted with incredulity.

Pursuing the matter, he was asked just *how* it was that he and this woman were so "compatible." What followed in reply was a recounting of very specific interaction episodes, including instances in which a witticism of his was understood and promptly returned, and a mention of the facts that they had played hours of gin rummy together, that they had jogged happily together, and that she had fixed sandwiches for him in preparation for his long car journey home. *That* was the sum total of his explanation! Even more disconcerting, however, was the fact that in his enthusiastic report of moments shared with the woman, it also emerged, in the most casual and incidental way, that: The woman is a chain-smoker. She drinks. She is Catholic. She is 43 years old. She has been married and divorced three times and recently terminated a three-year cohabitation relationship with a fourth man. She couldn't be less interested in antiques, in general, or pottery and Indian baskets, in particular; in fact, she heaped a pint of fresh strawberries in a $300 Indian basket he had just purchased, realizing neither its antiquity nor its value (this incident related with fond chuckles of amusement). She is largely uneducated, although she is, he said, "good-looking"—with dark hair, dark eyes, and a dark complexion! But— and for him this was the joyous bottom line—with no one, *ever*, had he been so "compatible"!

What does this man *mean* by compatibility? One thing he obviously means is that he has a good time in the presence of this person—that the relationship feels good to him and that it is devoid of friction, conflict, and bad feeling. Actually, according to most dictionaries, he has used the word correctly. The Random House Dictionary of the English Language (Unabridged, 1966), for example, gives the following preferred definition of "compatibility": "Capable of existing together in harmony: [as in] *the most compatible married couple I know.*" Existing together in harmony implies, of course, serenity and tranquility, an absence of negative emotion and feeling. Thus, when looked at apart from its assumed companions—such as the "healthiness" of the relationship or its "endurability"—what is left of compatibility and its meaning refers to the *emotional tenor of the relationship*.

So what conceptual problems does compatibility present? Well, even the most optimistic observer of human behavior, if not that beginning student of interpersonal attraction we referred to earlier, might suspect that in the happily blooming relationship described above, the seeds of dissension, of misery, of frustration, and of short life are already present. An intrepid friend might even go so far as to caution the man: "You must be crazy to be thinking of marriage! This will never last! You and she are basically incompatible, and it won't be long before the symptoms of that incompatibility will appear."

Thus, when people use the word compatibility, they, unlike the dictionary, are often referring to *more* than whether the couple is currently existing together in serenity and harmony; they are also making some predictions about how likely this state is to endure into the foreseeable future. And, in making such predictions, they are clearly concerned with something other than the current emotional tenor of the relationship. They are, in fact, making some guesses about the infrastructure of the relationship, and they are making the assumption that this latent structure will inevitably reveal itself in time.

In this chapter, we shall discuss the nature of this infrastructure. We will accept the proposition that compatible relationships are, indeed, relationships whose emotional tenor shows an absence of negative emotion and feeling. And we will also accept the corollary proposition that in order to predict the compatibility of a relationship between two people, it is necessary to predict the emotions and feelings they are likely to experience in association with each other. To discuss these issues, we shall draw upon the conceptualization of relationships drawn by Kelley, Berscheid, Christensen, Harvey, Huston, Levinger, McClintock, Peplau, and Peterson (1983) and the model of emotion-in-relationships advanced by Berscheid (1983; in press; Berscheid, Gangestad & Kulakowski, 1984), and we shall argue that:

1. Compatible relationships are not necessarily *close* relationships, although the reverse is probably true.
2. No amount of negotiation or "conflict resolution skills," no amount of relationship counseling or "working on" the relationship, may produce compatibility within a close relationship for some partners—despite a good deal of popular misconception to the contrary. Some people are simply and irrevocably incompatible with each other, and there is no human remedy that will allow the closeness of the relationship to be maintained while, at the same time, permitting compatibility to be achieved.
3. Compatible relationships do not necessarily *endure*, though they may, and we shall discuss the circumstances under which this is most likely to be true.
4. Compatible relationships are not necessarily healthy relationships.

Because all of these arguments rest upon an examination of the infrastructure of a relationship, we shall first consider the hidden underpinings that give rise to the relationship's more easily observable and salient characteristics, including the pyrotechnics of emotion that occur in some relationships.

The Anatomy of a Relationship

Like "compatibility," the word "relationship" also has an ephemeral quality to it. In fact, "relationship" is conceived and defined in so many different ways that sometimes even the principles in a relationship become confused and find themselves asking themselves and each other, "Do we still have a relationship?"—with, curiously enough, one person sometimes answering in the affirmative and the other in the negative. As Kelley et al. (1983) maintain, however, when all of its many conceptualizations are distilled, at the hard core of the term is the notion that two entities are in a relationship to the extent that they have *impact* on each other, or are *interdependent* with each other in that a change in the state of one causes a change in the state of the other. To determine if two people are in a relationship, then, it is necessary to determine if they are affected by, or *influence*, each other. To determine what *kind* of a relationship it is—whether it is a "close" relationship, or a "compatible" relationship, or a "healthy" relationship, for examples—it is necessary to know the nature of the influence that the partners have on each other. More precisely, it is necessary to

(1) identify the activities (e.g., the thoughts, the feelings and emotions, the overt actions, etc.) of each person that affect and are affected by the activities of the other, and (2) to specify the nature of the effects of each person's activities on those of the other. Thus, the descriptive analysis of a relationship, which precedes its classification as a "close" relationship, or a "compatible" relationship, or a "healthy" relationship, or anything else, focuses upon observing the number, nature, and temporal patterning of the causally interconnected activities of two people.

This pattern of causal interconnections between the activities of two people *is* the relationship. It is, at base, the relationship between two people as viewed by God, or Omniscient Jones, or the relationship researcher or therapist, regardless of whether the two persons involved *think* they have a relationship or not. For example, they may think they do not have a relationship because their interaction does not live up to *their* idea of what a relationship is or ought to be, whereas interactional analysis reveals that they have enormous influence on each other. Conversely, they may believe they have a relationship, even a "close" relationship, but interactional analysis reveals that the activities of each very rarely affect the activities of the other, and when they do, the degree of influence is slight.

Close Relationships

Some people are not merely in a relationship with each other, but their relationship is also characterized as a *close* one. In order to determine whether a relationship is close or not, Kelley et al. (1983) have argued that certain properties of the interaction pattern are important. Specifically, we have proposed that a relationship may be profitably described as close if the two people are highly interdependent on each other, where interdependence is revealed in four properties of their interconnected activities: (1) The partners have *frequent* impact on each other, (2) the degree of impact per each occurrence is *strong*, (3) the impact is upon *diverse* kinds of activities for each person, and (4) all of these properties characterize the partners' casually interconnected activity series for some *duration* of time.

Thus, to use an adult heterosexual relationship as an example, Joan's relationship with Bill might be classified as "close" if:

1. Bill's activities *frequently* influence Joan's. Physical proximity undoubtedly facilitates frequent influence. Communication through other means—such as phone calls and letters—also makes frequent influence possible, but long-distance relationships rarely stay close relationships. This is undoubtedly why the time-worn remedy used to weaken an undesirable close relationship by parents and others (and sometimes by one of the partners themselves) is to put physical distance between the partners. Conversely, match-makers and others who wish to facilitate the development of a close relationship between two people often contrive to "throw them together" for long

periods of time; indeed, physical proximity is usually considered to be a necessary (although not sufficient) condition for attraction between two people to develop (e.g., Berscheid, 1984).

2. The influence that Bill has on Joan's activities is not only frequent, but *strong*; that is, a single change in Bill's activities produces either numerous responses or responses of large amplitude in Joan's activities. Bill may idly mention that he thinks physical fitness programs are a good thing for anyone to undertake, whereupon Joan immediately rushes out to buy a jogging suit and running shoes, enrolls in a health club and exercise class, replaces ice cream with yogurt in the refrigerator, tunes out her favorite television program in favor of Howard Cosell and the Wide World of Sports, and eventually trades in her sedentary secretarial positon for a job delivering mail.

3. In this case, the impact upon Joan has been to *diverse* kinds of activities. Bill's remark has caused changes in Joan's recreational habits (and, undoubtedly, in her choices of social companions), as well as her eating habits and television-watching habits, not to mention immediate changes in the state of her bank account and subsequent changes in her work. Sometimes, of course, the influence is frequent and strong, but it is not to diverse kinds of activities. Sue and Tom, for example, may spend a good deal of time together, but all they ever do is play tennis or engage in sexual activities; beyond this limited realm, they may have little or no influence on each other, and, thus, their relationship would not be classified as close.

4. Finally, this kind of frequent, strong, and diverse impact of Bill's behavior on Joan has gone on for some time—so much so, in fact, that friends and associates may learn to forecast Joan's behavior simply by watching Bill and learning of his latest political convictions, his food preferences, his current enthusiasms, and so on.

It should be noted that the pattern of interdependence between Joan and Bill may be *symmetrical* or *asymmetrical*; that is, changes in Bill's activities may cause frequent, strong, and diverse changes in Joan's activities, but the reverse may not be true. While a mere frown on Bill's face may send Joan into a spin, the most heated diatribe of disapproval on Joan's part may leave Bill unmoved. In fact, to even discuss a matter of great concern to her, Joan may have to make a special appointment with Bill, only to find herself delivering her message to the top of his head as he is bending over the task of sorting out his fishing tackle. Furthermore, in reply to her communication, she may receive only random grunts and mumbles. Thus, as Jesse Bernard (1972) put it, there is *his* relationship, *her* relationship, and *their* relationship as viewed by an outsider. In Bill and Joan's case, "their" relationship appears to be asymmetrical, and, eventually, Joan may prefer to interact with someone more responsive and with whom she can develop a mutually close association.

Compatible Relationships

Compatible relationships are not necessarily close relationships. For example, an outside observer probably would not classify the relationship between Joan and Bill as close because of its lopsidedness (her relationship with him is close, but his with her is not). Still, the two of them may be compatible, at least for awhile, in that the emotional tenor of the relationship may be generally harmonious.

The emotional tenor of a relationship can be determined (see Berscheid, 1983) by simply observing, or by having the principals keep a diary, of the emotional events that occur *in* the relationship. To use our current example, there are changes in Bill's activities that cause changes in Joan's activities (or vice versa) such that we would term that particular pattern of change an "emotional" one. The scowl on Bill's face as Joan appears in her new dress for their dinner engagement may, for instance, cause a change in (1) Joan's *physiological state*, and she may feel the symptoms of that change as her face flushes, her heart pounds, and her hands tremble; (2) Joan's *thoughts*, which may abruptly switch from visions of the romantic evening ahead to "Now what have I done wrong?", or "Is my dress too tight?" and so on; and (3) Joan's *overt actions*, which may be to throw her hands up to her face, sob, and run out of the room.

All of these events, taken together, suggest that Joan's reaction to the scowl is an "emotional" one. Further, the emotion has occurred "in" her relationship with Bill, because it was a change in his activities (i.e., the scowl) that precipitated her emotional reaction. Bill may or may not understand that the precipitating cause of Joan's emotion occurred within their relationship. He may, in the latter case, incorrectly attribute it to something outside the relationship, such as to someone else in her social environment, perhaps her mother, with whom she had an argument earlier in the day, or to the physical environment, perhaps the oppressive heat and humidity to which she is sensitive, or to something internal to Joan, perhaps the onset of her menstrual period. In any event, a descriptive record of the frequency, intensity, and hedonic sign (positive or negative) of the emotional events occurring in the relationship allows one to classify it as "compatible" when there is an absence of negative emotion and feeling, or as "incompatible" when a substantial number of the couple's interactions are characterized by negative emotional events on the part of one or both partners.

Description, and subsequent classification, of the relationship along the dimension of compatibility does not, in itself, answer the question of *why* some people are incompatible, or why even forceful intervention is sometimes unsuccessful in transforming an emotionally negative relationship into a harmonious one. To discuss these questions, one has to recognize that the emotional events that bubble and swirl along the surface of turbulent relationships have their origin in the infrastructure of the relationship, the pattern of causal interconnections between the activities of the partners, as further elaborated below.

Emotion in Relationships

Berscheid (1983) has argued that if the substance of a relationship lies in the causal interconnections that exist between one partner's activities and the other's, and if physiological discharge of the autonomic nervous system (ANS) is a necessary condition for the experience of emotion, as most emotion theorists and researchers believe (e.g., see Strongman, 1978), and if we accept the proposal that *interruption* is a sufficient, and possibly necessary, condition for the occurrence of ANS discharge (e.g., see Mandler, 1975), then it follows that for the individual to experience emotion "in" the relationship, some event in the partner's (O's) series of activities must interrupt something in the individual's (P's) series of activities.

What is there to be interrupted? Mandler (1975) calls special attention to the individual's *highly organized behavior sequences* and *higher-order plans*. An organized action sequence is a series of actions that are emitted as a whole, or as a single unit; where the first action in the sequence occurs, the others in the series tend to follow. In addition to their inevitability of completion once started, the individual does not give full attention to the behaviors as they are being executed. The performance of each bit of behavior in organized behavior sequences tends to be "thoughtless," "automatic," or relatively "unconscious."

To illustrate, for many people the early-morning rising and breakfast routine is a highly organized action sequence. Triggered by the alarm clock, for example, Joan gets up, puts on her robe, yells at Johnny to get up, stumbles downstairs, makes the coffee, yells at Johnny to get up again, waits to hear his feet land on the floor, unloads the dishwasher, puts plates on the table, and so forth. The sequence has been performed so many times in the past, in just that invariant order and with each response in the intrachain sequence of activities serving as the stimulus for the next, that she can do it in her sleep—and often does. Interruption of the sequence, however, establishes the sufficient conditions for the occurrence of emotion. *This* morning, for example, Joan opens the coffee can only to find that Bill used it all for his poker group last night. She doesn't hear Johnny respond to the second call and so has to run back upstairs to shake him. She runs back down to unload the dishwasher and discovers that it is full of dirty dishes, undoubtedly because Johnny and his friends hooked up his homemade video game to the kitchen circuit and blew a fuse again. And so on. When Bill appears and asks, "Where the heck is my breakfast?" he is likely to find Joan in an emotional state.

Many organized action sequences are part of higher-order plans that are in the process of execution. Plans involve "goals," or objects or events that the person values and is also committed—at least in some degree—to striving for. Joan's highly organized morning routine, for example, may be part of several of her higher-order plans, including seeing to it that Johnny gets an education and arrives at school on time, as well as preserving her marriage to a man who believes a good wife and mother always provides a hardy breakfast for her family. Higher-order plans, then, are response sequences initiated and in some state of completion.

A large portion of a person's daily activities are organized response sequences and/or portions of higher-order plans that are in the process of being completed. Such activities are not discrete isolated responses, but rather part of a *chain* of responses, wherein the next response in the sequence is triggered by the prior response. These intrachained activities may be interrupted by the partner or by events outside the relationship. When they are interrupted by the partner, the sufficient condition for emotion to occur "in" the relationship is met.

Thus, Berscheid (1983) argues that *inter*chain causal connections from one partner's activities to the other partner's *intra*chain response sequences are a necessary condition for emotion to occur in the relationship. The existence of interchain causal connections to intrachain event sequences is a necessary but not sufficient condition for arousal and, thus, for emotion. For emotion to occur, the interchain causal connection must interrupt, or *interfere* with, the occurrence of the remainder of the events in the intrachain sequence (see Figure 6-1). That is, the events that would have occurred in P's activity chain (had O *not* performed o_1 and had o_1 not been causally connected to P_2) do *not* occur (or they occur more weakly, in distorted form, or otherwise show significant variance in strength or form from what would have been expected on the basis of P's previous performance of this intrachain sequence).

But interchain causal connections to intrachain event sequences are not always interruptive. Sometimes, in fact, they may *facilitate* and augment the performance of the next event in the sequence. Many relationship interactions are instances in which one person's intrachain sequence could not be performed well, if at all, were it not for the occurrence and appropriate timing of the other

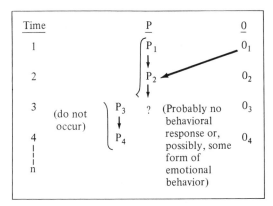

Fig. 6-1. Illustration of an interchain causal connection interrupting an intrachain sequence.

person's response that helps stimulate and make possible the next response in the individual's sequence. In adult marital relationships, these may include sexual activities, getting the kids ready for school, and so on.

Often, of course, especially in close relationships, *both* P and O are simultaneously executing highly organized intrachain sequences, and events in each person's chain facilitate the performance of the other's sequence (see Figure 6-2). In such cases, the two intrachain sequences are *meshed*, as contrasted to (1) *un-meshed* sequences, wherein there are no causal connections between the two intrachain sequences simultaneously occurring (when they are "disengaged," so to speak), and (2) *non-meshed* sequences, wherein the causal connections between the two intrachain sequences interfere with the enactment of one or both.

Meshed event sequences show all the characteristics of other highly organized behavior sequences: (1) Given the initial stimulus, the full chain of responses, on both P's and O's side, tends to run off, thereby revealing their character as a single unit rather than as discrete responses; (2) little variation in the nature of the sequence, and the form and timing of the responses, is observed; and (3) the behaviors are performed smoothly, rapidly, and without a great deal of conscious thought, sometimes allowing other activities to be pursued simultaneously. These characteristics, as well as their repetitive occurrence in P's and O's activity chains, permit their identification as meshed event sequences. Meshed sequences also often can be identified as having existed when one person, through sickness or absence or for other reasons, fails to do "his part" and the partner's sequences become disorganized. On these occasions, the failure of one person to provide the appropriate responses at the appropriate time in sequence is interruptive of the other person completing the sequence and probably constitutes a sufficient condition for emotional behavior.

If the relationship is characterized by a great number of meshed intrachain sequences, however, and if they stay meshed, there should be little occasion for

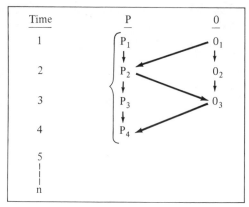

Fig. 6-2. Illustration of a meshed causally interconnected intrachain sequence.

the experience of intense emotion in the relationship, negative or positive. The two persons are clearly compatible, existing together in emotional harmony and tranquility. Such relationships, characterized by many meshed sequences, are also likely to be close relationships in that the interconnections between the partners are frequent, strong, and diverse.

In sum, that portion of the relationship's infrastructure (that is, again, the causal interconnections between the partners' activity chains) that is especially relevant to the relationship's compatibility or incompatibility is that portion that encompasses activities that are intrachained—or, in other words, that portion that represents each partner's organized action sequences and higher-order plans. Thus, whether—and how—the individual's sequences and plans impinge on the partner's sequences and plans (and vice versa) should determine the emotional tenor of the relationship. Where interchain connections between the partners interrupt one or both persons' intrachain activities, negative emotion should result; where interchain connections facilitate each person's perform-ance of intrachain activities, or where there are no interchain connections to these activities, harmony should prevail. In the beginning of a relationship, both persons bring with them a lifetime of organized behavior sequences as well as current plans in progress. How these two sets of intrachain activities fit together not only helps determine whether the relationship will be compatible or incompatible, close or distant, but also whether it shall live or die.

Close Relationships and Compatible Relationships

As previously mentioned, two people may be compatible with each other and yet not have a close relationship. For example, they may meet together only once a week to attend a play, and this interaction may proceed smoothly, each person facilitating the other's responses, thus contributing to emotional harmony in this limited relationship. Conversely, a close relationship may not always be, at least for a time, a compatible relationship. In fact, the closer the relationship—that is, the more interconnections between the partners' activity chains—the more opportunity there is for incompatibility, or for some of the interconnections to be interfering of the other person's organized behavior sequences and higher-order plans. Or, to put it another way, the more numerous the points of contact between two people, the more possible it is for one partner to *do* something that interferes with the other's execution of his or her sequences and plans, or *not* to do something which also interferes because the partner's failure to respond appropriately interrupts a previously meshed sequence. People in close relationships are usually, and in this way, "emotionally invested" in the relationship (see Berscheid, 1983); they are hostage to the other partner's activities and are vulnerable to interruptions from the other.

It follows, then, that close relationships may be, for a time, incompatible, with each person interfering a great deal with the other. This is not likely to continue indefinitely, however, since the most likely response to interruption is not only an emotional reaction, but also efforts to *complete* the interrupted sequence or plan. And, when the interruption is partner-inspired, the first of such efforts is likely to be directed toward persuading the partner to *stop* doing whatever he or she is doing that is interruptive or to *start* doing whatever it was that the individual expected, but which the partner failed to do. Such efforts, of course, may be unsuccessful.

The Difficulty of Achieving Compatibility While Maintaining Closeness

The effort to achieve compatibility may be unsuccessful largely for two reasons. First, the partner may not be *motivated* to preserve the relationship with the other. In order to perform responses that facilitate the other, or to refrain from performing responses that interfere with the other, the partner may have to interrupt his or her own sequences and plans, and some of these may have a higher priority than having a close and compatible relationship with the partner.

Second, the partner may be highly motivated to preserve the relationship and to maintain its closeness, but be *incapable* of performing the desired responses. It is undoubtedly one of the saddest facts of human affairs in general, and of interpersonal relationships in particular, that motivation without ability isn't enough. Some pairs are like the pot and the kettle floating down a stream in Aesop's fable; both would *like* to be close companions on their journey downstream, but the properties of the kettle make interaction injurious and interruptive to the pot, and since it is neither within the capacity of the kettle to make itself less hard nor within the capacity of the pot to make itself less breakable, a close *and* compatible relationship simply is not possible, however much both desire it. It is for this reason that in some adult relationships, no amount of "working on the relationship" produces the desired result. One or both partners simply are not capable of developing the requisite responses. For example, the poor hand-eye coordination that one partner was born with precludes that person becoming an acceptable tennis partner to the other, who is highly skilled and deeply fond of the sport. Or, one's limited intellect precludes making facilitative responses to the partner in discussing the play they have just seen. Or, to take yet another example, physical pain and ill health may preclude one partner's performing a wide variety of responses that the other partner needs in order to execute many of his or her sequences and plans. Hence, the plaintive cry, "I simply cannot be the person you want me to be!" Sometimes, indeed, they cannot.

In such cases, where motivation and/or ability to make (or not make) the relevant responses is absent, one can predict that the relationship will become *less close*, although it may become *more compatible*. There are at least three major routes by which compatibility may be achieved in cases where one partner interferes with the other's organized behavior sequences and plans, and where the partner either will not or cannot change his or her responses so as to facilitate, rather than interfere with, these sequences and plans:

1. The individual may *relinquish the sequences or plans* altogether. Tennis on Saturday mornings with the partner may be such a painful experience that the individual loses interest in the sport and takes up weight-lifting, which can be done without the aid of a partner. Or, since the partner's ill health precludes hiking and camping, the dream of building a cabin in the north woods may be abandoned.

2. The individual may retain the sequences and plans, but *develop additional skills or resources* that permit them to be completed without the aid or interference of the partner. For example, since the partner cannot, or will not, continue to chauffeur the individual to go shopping and to execute many other such sequences and plans, the individual may enroll in a driver's education class, obtain a driver's license and a car, and thus complete the original sequences and plans by her- or himself.

3. The individual may retain the sequences and plans, be unable to develop skills and resources to complete them without another's facilitation, but may search for and find a *substitute partner* who can, and will, provide the necessary facilitation. Sue may now spend Saturday mornings playing tennis with Joe, rather than with her husband, and Bill, the next-door neighbor, may be driving her to the grocery store.

All three of these remedies for incompatibility, or partner-inspired interference with the individual's sequences and plans, should restore some measure of harmony to the original relationship. However, harmony has been restored because the partner has been rendered *irrelevant* to the sequences and plans he or she previously interfered with, either because the sequences and plans have been completed by other means or because they have been abandoned. These remedies, then (as discussed also in Berscheid, 1983), have the effect of reducing the closeness of the original relationship by reducing the frequency, strength, and diversity of the causal interconnections between one partner and the other. And, because there are now fewer partner interchain connections to the individual's intrachain activities, the individual's emotional investment in the original relationship has also been reduced. The partner now has less power to interrupt the individual's currently facilitated sequences and plans by failing to perform the appropriate responses (and cause negative emotional reactions), and he or she also has less power to unexpectedly facilitate currently uncompleted sequences and plans (and cause positive emotion; see Berscheid, 1983) because the individual has found other means to complete the previously interrupted sequences and plans.

Thus, compatibility in a relationship is not infrequently purchased at the cost of the closeness of the relationship. In an effort to reduce negative emotion, relationships may be emotionally gutted over time. As one partner interferes with or fails to facilitate the other, the other finds alternate means of facilitation. In some cases, these "other means" may involve developing relationships with other people.

To summarize: (1) Compatible relationships are not necessarily close relationships; closeness, in fact, may have to be sacrificed in an effort to achieve or maintain compatibility; and (2) close relationships may be incompatible, but probably not for very long. Either compatibility will be achieved through the partner's developing the requisite facilitative responses and/or inhibiting interfering responses, thereby preserving the closeness of the relationship and the individual's emotional investment in it, or the individual will undertake other remedies, remedies that often have the side effect of reducing closeness with the partner.

Compatibility and the Endurance of Relationships

As previously noted, compatible relationships are frequently assumed to be "enduring" relationships. The notion that compatible relationships are enduring relationships carries the implicit assumption that *once* compatible, a relationship is *always* compatible. However, if one views compatibility as the extent to which two people facilitate, and/or fail to interfere with, each other's behavior sequences and plans, then the validity of that assumption seems dubious if only because, for one thing, people's plans change over time. Sometimes they change because they were relatively short-term and have been fulfilled, and sometimes they change because new information reveals that those goals are no longer as desirable as once thought and other plans and goals now appear to be more desirable.

Another reason that relationships might not remain compatible is because the skills and resources of one or both partners change over time such that the interlock between their own responses and the partner's current sequences and plans have changed. One partner, for example, may have greatly facilitated the other's highly cherished plan to obtain an M.D. degree through financial, social, and emotional support. But once the partner's plan to achieve the degree was completed, another plan, to build a thriving practice partially through social and recreational activities, took its place. The first partner, who was once so facilitative (and compatible), now may be interfering of the other partner's new plan. For example, in the case of a wife supporting her husband through medical school, the years spent at her secretarial job, scrimping to prepare low-budget meals and sew her children's clothes, may have left her ill-prepared to facilitate her husband's new dream. She doesn't know how to golf, to entertain, hates small talk, and finds decorating a bore. So, all of a sudden, they're "incompatible"; he says that he has outgrown her and the relationship.

The irony, and the poignancy, of the death of some such relationships is that they dissolve just because they are so successful. Because the partner so effectively succeeds in facilitating the other's goals, a point is reached at which the resources and skills of the partner are no longer needed; the individual has attained independence *because* of the relationship. Parents who succeed in facilitating their children's mental and physical health, their education, skills, and resources—who succeed in developing an independent, self-sufficient human being—often find that their child has outgrown the relationship, a bittersweet outcome, at best, for some parents. In any event, when one person in the relationship is rapidly changing, for maturational reasons or due to outside influence (e.g., schooling, the development of third-person relationships, etc.), and the other isn't, the chances of the first individual outgrowing the original relationship should be maximized.

Although it is easy to see why some compatible relationships may not endure indefinitely, it is sometimes harder to understand the endurance of incompatible relationships, or those of couples whose interaction is marked by conflict, anger, disappointment, and sadness, but who somehow continue to stumble on through time and space together. Following the analysis developed here, the "recipe" for such endurance in the face of incompatibility is:

1. The existence of sequences and plans whose completion requires facilitative responses from the partner (and/or the absence of interfering responses).
2. The partner's unwillingness or inability to perform the requisite facilitative responses (or refrain from performing interfering responses) relevant to some of these sequences and plans.
3. The individual's unwillingness or inability to relinquish the interrupted sequences and plans.
4. The individual's unwillingness or inability to find means to complete the interrupted sequences and plans through the development of his or her own skills and resources and/or with the aid of a substitute partner.

Although such incompatible relationships may endure because neither partner perceives (or perhaps *has*) any alternative to the present situation, they also may endure, despite the surface conflict and negativity, because each person does facilitate many *other* important sequences and plans for the other. Unfortunately, these facilitated sequences should not give rise to positive emotion if they have been meshed for a long time or, indeed, to any emotion at all (see Berscheid, 1983). Thus, and by default, the realm of activities in which the partners are incompatible accounts for the lion's share of their emotional life together—and it is negative in tone.

Compatible Relationships and Healthy Relationships

We noted earlier that it is often assumed that compatible relationships also tend to be healthy relationships. It is easy to understand why such an assumption might be made. First, if one assumes that individuals develop their organized behavior sequences and plans in an effort to maintain and enhance their welfare and survival, then it follows that partners who facilitate these, or at least do not interfere with their execution, are indeed helping to promote the others' welfare. Incompatible relationships, on the other hand, are fraught with interruption of individuals' organized behavior sequences and higher-order plans and, thus, also with negative emotion and feeling—or stress. Severe stress, in turn, has been well documented to be a major source of physical and mental disease (e.g., see Berscheid, 1983, for discussion of this point in the context of interpersonal relationships).

Further, and even beyond the physiological effects of stress on bodily organs and processes, the attentional and cognitive capacities of individuals coping with the stressful situations that chronically arise in their relationship with another are heavily engaged by the relationship. Thus, people caught in an incompatible relationship undoubtedly direct much of their limited attention, as well as their thoughts and actions, to dealing with relationship-inspired interruptions. For this reason, they tend to be distracted from problems that arise in their relationships with other people (e.g., an employer) or that arise in the physical environment (see Berscheid, Kulakowski, and Gangestad, 1984, for a discussion of this point), but which also constitute threats to their welfare. It is not hard, then, to see why compatible relationships are often assumed to be healthy relationships and incompatible relationships are assumed to be unhealthy.

Nevertheless, and again, compatibility can be, and probably ought to be, not entirely confused with this particular traveling companion. Compatible relationships, even very close compatible relationships, are not always healthy relationships; conversely, incompatible relationships are not always unhealthy. The "healthfulness" of a relationship to an individual may be conceptualized and measured in many different ways, but, for purposes of this discussion, we shall argue that it is useful to think of healthy relationships as those that maintain and/or promote both the individual's *immediate* survival and welfare and his or her *future* survival and welfare (see Berscheid, in press). When viewed in this way, it can easily be seen that many compatible relationships fail to meet the criteria for healthfulness.

Perhaps the most extreme, but unfortunately common, example of a compatible but unhealthy relationship is that between two drug addicts who support and enable each other's chemical dependency. "Days of wine and roses" relationships are clearly destructive of the partners' immediate welfare and their future welfare. More insidious, however, and not so commonly recognized as destructive, are enduring close relationships in which only one individual is chemically dependent, or has developed some other self-destructive behavior pattern, but, over time, the other partner has adapted to the individual's organized behavior sequences and plans that support and promote his or her ultimate destruction. Such gradual adaptation often comes about in an effort to achieve compatibility within the relationship.

For example, as an individual's chemical addiction grows stronger, those with whom the individual is in a close relationship often find their own behavior sequences and plans increasingly interrupted, and thus must find means to deal with these. Their alternatives are as outlined earlier. Again, they may seek, first, to implore the interrupting individual to *resume* doing what he or she is supposed to do (e.g., spend some time with his son after work) and *stop* doing what is interruptive (e.g., stop spending time in a bar every night). If, however, the addiction is stronger than the individual's motivation and/or ability to restore harmony to the relationship, then one can expect that the partners' alternatives are either to terminate the relationship or to: (1) relinquish those plans that require facilitative responses from the chemically dependent individual (e.g., gradually give up the hope of Daddy's ever taking them fishing again); (2) find a substitute partner (e.g., go fishing with a classmate and his father); or (3) develop skills and resources that permit the activities to be performed without the individual's aid (e.g., get a job delivering papers to buy a bicycle that will take him to the lake alone to go fishing).

Gradually, then, those surrounding the chemically dependent person will use, in one degree or another, all of these alternatives in various instances of interruption and so, over time, develop patterns of behavior that not only lessen the chances of interruption for themselves, but also lessen the chances that the individual's behavior sequences and plans associated with his or her addiction will be interrupted as well. In the end, then, the chemically dependent individual's interpersonal relationships (if they are not terminated earlier, during the period of incompatibility and interruption and before coping mechanisms are developed) may be quite compatible, and yet the individual's addiction may be alive and well—even thriving. It is for this reason that, increasingly, treatment programs for the chemically dependent, and those for other destructive behavior patterns, now treat the individual's family as well as the individuals themselves. They do so both for the sake of removing the individual's addiction and for the sake of the individual's children and spouse, who may themselves have developed behavior patterns that, while allowing them to maintain their relationship with the chemically dependent person, are destructive to their own welfare. Interestingly enough, many of these "treatments" are such that they would produce incompatibility within the old relationship; that is, children may be encouraged to restore some of their abandoned dreams and plans (e.g., "You have a right to want your Daddy to take you fishing and to spend some time with you"); spouses may be encouraged to, again, place household responsibilities on the shoulders of their mate rather than continue to "do it all" themselves; and coworkers may be enjoined against making excuses to cover up for the individual's lack of productivity.

Some compatible relationships are unhealthy not because they are currently destructive of the individual's welfare, but because they are destructive of the individual's *future* survival and welfare. For example, a husband may actively facilitate, through economic and social support, virtually all of his wife's activities and plans, and he may even actively encourage her to lean upon him for such facilitation and discourage her from finding alternative facilitative means (e.g., by developing her own skills and resources through education, employment, or by developing her own social network). Both may be happy and harmonious within such an arrangement. Indeed, in the eyes of observers, they even may be nominated for "The most compatible married couple I know." She needs him and he needs her in order to feel needed and powerful and important. Only one fact mars the happy scene, and that is that her life expectancy is a good deal longer than his. Without him, her welfare and survival is in doubt, for the end of their relationship will leave her bereft of the skills and resources that she will need to act in her own best interests.

Considerations of future welfare are, in fact, undoubtedly the prime precipitators of parents' actions that interrupt, and cause negative emotion, on the part of the child (e.g., "This hurts me worse than it does you!" and "You hate me for this now, but you're going to thank me when you're older"). That is (and discussed elsewhere, Berscheid, in press), many decisions that a parent makes concerning which of the child's behavior sequences and plans should be facilitated and which should be interrupted are based not only on considerations of the child's current welfare, but of the child's welfare in the future. The latter, of course, requires that some projections be made regarding the nature of the child's future social and physical environment.

In sum, incompatibility within a relationship, or partner-inspired interference with the individual's highly organized behavior sequences and plans, is not necessarily unhealthy for the individual. While perhaps painful for the individual at the time, and while it may result in negative emotions and bad feelings toward the interfering partner, such turmoil and disruption may be, in the long run, survival enhancing. Further, children, as well as adults, not infrequently do later feel gratitude for partners who precipitated painful but valuable learning experiences.

Summary

In this chapter, we have examined the concept of "compatibility" with the aim of distinguishing it from several of its assumed cohorts. We have taken the view that the core of the concept refers to the emotional tenor of an individual's relationship with another, with compatible relationships being characterized by emotional serenity and tranquility and with incompatible relationships being characterized by a negative emotional theme. We have argued that compatible relationships are not necessarily close relationships, but that close relationships that hope to remain so for any length of time are probably compatible relationships. We have also, however, attempted to illustrate how it is that compatible relationships do not always endure, largely because individuals and circumstances change over time such that the partner who was compatible at one point in time may be incompatible at another. We have also attempted to outline some of the likely responses to incompatibility and their effects upon the closeness of the relationship. Finally, we have argued that compatible relationships are not always healthy relationships and that, conversely, incompatible relationships not only are not always destructive of an individual's welfare, but that, in some circumstances, incompatibility within a relationship with another may actually promote the individual's future survival and welfare.

References

Bernard, J. S. (1972). *The future of marriage*. New York: World.

Berscheid, E. (1983). Emotion. In H. H. Kelley, E. S. Berscheid, A. Christensen, J. Harvey, T. L. Huston, G. Levinger, E. McClintock, L. A. Peplau, & D. R. Peterson, *Close relationships*. San Francisco: Freeman.

Berscheid, E. (1984). Interpersonal attraction. In G. Lindzey & E. Aronson (Eds.), *Handbook of social psychology* (3rd ed.). Reading, MA: Addison-Wesley.

Berscheid, E. (in press). Emotional experience in close relationships: Implications for child development. In Z. Rubin & W. Hartup (Eds.), *The effects of early relationships upon children's socioemotional development*. New York: Cambridge University Press.

Berscheid, E., Gangestad, S. W., & Kulakowski, D. (1984). Emotion in close relationships: Implications for relationship counseling. In S. D. Brown & R. W. Lent (Eds.), *Handbook of counseling psychology*. New York: Wiley.

Kelley, H. H., Berscheid, E. S., Christensen, A., Harvey, J., Huston, T. L., Levinger, G., McClintock, E., Peplau, A., & Peterson, D. R. (1983). *Close relationships*. San Francisco: Freeman.

Mandler, G. (1975). *Mind and emotion*. New York: Wiley.

Random House Dictionary of the English Language (Unabridged). (1966).

Strongman, K. T. (1978). *The psychology of emotion* (2nd ed.). New York: Wiley.

Chapter 7

Incompatibility, Loneliness, and "Limerence"

Phillip Shaver and Cindy Hazan

We have noticed, in ourselves and our acquaintances, a consistent pattern of feelings and behaviors that seem to appear as romantic ties dissolve. Excerpts from a recent conversation with a friend provide an example:

> We [he and his wife of 15 years] have become so defensive we can't talk to each other, we can't hold each other comfortably . . . and lately I've been so lonely. I feel like I'm dying inside, and I'm not going to be able to take it much longer. . . . My stomach is bothering me, and even though I've moved into the guest bedroom, I'm having a terrible time sleeping . . . [Much later in the conversation:] Have you noticed how graceful and good-humored N [an attorney in his firm] is? She's so undefensive, so open and free—just the opposite of my wife.

The pattern we observe is this: As a once-intimate relationship declines in quality, one or both partners begin to long for intimacy (perhaps also for sexual gratification)—a longing that is often labeled "loneliness"—and to fantasize about alternative partners. Very often these potential partners are idealized to the point of seeming to embody perfect "lovability." Soon after, the intimacy-hungry person "falls in love" with one of these perfect people (perfect especially in ways that the previous partner was not).

Our goal in the present chapter is to shed some light on this familiar sequence of events and at the same time reveal what we believe are gaps or misleading emphases in current theories of emotion and close relationships. How can it be that people who once loved each other, who have happily shared their lives for years, arrive at a point where they feel so incompatible that psychological and physical intimacy are impossible? When this happens, why do one or both partners feel lonely? What is the connection between loneliness and falling in love? Why does the lonely person seem so ready to view potential new partners as fulfillments of a romantic fantasy? Although focusing on the dynamics of relationship decline helps to reveal some important connections between incompatibility, loneliness, and love (which, for reasons to be disclosed later, we will call "limerence"), most of our analysis applies as well to totally unattached individuals who are searching for a compatible love partner.

As for our critique of existing theories, we will repeatedly emphasize the neglect of needs or desires in recent approaches—the recurrent drift toward behavioral conceptions which, though not wrong in themselves, ignore the central role of motivation, of yearning or desire. We begin by considering ways in which this pervasive bias affects the very definition of compatibility and incompatibility.

Incompatibility Defined

The term incompatibility implies a lack of harmony, a failure of parts to mesh. What is it, exactly, that fails to mesh when two people cannot get along? Psychologists, especially those who are behaviorally inclined, tend to conceptualize and examine compatibility or complementarity at the *behavioral* level. The harmony or meshing at issue is viewed in terms of interlocking actions or behavioral patterns, as if interpersonal relations were equivalent to a dance having no meaning or emotional significance beyond the mutual coordination of steps.

In recent years, considerable progress has been made in identifying the major categories of interpersonal behavior and in demonstrating empirically that the complete set of categories forms a circular array or circumplex (e.g., Carson, 1969; Kiesler, 1983; Wiggins, 1979, 1980). (See Figure 7-1.) According to these circumplex models, two people's interpersonal behaviors are compatible ("complementary" in Kiesler's terms) if they are reciprocal (opposite) on the dominance-submission dimension and correspondent (the same) on the love-hate dimension.

A fundamental postulate of the circumplex approach is, in Kiesler's words, that "a person's interpersonal actions tend . . . to initiate, invite, or evoke from an interactant complementary responses" (pp. 200–201). Another assumption, which quietly smuggles feelings into the behavioral picture, seems to be that "a complementary interaction is in itself mutually rewarding to at least some degree" (p. 200). In other words, it is assumed—often implicitly—that a person who initiates, say, loving-dominant behaviors *feels gratified* (at least "to some degree") when his or her partner responds with loving-submissive behaviors. Finally, to the extent that people can be said to possess interpersonally relevant personality traits, these traits are, according to circumplex theorists, preferred positions around the circle which each person has adopted because of some combination of inherited temperament and social reinforcement (Carson, 1969).

In terms of circumplex theory, then, a compatible couple is one that has naturally fallen into, or over time has created, a smoothly meshed set of interpersonal behaviors. An advantage of this approach is that it helps explain how a couple can seem to be well matched for years, only to move rather suddenly into a period of conflict and hostility. All that is required is for one person to change—say, from a loving-submissive partner to either a more

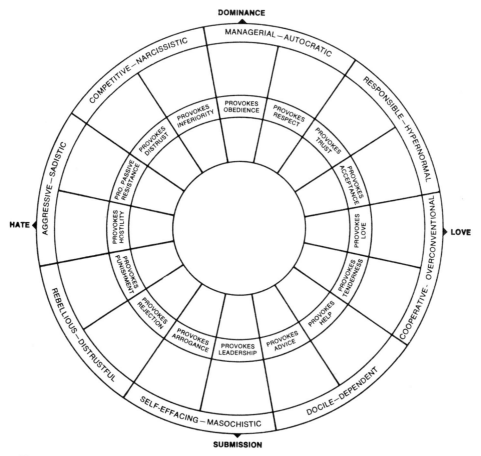

Figure 7-1. Circumplex of interpersonal traits. (Adapted from Carson, 1969, and Leary, 1957.)

assertive or a more hostile one—and for the other partner to be unwilling or unable to change in an accommodating fashion. To the extent that trust and intimacy are based on a predictable and initially comfortable interaction pattern, they can be threatened by one person's behavioral changes; thus, what looked and felt like compatibility can fairly easily become incompatibility.

The trouble with a strictly behavioral view of complementarity is that interviews (e.g., Rubenstein & Shaver, 1982b; Weiss, 1973), as well as our own casual observations and introspections, suggest that some couples who seem behaviorally complementary—and who are in that sense compatible—contain severely lonely members. In contemplating this paradox we have come to the conclusion that although behavioral compatibility is important, still more important and lying at the heart of the matter is *personal need satisfaction*. The often implicit assumption that need satisfaction follows automatically from behavioral complementarity is false; most people, at least in this society and at this time, want more from a close relationship than behavioral synchrony (Veroff, Douvan, & Kulka, 1981).

Interestingly, 25 or 30 years ago, when categories of interpersonal behavior were first being identified and measured, and circumplex models were beginning to be elaborated, the concept of need occupied a much more central position in psychological theory than it does today. For example, Sullivan (1953) originated the notion of interpersonal reciprocity with a "theorem of reciprocal emotion" stating that "integration in an interpersonal situation is a process in which (1) *complementary needs* are resolved (or aggravated); (2) reciprocal patterns of activity are developed (or disintegrated); and (3) foresight of *satisfaction (or rebuff) of similar needs* is facilitated" (p. 129, our italics). Schutz (1958) defined compatibility in terms of three classes of needs: inclusion, control, and affection. "Reciprocal compatibility" was achieved when each partner's level of expressed behavior matched the other partner's level of desired behavior in each of the three need areas. "Interchange compatibility" was determined by the degree to which both partners agreed on the relative importance of the three need categories. Finally, and most important for our purposes, Leary (1957) argued that the interpersonal circumplex exists at *multiple levels*, including both the "level of public communication" and the "level of private perception" (i.e., the level of *need* or *desire*).[1]

The public level in Leary's analysis is essentially the same as the *only* level dealt with by current circumplex theories. The private level, in contrast, has to do with the "interpersonal motives and actions attributed to the figures who people [the individual's] fantasies, creative expressions, wishes, [and] dreams" (p. 154). This level often reveals needs and desires that are not being met at the level of actual interpersonal relations. Leary used the famous "Secret Life of Walter Mitty" (Thurber, 1945) as an example. Mitty's actual behavior is exemplified in the following excerpt, which Leary coded as involving "passive resistance" and "obedience" on Mitty's part and "giving directions," "patronizing," "ridiculing," and "making accusations" on the part of Mitty's wife:

> Walter Mitty stopped the car in front of the building where his wife went to have her hair done. "Remember to get those overshoes while I'm having my hair done," she said. "I don't need overshoes," said Mitty. She put her mirror back into her bag. "We've been all through that," she said, getting out of the car. "You're not a young man any longer." He raced the engine a little. "Why don't you wear your gloves? Have you lost your gloves?" Walter Mitty reached into a pocket and brought out the gloves. He put them on, but after she had turned and gone into the building and he had driven on to a red light, he took

---

[1] Leary actually defined five levels, of which we mention only two. The other three are not relevant to the present chapter.

them off again. "Pick it up brother!" snapped a cop as the light changed, and Mitty hastily pulled on his gloves and lurched ahead.[2]

Compare that slice of reality with the following excerpt from one of Mitty's fantasies, in which his alter ego, the Commander, is coded by Leary as "dominant," "confident," etc.:

> "We're going through!" The Commander's voice was like thin ice breaking. He wore his full-dress uniform, with the heavily braided white cap pulled down rakishly over one cold gray eye. "We can't make it, sir. It's spoiling for a hurricane, if you ask me." "I'm not asking you, Lieutenant Berg," said the Commander. "Throw on the power lights! Rev her up to 8,500! We're going through!" . . . "Full strength in No. 3 turret!" The crew, bending to their various tasks in the huge, hurtling eight-engined Navy hydroplane, looked at each other and grinned. "The Old Man'll get us through," they said to one another. "The Old Man ain't afraid of Hell!" (see Footnote 2)

How might it happen that a person's desires would not be translated into need-gratifying interpersonal behaviors? In other words, why are the circumplexes at the behavioral level and at the level of desire not perfectly congruent? There are several possibilities: (1) The person might not know how (i.e., might not be sufficiently socially skilled) to move interactions in directions that would better meet his or her needs (Shaver, Furman, & Buhrmester, 1984). (2) Even if the person knew how to initiate such moves, the partner might resist them. (3) The person might be afraid of the imagined negative consequences of acting in new and (to the partner) unexpected ways. (4) The person might be at the mercy of behaviorally incompatible desires. (5) The person might, in previous relationships, have so overlearned behavioral patterns that fail to meet his or her current needs that other behavioral possibilities seem quite foreign (Bowlby, 1969; Shaver & Rubenstein, 1980; Sroufe & Fleeson, in press).

Obviously, several of these possibilities can coexist and in most cases probably do. The main point is that, for a variety of reasons, behavioral compatibility and mutual need-satisfaction are not necessarily the same.

Desire and Emotion

The needs-oriented view of compatibility is closely linked to the assumption that people initiate interpersonal behaviors and maintain close relationships in order to experience certain feelings and avoid experiencing others. In other words, needs and desires (along with associated fantasies) impel interpersonal behavior, and feelings or emotions inform the behaving person about whether the needs are being met (Klinger, 1977). To borrow and adapt an economic metaphor common in social psychology, emotion is the currency in terms of

---

[2]Copr. © 1942 James Thurber. Copr. © 1970 Helen W. Thurber and Rosemary T. Sauers. From *My World—and Welcome to It*, published by Harcourt Brace Jovanovich.

which close-relationship balance sheets are tallied. The "bottom line," as Thibaut and Kelley (1959; Kelley & Thibaut, 1978) have argued, records the balance of positive over negative emotions.

Since emotions are essential to a needs-oriented view of compatibility, we must pay some attention to contemporary theories of emotion. For purposes of this chapter, we want to choose one that fits with our intuitive notion that loneliness is a feeling, a feeling that indicates that one's relationships are failing to provide what is wanted or needed.

The most extensive recent examination of emotion in the context of close relationships is Berscheid's (1982, 1983, and Chap. 6 of this volume). Unfortunately, from our point of view, she relies too heavily on Mandler's (1975) interruption theory of emotion, according to which emotions are initiated by interruptions of well-learned behavior sequences. Admittedly, this theory offers certain advantages to the relationship theorist; it helps explain, for example, why the beginnings and endings of relationships, with their unfamiliar and unpredictable interactions, are so emotionally tumultuous, while the middles (which may last for decades) can be fairly placid. An extreme statement of the Berscheid-Mandler view is that there are no emotions as long as everything is predictable and compatible at the behavioral level.

This approach is to emotion theory what the behavioral-level circumplex is to the theory of interpersonal complementarity. Just as the behaviorally oriented interpersonal relations theorist ignores the desires and wishes that underlie people's satisfaction or dissatisfaction with their relationships, Berscheid neglects the central role of need or desire in emotion—the wishes and values that lie behind goal-directed behavior and gratification-directed fantasy.[3]

More useful for our purposes is Roseman's (1979, 1984) theory of emotion-generation. According to this theory, all emotions are reactions to the match or mismatch between "wants" and "outcomes." Figure 7-2 displays the four basic emotional possibilities: joy (getting what you want, in Roseman's terms), sadness (not getting what you want), distress (getting what you do not want), and relief (not getting what you do not want). Three additional aspects of the judgments that determine emotional reactions—besides "wants" and "out-comes"—are: (1) "probability"; some emotions are future-oriented rather than past-oriented (e.g., fear involves an imagined future mismatch between desire and outcome; hope, an imagined future match); (2) "agency"; some emotions are based on self-oriented rather than other-oriented or circumstance-oriented attributions (agency distinguishes, for example, between shame, hostility, and distress); and (3) "legitimacy," which distinguishes anger and guilt from other

---

[3]Berscheid (1982) *did* occasionally mention desire in her first essay on emotions and relationships, but only as an unanalyzed cause of goal-directed behavior. In subsequent papers she has placed more and more attention on interrupted behavior sequences as the cause of emotional arousal, leaving desires and their connections with specific discrete emotions far in the background.

OUTCOME

		Getting	Not Getting
DESIRE	What is Wanted	Joy, Pleasure	Sadness, Sorrow
	What is Not Wanted	Distress	Relief

Figure 7-2. The four fundamental desire-outcome conjunctions according to Roseman's theory of emotion.

forms of distress. All together, these five factors—desire, outcome, probability, agency, and legitimacy—account for what Roseman calls the "13-or-so" basic emotions.[4]

Similar in certain respects, although not as detailed, is Dahl's (1979) "appetite hypothesis of emotions." According to Dahl, certain emotions—fear, anger, and love, for example—are similar to appetites such as hunger and thirst in that they share three structural components: "(1) a perception (e.g., of thirst); (2) a wish to achieve perceptual identity with the previous experience of satisfaction (e.g., the taste of water); and (3) a consummatory act (e.g., drinking water)." Dahl reasons as follows:

> If emotions with objects were like appetites, then we might understand that the perception of an emotion is comparable to the perception of an appetite. We would expect to find a consummatory act and we would expect to be able to infer an implicit wish. Thus, if anger were an appetite, ... repulsion of the object of anger would be its consummation. ... And if tenderness [or love] were an appetite, the implicit wish would be tender touching and holding, and carrying out that wish would be its consummation. (pp. 212–213)

This line of thinking led Dahl to "redefine pleasure as satisfaction of a wish and unpleasure as nonsatisfaction of a wish" (p. 206). After making allowance for the creative potential of human symbolic capacity, he defined a wish as "an attempt to achieve perceptual identity and/or symbolic equivalence with a previous experience of satisfaction" (p. 209). ("Symbolic equivalence" helps explain why adult fantasies of interpersonal gratification are not perfect replicas of memories of satisfying childhood relationships.)

---

[4]In his 1984 paper, Roseman altered the theory slightly—making legitimacy a subtype of "control," for example— but for our purposes the 1979 version of the theory is adequate and easier to summarize briefly.

The advantage of the approaches outlined by Roseman and Dahl, in comparison with the approach advocated by Mandler and Berscheid, is that the former push the analysis back to a deeper level, the level of need, value, and desire. Like the behavioral-circumplex model of compatibility, the Berscheid-Mandler interruption approach to emotion is not necessarily incorrect, just incomplete. Since goal-directed behavior is generally initiated by desire (as the term "goal" implies), interruption of an action sequence generally produces an unexpectedly sudden outcome—one that the person in question either wants or does not want—and this produces an emotion. Unfortunately, unless the psychological analyst knows something about the values, needs, or desires lying behind the action-outcomes sequence, it is often impossible to understand the emotional reaction. Moreover, the interruption approach offers no easy explanation for long-term relationships in which well-synchronized partners gain considerable pleasure from each other's company, whereas Roseman's and Dahl's approaches imply that pleasure is always possible as long as one partner is obtaining desirable outcomes.

Loneliness and Social Needs

"Loneliness is an emotional state, like anger or fear" (Shaver & Buhrmester, 1983). In terms of Roseman's framework (refer back to Figure 7-2), loneliness is a form of *sadness* or *distress*—a consequence of not getting something a person needs or wants (intimacy, affection) or of experiencing unwanted outcomes (rejection, intense criticism, being ignored, etc.). In his pioneering book on loneliness, Weiss (1973) seems to agree. In some places he refers to "relational deficits" (the absence of something that the lonely person wants); in another place he says, "Loneliness is among the most common *distresses*" (p. 1, our italics). He also mentions the *appetitive* quality of loneliness, quoting Sullivan (1953), who called loneliness a "driving force," as follows: "The fact that loneliness will lead to integrations in the face of severe anxiety automatically means that loneliness in itself is more terrible than anxiety" (p. 262).[5] Moreover, Weiss suggests, on the basis of interviews with lonely and formerly lonely people, that surface compatibility (i.e., interaction compatibility judged solely at the behavioral level) is not a sufficient antidote to loneliness:

> Loneliness is not simply a desire for company, any company; rather it yields only to very specific forms of relationship. *Loneliness is often uninterrupted by social activity; the social activity may feel "out there," in no way engaging the individual's emotions.* It can even make matters worse. However, the responsiveness of loneliness to just the right sort of relationship with others is

---

[5] Sullivan's phrase, "automatically means," is not logically compelling. In reality, some people are so anxious that they are willing to tolerate chronic loneliness; other people, as Sullivan claims, are lonelier than they are anxious, so to speak, and so seek social contact despite their discomfort.

absolutely remarkable. Given the right establishment of these relationships, loneliness will vanish abruptly and without a trace, as though it had never existed. (1973, pp. 13–14, our italics)

Loneliness is, according to Sullivan (1953, p. 290), "the exceedingly unpleasant and driving experience connected with inadequate discharge of the need for human intimacy"—a definition close to the one we will be adopting here. Weiss (1973), without contradicting Sullivan, offers a more differentiated conception of the causes of loneliness: "Loneliness appears always to be the absence of some particular type of relationship or, more accurately, a response to the absence of some particular relational provision. In many instances it is a response to the absence of the provisions of a close, indeed intimate, attachment. It may also be a response to the absence of the provisions of meaningful friendships, collegial relationships, or other linkages to a coherent community" (p. 17). Weiss returns to Sullivan's notion of a driving force in the following sentence: "All loneliness syndromes would seem to give rise to *yearning* for the relationship—an intimacy, a friendship, a relationship with kin—that would provide whatever is at the moment insufficient" (p. 18, our italics).

Peplau and Perlman (1982; Perlman & Peplau, 1981) have broadened the conception of loneliness by hypothesizing that it "exists to the extent that a person's network of social relationships is smaller or less satisfying than the person desires" (1981, p. 32). As Shaver and Buhrmester (1983) have pointed out, however, the precise nature of "desire" remains unclear in this formulation. Peplau and Perlman have taken what they call a "cognitive approach" to loneliness: "Cognitive approaches propose that loneliness occurs when the individual *perceives a discrepancy between two factors*, the desired and the achieved patterns of social relations" (1982, p. 5, our emphasis). They contrast this cognitive approach with the "social needs" approach, which is the one we are elaborating here: "The social needs approach emphasizes the affective aspects of loneliness; cognitive approaches emphasize the perception and evaluation of social relations and social deficits" (1982, p. 5).

In our opinion, once an emotion theory like Roseman's or Dahl's is accepted, it is no longer possible to distinguish clearly between cognitive and social-needs approaches. According to Dahl (1979), the first structural component of emotion is a "perception"—what other theorists, following Arnold (1960), have called an *appraisal*. Roseman, in his theory, deals explicitly with this perceptual or cognitive appraisal process and finds it impossible to do so without referring to needs and desires ("wants"). In other words, behind concepts such as "less satisfying" and "desires"—terms used in Peplau and Perlman's cognitive approach—there lurk motivational and emotional constructs of some kind, one of which is likely to be "social needs."

On the basis of his research, Weiss (1973) distinguished between two different types of loneliness, which he called emotional isolation and social isolation. In line with his claim that loneliness is due to the absence of "relational provisions," he suggested that emotional isolation is due to the absence of a secure, intimate "attachment" (Bowlby, 1969), whereas social isolation is due to the absence of a supportive, engaging, wider social network Empirical support for this distinction has been obtained by Brennan and Auslander (1979) and Rubenstein and Shaver (1982a, 1982b).

Shaver and Buhrmester (1983) elaborated this distinction by examining lists of social provisions corresponding loosely with the two major forms of loneliness (see also Weiss, 1974). Table 7-1 summarizes these lists. In this chapter, because we are focusing on close romantic relationships, our concern is primarily with the set of provisions constituting "psychological intimacy." Intimate attachment, whether between human infants and their caretakers or between adult lovers, involves feelings of trust, familiarity, safety, and warmth. The infant is presumably without defenses; adult lovers are usually less defensive with each other than they are in any of their other relationships. Related to this lack of defensiveness is mutual self-disclosure (Archer & Earle, 1983; Jourard, 1971) and free expression and release of feelings (Scheff, 1979). The prototypical intimate relationship is also marked by affection, warmth, and what Rogers (1959) called "unconditional positive regard." (For further elaboration, see Shaver & Buhrmester, 1983, and discussions of love and caring in Kelley, 1983, and Rubin, 1973.)

Several empirical studies support the idea that loneliness involves an absence of and a desire for psychological intimacy (e.g., Cutrona, 1982; Rubenstein & Shaver, 1982a, 1982b; Wheeler, Reis, & Nezlek, 1983; Williams & Solano, 1983.) But just what form(s) does this desire for intimacy take? Unfortunately, few researchers have addressed this question. However, if Dahl (1979), Leary (1957), and other psychodynamically oriented thinkers are correct, desire should manifest itself in wishes, fantasies, or dreams (Atkinson, 1982; Klinger, 1977). Dahl (1979, p. 205) quotes authorities as diverse as Sigmund Freud and Helen Keller to make this point. Freud: "As a result of the link that has thus been established, next time this need arises a psychical impulse will at once

Table 7-1. Two Categories of Social Provisions

Psychological Intimacy	Integrated Involvement
Affection and warmth	Enjoyable and involving projects and
Unconditional positive regard	activities (alleviation of boredom)
Opportunity for self-disclosure and	Social identity and self-definition
emotional expression	Belongingness, not being a "loner"
Lack of defensiveness and concern for	Social comparison information
social presentation	Opportunity for power and influence
Giving and receiving nurturance	Conditional positive regard (approval
Security and emotional support	for contributions to group goals)
	Support for one's beliefs and values

Note. From "Loneliness, sex-role orientation, and group life: A social needs perspective" by P. Shaver and D. Buhrmester, in P. B. Paulus (Ed.), *"Basic group processes,"* Springer-Verlag, 1983.

emerge which will seek to re-cathect the mnemic image of the perception and to re-evoke the perception itself, that is to say, to re-establish the situation of the original satisfaction. An impulse of this kind is what we call a wish; the reappearance of the perception is the fulfillment of the wish" (1900/1953, pp. 565–566). Keller: "When I wanted anything I liked—ice cream, for instance, of which I was very fond—I had a delicious taste on my tongue . . . and in my hand I felt the turning of the freezer. I made the sign, and my mother knew I wanted ice cream" (1908, p. 115).

Are there intimacy-oriented equivalents of the wishes and images discussed by these writers? We think so, and believe that their nature has been well captured in the provocative interviews reported in Tennov's (1979) book *Love and Limerence*.

Limerence: Fantasy Meets Reality

In *Love and Limerence*, Tennov contrasts "love," which other writers (e.g., Berscheid & Walster, 1974; Kelley, 1983; Walster & Walster, 1978) have called "companionate love," with "limerence"—passionate or romantic love— a phenomenon so remarkable when examined in detail that Tennov felt compelled to coin a new name for it.

Limerence begins, according to Tennov, when "you suddenly feel a sparkle of interest in somebody else, an interest fed by the image of returned feeling" (p. 18). She does not say why a particular person would be subject to just that sparkle at just that moment, or why anyone would be so eager for "returned feeling," but it will be our hypothesis that limerence begins when an intimacy-hungry, lonely person encounters someone who is apparently "compatible" with his or her wishes and fantasies. As in Roseman's (1979, 1984) theory of emotion, we will assume that the limerent person can either be consciously looking for a certain kind of partner (like our friend who revealed his attraction to someone who is, in certain respects, unlike his wife) or be very pleasantly surprised by someone who offers provisions that the person values and perhaps needs but has not consciously been seeking.

In one of Tennov's examples, a middle-aged college professor, Dr. Vesteroy, tells with a sense of wonder how he began to fall in love with Dr. Ashton, a new faculty member in his department:

> [At first] I was much more interested in her research findings than in the way the sunlight caused those little sparkles in her hair. ([Although] obviously I had noticed them.) And I was rather taken by the intensity of her concentration as she wrote. . . . She flushed a bit and gathered her things, saying that she hoped she had not kept me. Then just before she went, she looked at me and smiled! It was that smile and that look that started the whole thing off . . . I had this flash, this thrill, a running sensation of excitement. . . . *I felt strongly at the time, even that first time, that some spark of communication had passed between us and that it was communication of a very personal and delightful sort.* (pp. 19–20, our italics)

Notice how quickly Dr. Vesteroy jumped to the conclusion that Dr. Ashton intended to establish "personal" (i.e., intimate) communication. We believe this rapid "spark" is a sign that the person who experiences it has been prepared by desire to spin a fantasy of idyllic reciprocation. In a novel about the deceptiveness of romantic love, writer John Fowles (1978) comments on this suddenness:

> One doesn't fall in love in five seconds; but five seconds can set one dreaming of falling in love.... The more I thought of that midnight face, the more intelligent and charming it became; and it seemed too to have had a breeding, a fastidiousness, a delicacy [evidently all part of an Oxford graduate's romantic ideal], that attracted me as fatally as the local fisherman's lamps attracted fish on moonless nights. (pp. 161–162)

Walster and Walster (1978) quote an interview with actor Robert Redford, which reveals a common subsequent step in the establishment of intimacy (at least for highly verbal people):

> I was completely alone and I felt like I'd aged and become an old man. No one I knew could relate to the feeling of isolation I had and I started drinking worse than ever. . . . Lola was just out of high school and her attitude was so fresh and responsive. I had so much to say to her, that I started talking, sometimes all night long. She was genuinely interested in what I had to say, at a time when I really needed to talk. There were nights when we would walk around Hollywood Hills and start talking, like after dinner; walk down Hollywood Boulevard to Sunset, then up Sunset to the top of the Hills, then over to the Hollywood Bowl and back to watch the dawn come up—and we'd still be talking. I had always said I'd never get married before I was 35, but my instincts told me that this was a person I'd like to go through life with.[6]

When interactions between the limerent person and what Tennov calls his or her "limerent object" (LO) escalate successfully toward intimacy, the person often experiences what Simone de Beauvoir called "ecstatic union." One of the women interviewed by Tennov made this literary connection, and went on to say:

> I thought that word. "Ecstasy." After our first night together, I woke up with this strange and wonderful feeling like nothing describable or nothing I had ever felt before. Problems, troubles, inconveniences of living that would normally have occupied my thoughts became unimportant. I looked at them over a huge gulf of sheer happiness. . . . I literally could scarcely feel the ground as I walked. . . . I relived our moments of intimacy as I drove—the loving pressure of Rick's arms around me, the softness of his lips, and, most of all, his eyes. His look was an embrace. (p. 22)

This example raises the question of whether limerence is simply another name for sexual attraction. According to Tennov, "Sex is neither essential nor, in itself, adequate to satisfy the limerent need. But sex is never entirely excluded in the limerent passion, either. Limerence is a desire for *more* than sex, and a

---

[6]Reprinted by permission of Redbook Magazine. Copyright © 1977 by The Hearst Corporation. All rights reserved.

desire in which the sexual act may represent the symbol of its highest achievement: reciprocation" (p. 20). We suspect that sex is part of limerence just to the extent that sexual dissatisfaction is part of the limerent person's sense of incompatibility with his or her unsatisfactory partner, or is part of an unattached person's limerent ideal. If sex with LO fails to live up to the limerent person's fantasy, as actually happened in several of the cases that Tennov studied, it can destroy limerence. If sex *fulfills* the fantasy, however, limerence blazes all the brighter.

Our discussion of sex begins to reveal the negative side of limerence. Needless to say, it is difficult for reality to match most people's fantasies. Walster and Walster (1978) illustrate this sad fact by quoting an interview with actor Marcello Mastroianni:

> That's my trouble. I believe I'm having a great love, but it's only on a plane of fantasy. I can't bring it down to the acts, the gestures, the attitudes of one who's really in love. Maybe one should love without imagining too much. But I can't, and it becomes a game where I'm left with the fantasy while the reality, the woman I love, is eventually gone ... destroying any chance [I have] for a happy life. (Copyright © 1977 by the Condé Nast Publications Inc.)

Once a person opens himself or herself to intimacy and acknowledges a personal investment in the potential fantasy-come-true, the possibility of rejection is a constant torment (Walster & Walster, 1978, Chap. 5). "When I was intensely in love with Barry," a young woman told Tennov, "I was *intensely* in love. When I felt he loved me, I was intensely in love and deliriously happy; when he seemed rejecting, I was still intensely in love, only miserable beyond words" (p. 45). A 28-year-old man revealed: "I'd be jumpy out of my head. It was like what you might call stage fright, like being up in front of an audience" (p. 49).

The intense mental battle between images of ecstasy and images of rejection pretty well rules out thinking about anything else: "Thoughts of Laura intruded while I was working, and it was that struggle with myself that, I suppose, was one of the most unpleasant aspects of the thing. As far as free time was concerned, while shaving, walking about, waiting for sleep to come at night— [the mental intrusion] was often at 100 percent" (p. 42).

Table 7-2 lists some of the main features of limerence gleaned from Tennov's hundreds of questionnaire responses and interviews. Although she made no attempt to weave all of the features into a coherent model, the features fit well with our analysis of the interrelations among social needs, loneliness, and fantasied gratification. If we consider a prototypical needy, lonely person, someone without close relationships or perhaps languishing in an "empty" (Levinger, 1979) or incompatible one, it is easy to see why he or she would be quick—perhaps too quick—to seize upon a potential new love as the perfect LO. When LO seems likely to reciprocate, the limerent person dwells on the signs of reciprocation, concocts imagined scenarios of gratification, and feels buoyed up ("on air," "on cloud nine"). When LO seems less than fully interested, the limerent person either invents an elaborate excuse or becomes

Table 7-2. Key Features of Limerence

Intrusive thinking about "limerent object" (LO)

A general intensity of feeling that leaves other concerns in the background

Acute longing for reciprocation and dependency of mood on LO's actions

Vivid imagination of action by LO that means reciprocation

Acute sensitivity to any act or thought or condition that can be interpreted favorably, and an extraordinary ability to devise or invent "reasonable" explanations for why the neutrality that the disinterested observer might see is in fact a sign of hidden passion in the LO

Fear of rejection

An aching of the "heart" when uncertainty is strong

Bouyancy when reciprocation seems evident

A remarkable ability to emphasize what is admirable in LO

Note. Adapted from *"Love and limerence: The experience of being in love"* (pp. 23–24) by D. Tennov, Stein and Day, 1979.

terrified of rejection. Obviously, this places him or her on an emotional roller coaster, especially if LO is not inclined to reciprocate. To an outside observer, the intensity of the process often seems way out of line with reality; but if we take into account the limerent person's desires, wishes, and fears, the intensity is more understandable.

Figure 7-3 summarizes the process we have outlined—the hypothesized pathway from incompatibility (or total absense of close relationships), through loneliness and fantasied gratification, to limerence. According to the model and in line with Roseman's (1979, 1984) emotion theory, negative emotions—including loneliness—arise when real relationships (real-world "outcomes," in Roseman's terms) fail to correspond with what one needs or wants; hope sustains the person's search for future romantic and sexual gratification. The lonely person is constantly on the lookout for new relationship partners, easily "falling in love" or becoming limerent in the presence of someone who seems capable of gratifying urgent needs. Since limerence in itself is not the same as need gratification (although for a while it may seem to be), we have hypo-thesized a final step in which either the limerent person gets to know LO intimately and develops a more realistic, need-gratifying companionate rela-tionship or the fantasy crumbles, as obvious incompatibility or outright rejection causes the lonely person to give up in despair or begin searching again for a compatible partner. (In the latter case, the person starts the whole process over again—a development that could be represented by an arrow returning from the box in the lower right-hand corner of the figure to the box in the upper left-hand corner.)

Issues for Research

The model presented in Figure 7-3 raises several questions for research. In this final section we outline a few of these, following the major steps in the model from left to right.

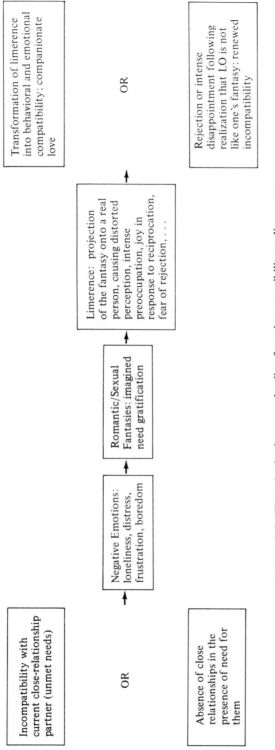

Figure 7-3. Hypothesized process leading from incompatibility to limerence.

Incompatibility. Informal observation suggests that unmet needs can operate either consciously or unconsciously. While scientifically troublesome, this distinction seems essential here (see also Klinger, 1977). When conscious, social needs can be articulated by a respondent in an interview or open-ended questionnaire. The friend quoted at the beginning of this chapter, for example, knows that he is dissatisfied with his marriage and can readily say why. (Whether his reasons are either complete or completely accurate is another matter.) But cases of limerence like the one involving Drs. Vesteroy and Ashton suggest that a person can be "available" for limerence without consciously realizing it.

Can psychological measurement detect this "availability"? We think so. One approach might be to interview people in some detail about their current close relationship: Is there anything disappointing, frustrating, or dull about it? If so, what is the interviewee's attitude about this? Limerence-prone individuals could probably begin to articulate their unmet needs if encouraged in this way by an interviewer.

Another tactic would be to sample the "stream of thought" (Atkinson, 1982; Klinger, 1977), for example by administering projective measures such as the Thematic Apperception Test (TAT). McAdams (1982, 1983) has recently developed a procedure for scoring "need for intimacy" in TAT stories. While he has concerned himself primarily with stable individual differences in intimacy needs, it seems likely that similar methods could be used to study short-term fluctuations in these needs, just as achievement motivation researchers measure both personality-based and situationally manipulated need for achievement from the same kinds of TAT stories (Atkinson, 1958, 1964). Of course, it would take some experience with both interview and projective methods to distinguish normal degrees of relationship dissatisfaction from needs strong enough to evoke loneliness and limerence.

Loneliness and other negative emotions. The most widely used measures of loneliness do not distinguish between emotional and social isolation (Russell, 1982), nor do they reveal precisely what it is that a particular lonely person needs or wants. Just as interviews, open-ended questionnaires, and projective measures could reveal the form of a person's relationship dissatisfaction, they could also be used to discover what lonely people want from their relationships—i.e., what they long for. (See Rubenstein and Shaver, 1982b, for several informal examples.)

If Roseman's (1979, 1984) approach to emotion is correct, we would expect loneliness to go hand in hand with other negative emotions, the particular emotions depending on the lonely person's appraisals of his or her unsatisfactory social situation. Rubenstein and Shaver (1982a, 1982b) found, in fact, that feelings as diverse as sadness, insecurity, fear, boredom, vulnerability, emptiness, resignation, and anger or resentment were associated with loneliness. Peplau and her colleagues (e.g., Peplau & Perlman, 1982; Peplau, Russell, & Heim, 1979), following the approach pioneered by Weiner (1974) in studies of achievement attributions, have shown how feelings as distinct as depression and anger can arise in conjunction with a person's causal attributions for loneliness. Attributing loneliness to inadequacies in oneself predisposes a person to depression; attributing it to other people's inconsiderateness or inadequacies results in anger, for example. Because the details of a lonely person's emotional appraisals and attributions are likely to be relevant to his or her specific wishes for a better relationship, it would be useful to examine these more carefully than loneliness or relationship researchers have to date.

Limerence. A disappointing feature of Tennov's (1979) otherwise admirable book is that she was unable to determine why some people experience limerence while others apparently do not, and why even people who have this propensity express it only at certain times and with certain relationship partners. Reaching the end of Tennov's book, the curious reader is as mystified by the appearance of limerence in particular cases as cave dwellers must once have been about the timing and targets of lightning bolts.

The approach we have been outlining suggests some promising avenues for research into these matters. Limerence-prone people, like subjects in Klinger's (1977) studies of the effects of "current concerns" (needs, desires, goals) on perception, cognition, and dreams, should be measurably quick to incorporate seemingly neutral "stimuli" into their goal-oriented strivings. We suspect, for example, that experimental subjects—preselected on the basis of loneliness or need for intimacy scores—could be presented with pictures or descriptions of potential relationship partners, and when they came upon one that struck them as personally appealing (i.e., as someone they could probably fall in love with), they could be asked to expand on the information given and describe in detail this person's traits, interests, habits, and so forth. In so doing, the subjects would presumably disclose the fantasy they have waiting for the first unsuspecting person who minimally meets their requirements for LO.

Perhaps a more naturalistic version of the same study could be done by following a group of divorcing individuals through their various infatuations, attachments, and (eventually, in most cases) remarriages. Given a reasonably large sample of such people, one would surely be able to document several cases of "mistaken identity"—i.e., attractions based more on projection than on realistic perception of a potential partner's actual qualities. In a large proportion of these cases, it would also be possible to record the disappointment and disillusionment that sets in when the mismatch between fantasy and reality becomes evident.

One of the most interesting issues for future research is the frequently observed discrepancy between a lonely person's conscious list of qualifications for his or her next partner and the unconscious forces that impel the person toward LOs who do not seem to meet these qualifications at all (see Berscheid, Chap. 6 in this volume). The friend mentioned at the outset of the present chapter repeatedly finds, for example, that he is attracted to women who look like his wife, even though he believes consciously that it would be dangerous to get involved with "a Sarah look-alike." Evidently, the feelings of attraction are based on appraisal mechanisms that operate outside of awareness. This is what makes us suspect that projective or free-associative measures of some kind will be necessary for researchers who wish to study these mechanisms.

Finally, if Tennov's observations are correct, there are many people who have reached at least middle age without ever having experienced limerence. In fact, it was in deference to them that she decided to call the phenomenon of interest limerence rather than love; the nonlimerents insisted that they *had* experienced love, just not the crazy kind depicted in romantic movies—and in many of Tennov's other interviews! One possible explanation of this finding is that people differ in what might be called their love ideologies, some being "romantics" or "limerents," others being more practical and down to earth. This possibility, which is consistent with existing research (e.g., Athanasiou, Shaver, & Tavris, 1970; Averill, in press; Cunningham & Antill, 1981), was illustrated in a recent social psychology class taught by Shaver. Students, who had read about both limerence and research on mother-infant attachment, were asked in an essay examination to speculate about the attachment histories of people who, on the one hand, readily succumbed to limerence as compared with those who rarely, if ever, had had the experience. Some students—almost surely the ones who were prone to limerence themselves—extolled the virtues of the limerents, guessing them to have come from secure, loving family backgrounds and therefore being "open" to the healthy joys of limerence. Other students— the perpetual nonlimerents, we suppose—portrayed the poor limerents as victims of insecure attachment, ever ready to plunge into romance in a desperate attempt to find stable love and security.

Whether either of these ideologies is close to the truth remains to be seen. That the prolimerents' ideology has serious adherents among research-oriented psychologists is evident in the following comments on "Intimacy Motivation" by McAdams (1982, p. 166):

> An hypothesis is beginning to take form: The secure mother-infant attachment relationship is the prototype of a particular quality of interpersonal experience that, throughout the life cycle, assumes great salience for a person with a particular motive profile. The key component in the profile is the relative strength of intimacy motivation for a given individual. . . . One might further speculate that the secure attachment relationship characterized by mutual delight and reciprocal harmonious dialogue (generally nonverbal) provides a set of experiences for both partners that beckons to be found again in interpersonal relationships throughout life.

According to this line of argument, the limerence-prone among us are those who have experienced idyllic reciprocation in the past. However, just as plausible at the moment is the possibility that limerence "happens" to people who have perpetually longed for reciprocation but never attained it. This view is consistent with the generally distressing quality of the relationships documented by Tennov and with our own informal observations of acquaintances who seem so "needy"—so hungry for love—that a new infatuation develops at least once a month.

For the time being, no conclusion about the healthiness or desirability of limerence is warranted. The evidence is still too sketchy.[7]

Conclusion

When a close relationship, such as a marriage, becomes incompatible, it does so partly because it no longer meets at least one of the partners' needs, or no longer satisfies at least one person's desires. Such a situation causes the dissatisfied partner(s) to feel a host of negative emotions, often including loneliness and related feelings such as emptiness. Loneliness can be thought of as a social-psychological hunger. Although the social provisions for which people hunger vary from situation to situation and from person to person, when one's closest relationships are deficient, the provisions of greatest importance can be summarized by the term "intimacy." The intimacy-hungry person, like a person "hungry" for any of life's other major incentives, is likely to fantasize the perfect embodiment of the desired provisions—in this case, the ideal lover defined with reference to current or recent unsatisfactory ones. The intimacy-hungry person is therefore ripe for limerence, an intense form of love in which a real person is temporarily perceived as exemplifying the ideal. In order to understand this process, which we take to be typical of human neediness in all of life's domains, we must go beyond the behavioral level of analysis to the level of feelings, needs, and desires. This "going beyond" will probably involve some "going back," at least temporarily, to recapture some of the rich insights of psychodynamic and motivational approaches to psychology.

Acknowledgments. The authors are grateful to Bill Ickes, Sandy Pipp, Howie Markman, and Carol Bormann for helpful comments on an earlier draft of this chapter.

---

[7]One complication, which we do not have space to deal with here, is that McAdams (1982, 1983) has designed his need-for-intimacy measure in a way that emphasizes the pleasures of intimacy rather than the painful and ambivalent striving for it. Researchers interested in loneliness and limerence may find it necessary to design their own more appropriate projective measures, perhaps based on the example provided by achievement motivation researchers who developed measures of both "motive to approach success" (need for achievement) and "motive to avoid failure" (fear of failure). Apparently, McAdams has not developed a measure of motive to avoid the absence of intimacy, fear of separation, or whatever it should be called. Since limerence clearly involves both hope of reciprocation and fear of rejection, a two-motive approach to intimacy motivation (as related to limerence-proneness) seems especially appropriate.

References

Archer, R. L., & Earle, W. B. (1983). The interpersonal orientations of disclosure. In P. B. Paulus (Ed.), *Basic group processes* (pp. 289–314). New York: Springer-Verlag.

Arnold, M. B. (1960). *Emotion and personality (Vol. 1): Psychological aspects*. New York: Columbia University Press.

Athanasiou, R., Shaver, P., & Tavris, C. (1970). Sex: Attitudes and behavior. *Psychology Today, 4,* 37–52.

Atkinson, J. W. (Ed.) (1958). *Motives in fantasy, action, and society*. Princeton, NJ: Van Nostrand.

Atkinson, J. W. (1964). *An introduction to motivation*. Princeton, NJ: Van Nostrand.

Atkinson, J. W. (1982). Motivational determinants of thematic apperception. In A. J. Stewart (Ed.), *Motivation and society* (pp. 3–40). San Francisco: Jossey-Bass.

Averill, J. R. (in press). The social construction of emotion: With special reference to love. In K. J. Gergen & K. E. Davis (Eds.), *The social construction of the person*. New York: Springer-Verlag.

Berscheid, E. (1982). Attraction and emotion in interpersonal relations. In M. S. Clark & S. T. Fiske (Eds.), *Affect and cognition* (pp. 37–54). Hillsdale, NJ: Erlbaum.

Berscheid, E. (1983). Emotion. In H. H. Kelley et al., *Close relationships* (pp. 110–168). New York: W. H. Freeman.

Berscheid, E., & Walster, E. (1974). A little bit about love. In T. L. Huston (Ed.), *Foundations of interpersonal attraction* (pp. 355–381). New York: Academic Press.

Bowlby, J. (1969). *Attachment and loss (Vol. 1): Attachment*. London: Hogarth Press.

Brennan, T., & Auslander, N. (1979). *Adolescent loneliness* (Vol. 1). Boulder, CO: Behavioral Research Institute.

Carson, R. C. (1969). *Interaction concepts of personality*. Chicago: Aldine.

Cunningham, J. D., & Antill, J. K. (1981). Love in developing relationships. In S. Duck & R. Gilmour (Eds.), *Personal relationships 2: The development of personal relationships*. London: Sage.

Cutrona, C. E. (1982). Transition to college: Loneliness and the process of social adjustment. In L. A. Peplau & D. Perlman (Eds.), *Loneliness: A sourcebook of current theory, research and therapy* (pp. 291–309). New York: Wiley-Interscience.

Dahl, H. (1979). The appetite hypothesis of emotions: A new psychoanalytic model of motivation. In C. E. Izard (Ed.), *Emotions in personality and psychopathology* (pp. 201–225). New York: Plenum.

Fowles, J. (1978). *The magus* (rev. ed.). New York: Dell.

Freud, S. (1900/1953). The interpretation of dreams. *Standard edition of the complete psychological works of Sigmund Freud* (Vol. 5). London: Hogarth Press.

Jourard, S. M. (1971). *The transparent self* (2nd ed.). New York: Van Nostrand Reinhold.

Keller, H. (1908). *The world I live in*. New York: Century.

Kelley, H. H., & Thibaut, J. W. (1978). *Interpersonal relations: A theory of interdependence*. New York: Wiley-Interscience.

Kelley, H. H. (1983). Love and commitment. In H. H. Kelley et al., *Close relationships* (pp. 265–314). New York: W. H. Freeman.

Kiesler, D. J. (1983). The 1982 interpersonal circle: A taxonomy for complementarity in human transactions. *Psychological Review, 90,* 185–214.

Klinger, E. (1977). *Meaning and void: Inner experience and the incentives in people's lives*. Minneapolis: University of Minnesota Press.

Leary, T. (1957). *Interpersonal diagnosis of personality*. New York: Ronald.

Levinger, G. (1979). A social psychological perspective on marital dissolution. In G. Levinger & O. C. Moles (Eds.), *Divorce and separation: Context, causes, and consequences* (pp. 37–60). New York: Basic Books.

Mandler, G. (1975). *Mind and emotion*. New York: Wiley.

McAdams, D. P. (1983). Intimacy and affiliation motives in daily living: An experience sampling analysis. *Journal of Personality and Social Personality*, *45*, 851–861.

McAdams, D. P. (1982). Intimacy motivation. In A. J. Stewart (Ed.), *Motivation and society* (pp. 133–171). San Francisco: Jossey-Bass.

Peplau, L. A., & Perlman, D. (Eds.) (1982). *Loneliness: A sourcebook of current theory, research and therapy*. New York: Wiley-Interscience.

Peplau, L. A., Russell, D., & Heim, M. (1979). The experience of loneliness. In I. Frieze, D. Bar-Tal, & J. Carroll (Eds.), *New approaches to social problems: Applications of attribution theory*. San Francisco: Jossey-Bass.

Perlman, D., & Peplau, L. A. (1981). Toward a social psychology of loneliness. In S. Duck & R. Gilmour (Eds.), *Personal relationships 3: Personal relationships in disorder*. London: Academic Press.

Rogers, C. R. (1959). A theory of therapy, personality, and interpersonal relationships, as developed in the client-centered framework. In S. Koch (Ed.), *Psychology: A study of a science* (Vol. 3, pp. 184–256). New York: McGraw-Hill.

Roseman, I. (1984). Cognitive determinants of emotion: A structural theory. In P. Shaver (Ed.), *Review of personality and social psychology* (Vol. 5). Beverly Hill, CA: Sage.

Roseman, I. (1979). Cognitive aspects of emotion and emotional behavior. Paper presented at the annual meeting of the American Psychological Association, New York City.

Rubenstein, C., & Shaver, P. (1982a). The experience of loneliness. In L. A. Peplau & D. Perlman (Eds.), *Loneliness: A sourcebook of current theory, research and therapy* (pp. 206–223). New York: Wiley-Interscience.

Rubenstein, C., & Shaver, P. (1982b). *In search of intimacy*. New York: Delacorte.

Rubin, Z. (1973). *Liking and loving: An invitation to social psychology*. New York: Holt, Rinehart, & Winston.

Russell, D. (1982). The measurement of loneliness. In L. A. Peplau & D. Perlman (Eds.), *Loneliness: A sourcebook of current theory, research and therapy* (pp. 81–104). New York: Wiley-Interscience.

Scheff, T. J. (1979). *Catharsis and healing, ritual and drama*. Berkeley, CA: University of California Press.

Schutz, W. C. (1958). *FIRO: A three-dimensional theory of interpersonal behavior*. New York: Holt, Rinehart, & Winston.

Shaver, P., & Buhrmester, D. (1983). Loneliness, sex-role orientation, and group life: A social needs perspective. In P. B. Paulus (Ed.), *Basic group processes* (pp. 259–288). New York: Springer-Verlag.

Shaver, P., Furman, W., & Buhrmester, D. (1984). Aspects of a life transition: Network changes, social skills, and loneliness. In S. Duck & D. Perlman (Eds.), *The Sage series in personal relationships* (Vol. 1). London: Sage.

Shaver, P., & Rubenstein, C. (1980). Childhood attachment experience and adult loneliness. In L. Wheeler (Ed.), *Review of personality and social psychology* (Vol. 1, pp. 42–73). Beverly Hills, CA: Sage.

Sroufe, L. A., & Fleeson, J. (in press). Attachment and the construction of relationships. In W. Hartup & Z. Rubin (Eds.), *The development of relationships*.

Sullivan, H. S. (1953). *The interpersonal theory of psychiatry*. New York: Norton.

Tennov, D. (1979). *Love and limerence: The experience of being in love*. New York: Stein and Day.

Thibaut, J. W., & Kelley, H. H. (1959). *The social psychology of groups*. New York: Wiley.

Thurber, J. (1945). The secret life of Walter Mitty. In *The Thurber carnival* (pp. 47–51). New York: Harper.

Veroff, J., Douvan, E., & Kulka, R. A. (1981). *The inner American: A self portrait from 1957 to 1976*. New York: Basic Books.

Walster, E., & Walster, G. W. (1978). *A new look at love*. Reading, MA: Addison-Wesley.

Weiner, B. (1974). *Achievement motivation and attribution theory*. Morristown, NJ: General Learning Press.

Weiss, R. S. (1973). *Loneliness: The experience of emotional and social isolation*. Cambridge, MA: MIT Press.

Weiss, R. S. (1974). The provisions of social relationships. In Z. Rubin (Ed.), *Doing unto others* (pp. 17–26). Englewood Cliffs, NJ: Prentice-Hall.

Wheeler, L., Reis, H., & Nezlek, J. (1983). Loneliness, social interaction, and sex roles. *Journal of Personality and Social Psychology, 45*, 943–953.

Wiggins, J. S. (1980). Circumplex models of interpersonal behavior. In L. Wheeler (Ed.), *Review of personality and social psychology* (Vol. 1, pp. 265–294). Beverly Hills, CA: Sage.

Wiggins, J. S. (1979). A psychological taxonomy of trait-descriptive terms: The interpersonal domain. *Journal of Personality and Social Psychology, 37*, 395–412.

Williams, J. G., & Solano, C. H. (1983). The social reality of feeling lonely: Friendship and reciprocation. *Personality and Social Psychology Bulletin, 9*, 237–242.

Part IV
Personality and Cognitive Interdependence

Chapter 8

Sex-Role Influences
on Compatibility in Relationships

William Ickes

The theme of this chapter can be encapsulated in a little story called "Felicia Femme Falls In and Out of Love." The story goes like this:

One warm day in June, Felicia Femme is married to Michael Manley. Felicia is very happy and very much in love. "Mike is the ideal man," she feels. "He is strong, capable, and ambitious. He will take good care of me and will be a good provider for our children. I made the right decision when I agreed to marry him."

Mike is happy too. "Felicia is the ideal woman," he tells himself. "She is warm and caring. She gives my ego a boost when I'm down. She will be there when I need her and will be a wonderful mother to our children. I did the right thing when I asked her to marry me."

Following a blissful honeymoon, time passes.

Ten years later, on a hot day in July, the former Felicia Femme is in a marriage counseling session with Michael Manley. In the privacy of her own mind, between the rounds of reciprocated accusations, Felicia feels very unhappy and very much *out* of love. "Mike is an insensitive, self-centered jerk," she thinks. "He is married to his job, and even when his body is at home, his mind and feelings are somewhere else. He's a good provider, but that's it; our emotional life is nil. He thinks it should be 90% sex and 10% love, but I'd be happier if it were the other way around. If I weren't so dependent on him financially, I would get a divorce. I made the wrong decision when I agreed to marry him."

Mike is irritated and somewhat confused. "Felicia doesn't understand or appreciate how hard I have to work," he thinks. "She nags me when I'm home and says she feels neglected. But that's not true; I make love to her all the time. Things may not be as good as they were before we were married, but they're not as bad as she says. I can't see what she's so unhappy about. Maybe I did the wrong thing when I asked her to marry me."

The characters in this little story—Felicia Femme and Michael Manley—are intended to symbolize all women and men who have internalized the traditional, stereotypic sex-role orientations that have long been regarded as "gender appropriate" in our culture: a traditionally feminine sex-role orientation for women and a traditionally masculine sex-role orientation for men. The story itself is intended to illustrate the theme of this chapter: that these societally prescribed sex-role orientations, which have ostensibly evolved in order to facilitate the *compatibility* of male-female relationships, may actually be responsible for much of the *incompatibility* upon which divorce statistics are based.

In the first section of this chapter, data are reviewed from the author's laboratory studies of the influence of sex-role orientations on dyadic interaction. This research was the first to suggest that the behavioral enactment of stereotyped sex roles by men and women may actually produce incompatibility, rather than compatibility, in their personal relationships. The findings from this research also provided the basis for a general theory of sex-role influences on dyadic interaction that is briefly summarized in the second section of the chapter. A potential problem with the theory is explored in the third section, which focuses on the results of two large-scale survey studies that relate the sex-role orientations of married couples to their ratings of marital satisfaction. An inconsistency between the theory and an "anomalous" finding from these survey studies is considered, and a theoretical resolution is proposed. In the final section, some important implications of these findings are discussed. This discussion focuses on the dynamic processes that may underlie "sex-role incompatibility" and goes on to propose a number of specific hypotheses for future research.

Sex Roles and Dyadic Compatibility in the Laboratory

A laboratory study conducted by Ickes and Barnes (1978) provided the first clear-cut evidence that the enactment of traditional sex roles by men and women might contribute to incompatibility in their relationships. This was one of the first studies in a continuing series designed to explore the role of personality variables in the formation of compatible and incompatible relationships. Like the other studies in the series, it employed a research paradigm that the present author developed to examine the influences of personality factors on the behavior occurring in initial, unstructured dyadic interactions (for reviews, see Ickes, 1982, 1983).

The immediate purpose of the study was to determine how the sex-role orientations of male and female participants would affect their initial interactions in mixed-sex dyads. Its broader purpose was to develop some testable hypotheses about the compatibility/incompatibility of dyads composed of men and women with traditional (i.e., masculine, feminine) or nontraditional (i.e., androgynous) sex-role orientations. The results were expected to have implications for clinical psychology (specifically, for marital counseling) if socially "compatible" versus "incompatible" dyad types could be identified.

The subjects in the study were 40 male and 40 female undergraduates whose sex-role orientations had been assessed earlier in the semester by means of the Bem Sex-Role Inventory (BSRI) (Bem, 1974). Within the constraints imposed by their gender and sex-role orientation, the subjects were randomly (and without their prior knowledge) assigned to one of four different types of mixed-sex dyads. These dyad types were based on the systematic pairing of (1) a "masculine" man and a "feminine" woman, (2) a masculine man and an androgynous woman, (3) an androgynous man and a feminine woman, and (4) an androgynous man and an androgynous woman.[1]

After being contacted by telephone and scheduled to participate at the same time, the subjects in each dyad reported to separate waiting areas—a procedure designed to ensure that they would not meet or interact before the session began. The experimenter met them, established that they did not know each other, and escorted them into a "waiting room." There, they were invited to be seated on a large couch. The experimenter left them alone together, ostensibly to collect some questionnaires to be used in the study, and timed a 5-min interval in which the subjects' behavior was covertly audiotaped and videotaped. Upon returning to the room, the experimenter explained the need for deception and obtained the subjects' written permission releasing the tapes for use as data. The subjects were then asked to complete posttest questionnaires concerning their perceptions of self and other during the 5-min interaction period. Following the collection of these self-report data, the subjects were thanked for their participation and released.

Several behavioral measures were subsequently coded from the videotapes by raters who were kept "blind" to the subjects' sex-role orientations. Analyses of the resulting behavioral and self-report data revealed that the most "traditional" dyad type—the one composed of a masculine man and a feminine woman—had interactions that were significantly less involving and rewarding than those occurring in dyads in which one or both participants were androgynous. Subjects in the "masculine man–feminine woman" dyads not

---

[1]As defined by such measures as Bem's (1974) Sex Role Inventory or Spence, Helmreich, and Stapp's (1975) Personal Attributes Questionnaire, the *masculine* sex role represents an active, controlling, and instrumental orientation toward social interaction, whereas the *feminine* sex role represents a more reactive, emotionally responsive, and expressive orientation. *Androgyny* is an orientation toward social interaction that combines the agentic-instrumentality of the traditionally masculine orientation with the communal-expressivity of the traditionally feminine one (cf. Ickes, 1981, pp. 96–101). A final orientation, labelled *undifferentiated* by Spence et al. (1975), is essentially the opposite of the androgynous one. Undifferentiated individuals are neither agentic-instrumental nor communal-expressive in their orientation toward social interaction, and they appear to be deficient in both of those sets of skills which Ickes (1981) assumed to be necessary for effective interaction with others.

William Ickes

only spoke, looked, gestured, and smiled toward each other less than did subjects in the remaining dyad types, but expressed less liking for each other as well (see Table 8-1).

At first glance, these findings struck many people (the authors included) as somewhat surprising and counterintuitive. Many of us have been socialized to believe that society prescribes and reinforces the adoption of stereotyped sex roles because of their time-tested utility in promoting the effective social integration of its members. In other words, we may believe that men should adopt a traditionally masculine sex-role orientation and women a traditionally feminine one because our implicit assumption is that everyone will get along together much better that way. The Ickes and Barnes (1978) data suggested, however, that this assumption may at least be questionable, if not completely wrong—that, in fact, some degree of social incompatibility between males and females may be the result of their *adherence* to these socially endorsed sex

Table 8-1. Differences in Liking and Behavior Between the ♂ST-♀ST Dyad Type and the Other Dyad Types over a 5-Min Interaction Period

Dependent Measure	Dyad types				$F(1, 36)^a$
	♂ST-♀ST	♂ST-♀A	♂A-♀ST	♂A-♀A	
Liking	19.2	43.0	42.6	40.8	15.98****
Verbalizations					
Total frequency	21.0	29.7	34.6	28.3	3.03*
Total duration	46.7	90.2	87.3	67.0	4.80**
Directed gazes					
Total frequency	12.9	19.7	21.7	20.8	2.99*
Total duration	34.9	75.2	74.7	61.1	4.69**
Expressive gestures					
Total frequency	1.6	7.2	4.7	4.0	4.41**
Total duration	1.3	11.4	6.1	4.0	3.58*
Positive affect					
Total frequency	4.0	8.2	9.8	8.4	6.59***
Total duration	11.4	21.5	29.1	23.0	4.10**
Negative affect					
Total frequency	1.2	0.7	0.9	1.1	<1
Total duration	1.9	0.6	1.9	1.2	<1
Pos-Neg affect					
Total frequency	2.8	7.5	8.9	7.3	7.26***
Total duration	9.5	20.9	27.2	21.8	4.41**

Note. From "Boys and girls together—and alienated: On enacting stereotyped sex roles in mixed-sex dyads" by W. Ickes and R. D. Barnes, *Journal of Personality and Social Psychology*, 1978, *36*, 669–683. Copyright 1978 by the American Psychological Association. Reprinted by permission.
ST, sex-role stereotyped; A, androgynous.
[a]Contrast comparing the mean of the ST-ST dyads with those of the remaining dyad types.
*$p < .10$.
**$p < .05$.
***$p < .02$.
****$p < .001$.

roles, not their lack of adherence to them. The data also supported the claim of many feminist writers that stereotyped sex roles are a fundamental cause of problems in the relationships between men and women.

If the enactment of stereotyped sex roles could produce relatively low social involvement in mixed-sex (i.e., male-female) dyads, would it produce a similar outcome in same-sex (i.e., male-male, female-female) dyads as well? This question was addressed in a follow-up study by Ickes, Schermer, and Steeno (1979). In this study, the initial interactions of 30 male-male dyads and 30 female-female dyads were studied in the laboratory using the same procedure employed by Ickes and Barnes (1978). Comparisons of dyad types of differing sex-role compositions again revealed relatively low social involvement in dyads whose members were both stereotypically sex-typed (i.e., in dyads composed of two masculine men or two feminine women). Members of these dyad types talked, looked, and gestured toward each other significantly less than members of dyad types in which the two men or the two women were both androgynous. This pattern of differences was later replicated in a study of female-female dyads conducted by Lamke and Bell (1981). In this study, dyads composed of two androgynous women talked, looked, gestured, and displayed more positive affect than dyads composed of two stereotypically sex-typed women.

A Theoretical Integration

The findings from the three studies described above are consistent with the notion that masculinity, femininity, and androgyny do indeed constitute different orientations toward social interaction. But how, exactly, do these orientations differ in their influences on social behavior? In attempting to answer this question, the author (Ickes, 1981) began by considering some important leads found in previous theoretical work.

A number of writers (e.g., Bakan, 1966; Bales, 1955, 1958; Block, 1973) have proposed that social systems are optimally functional to the degree that both instrumental (i.e., masculine) and expressive (i.e., feminine) capabilities are integratively applied (for a review, see Spence and Helmreich, 1978). With regard to the process of social interaction, this reasoning suggests that an androgynous orientation may be particularly effective, because androgynous individuals possess both instrumental and expressive capabilities and can presumably apply both sets of capabilities in their interactions with others. Other writers (e.g., Bem, 1974; Deaux, 1976; Kaplan & Sedney, 1980) have complemented this argument by proposing that the behavior of androgynous individuals is more flexible and situationally adaptive than that of sex-role-stereotyped individuals. Because they can draw upon both instrumental and expressive capabilities, androgynous individuals are not constrained, as masculine and feminine individuals are, to operate within a narrow range of sex-role-appropriate behaviors. For this reason, they should be more likely to make effective and situationally appropriate responses to particular social situations.

Although most writers appear to agree that androgyny constitutes a more flexible and effective orientation toward social interaction than either masculinity or femininity, this conclusion has not gone unchallenged. In fact, at least one critic (Sampson, 1977) has argued that "androgyny, as a valued individual synthesis of masculine and feminine characteristics," is potentially a threat to social relatedness and cooperation because it is inherently "incongruent with the thesis of interdependence" (p. 771). In other words, Sampson proposes that androgyny threatens interdependence and discourages social interaction because instrumental and expressive functions are synthesized within a given individual rather than within an interdependent social system.

Sampson's view appears to be based on two assumptions: (1) Bales' (1955, 1958) initial assumption that effective interaction depends on the integration of instrumental and expressive functions; and (2) Sampson's (1977) additional assumption that the integration of these functions at a personal level (in the form of androgyny) must somehow preclude their integration at an interpersonal level. Unfortunately for his argument, however, only the first of these assumptions has been supported by relevant empirical research (Bales, 1958; Parsons & Bales, 1955). Sampson's additional assumption, that androgyny somehow threatens interdependence and discourages social interaction, is flatly contradicted by the results of the three studies of sex-role influences on dyadic interaction reviewed earlier in this chapter. Far from supporting Sampson's position that androgyny is alienating and antithetical to social involvement, these data instead support the earlier and more widely held position that androgyny is a particularly flexible and effective orientation to social interaction.

With these considerations in mind, the present author proposed a general model of sex-role influences in dyadic interactions (Ickes, 1981). In its simplest form, the model can be reduced to the following set of theoretical postulates:

I. Dyads, as simple social systems, are optimally functional to the degree that both instrumental and expressive capabilities are integratively applied. It is assumed (a) that these instrumental and expressive capabilities have their locus in the individual members of the dyad, and (b) that these capabilities are applied in an interaction through the overt, socially-available behavior of the dyad members.

II. The sex-role orientations of the dyad members determine the degree to which instrumental and expressive capabilities can be applied and integrated within their interaction. Specifically: (a) Individuals with *masculine* orientations can apply a high level of instrumental capabilities, but only a low level of expressive capabilities, to an interaction; (b) Individuals with *feminine* orientations can apply a high level of expressive capabilities, but only a low level of instrumental capabilities, to an interaction; (c) Individuals with *androgynous* orientations can variably apply their instrumental or expressive capabilities to an interaction, depending on their perceptions of the situational appropriateness of displaying or not displaying either or both sets; and (d) Individuals with *undifferentiated* orientations (i.e., neither masculine nor feminine) can apply only low levels of both instrumental and expressive capabilities to an interaction.

III. A major aspect of the functioning of the dyad as a social system can be assessed by various measures of interactional involvement. These measures may include self-reports of perceived involvement as well as behavioral measures of the amount of talking, looking, smiling, gesturing, mutual gaze, etc.

IV. In addition to determining the level of interactional involvement in the dyadic interaction (an *interpersonal* outcome), the sex-role orientations of the dyad members help determine the subjective reaction of each dyad member to that level of interactional involvement (a *personal* outcome). In general, the degree of satisfaction dyad members experience regarding an interaction depends upon the degree to which the level of interactional involvement was consistent with their own dispositions to be *expressive*. Thus, (a) individuals with *masculine* orientations, having relatively little capability and motivation to be expressive, should be satisfied with relatively low levels of interactional involvement; whereas (b) individuals with *feminine* or *androgynous* orientations, having a relatively greater capability and motivation to be expressive, should be satisfied only with relatively high levels of interactional involvement.

V. The integration within an interaction of instrumental and expressive capabilities need not take the form of an interdependent integration. In dyadic interactions, each dyad member can apply neither, one, or (in the case of androgynous individuals) both sets of capabilities. Moreover, because the conditions for an interdependent integration of instrumental and expressive capabilities have not yet been specified, either by Sampson (1977) or anyone else, the status of this phenomenon must remain an open question.

Implications for Heterosexual Dyads

From the theoretical postulates just presented, a large number of specific hypotheses can be derived (see Ickes, 1981, pp. 104–107, 119–122). Here we will consider only those hypotheses of direct relevance to the topic of this chapter: those concerning the influences of sex-role-stereotyped (ST) versus androgynous (A) orientations on the interactions of male-female dyads. These hypotheses are numbered sequentially, beginning with Hypothesis 5a, just as they appeared in the paper by Ickes (1981).

Hypothesis 5a: In dyads composed of a stereotypically masculine male and a stereotypically feminine female (an ST-ST dyad type), the level of interaction should depend on whether or not the male's instrumental capabilities and the female's expressive capabilities can be independently integrated, as Sampson (1977) has asserted. If such an integration occurs, the level of interaction in these dyads should be relatively high; if not, the level of interaction should be relatively low (see Postulate V).

Hypothesis 5b: If the level of interactional involvement is high (an interdependent integration of capabilities occurs), the feminine-oriented females in these ST-ST dyads should be generally satisfied with the interaction because their strong expressive needs have been met. Their masculine male partners should be somewhat less satisfied, however, because the level of involvement was higher than (i.e., positively discrepant from) the level needed to satisfy their weaker expressive needs.

If the level of interactional involvement is low (an interdependent integration of capabilities does not occur), the reverse outcome should obtain: The masculine-oriented males should be somewhat more satisfied than their feminine-oriented partners.

Hypothesis 6a: In dyads composed of an androgynous male and an androgynous female (an A-A dyad type), the level of interaction should be relatively high. Because both instrumental and expressive capabilities can be applied by both members of these dyads, the participants should have little difficulty maintaining a high level of interactional involvement.

Hypothesis 6b: Both the androgynous male and the androgynous female should be generally satisfied with the high level of involvement of their interaction, because it allows them to fulfill their strong expressive needs.

Hypothesis 7a: In dyads composed of a stereotypically masculine male and an androgynous female or those composed of a stereotypically feminine female and an androdynous male (ST-A dyad types), the level of interaction should depend on the androgynous individual's mode of adaptation to his or her partner. Assuming that the androgynous individual considers it appropriate to display both instrumental and expressive capabilities in interaction with a sex-role-stereotyped partner of the opposite sex (see Ickes, 1981, p. 107), the level of interaction in these ST-A dyads should be relatively high. This predicted high level of interaction need not depend on the additional assumption of an interdependent integration of capabilities, since it is sufficient merely to assume that the androgynous individual can apply both sets (see Postulate V).

Hypothesis 7b: Because of the high level of interactional involvement expected in these ST-A dyads, differences in expressive needs should cause masculine-oriented males to be somewhat less satisfied with the interaction than their androgynous female partners. However, in dyads where feminine-oriented females are paired with androgynous males, both the male and the female should be generally satisfied with their high level of interactional involvement.

The results of the study by Ickes and Barnes (1978), described earlier in this chapter, are obviously relevant to the set of hypotheses listed above. It is worth reminding the reader that these data appear to discredit both implications of Sampson's (1977) "interdependence assumption." First, they indicate that the interdependent integration of functions which Sampson has proposed may not have occurred in the "masculine man–feminine woman" dyads. The level of interactional involvement was clearly the lowest in these dyads (see Table 8-1), suggesting that the members of these dyads were unable to apply their respective instrumental and expressive capabilities in an interdependent manner. Second, the results belie Sampson's corollary assumption that androgyny is alienating and discourages interactional involvement. On the contrary, the data in Table 8-1 reveal that in the dyads in which one or both members were androgynous, the level of interaction was consistently quite high.

Because these data appear to contradict the interdependence assumption, they are consistent with only the last proposition stated in Hypothesis 5a, but are entirely consistent with the reasoning proposed in Hypotheses 6a and 7a. The consistency between data and theory in each of these cases may not mean much, however, when one considers that the data from the Ickes and Barnes (1978) and Ickes et al. (1979) studies not only predated the theory but provided the primary basis for the theory's inductive development. An additional limitation is that the data from these studies concern only the initial, short-term interactions of pairs of strangers. If the theory is to have any meaningful implications for compatibility in long-term heterosexual relationships, it is important that its implications be tested directly in the context of such relationships. A final limitation of these data is that no measures were taken of the dyad members' satisfaction with the relationships. For this reason, Hypotheses 5b, 6b, and 7b could not be tested in the Ickes and Barnes (1978) study.

Sex Roles and Marital Satisfaction: Survey Research

Fortunately, the data from two recent survey studies help to address these concerns about the theory's predictive validity and its generalizability to long-term dyadic relationships. The first of these studies was a magazine survey conducted in the United States, in which more than 30,000 readers of the *Ladies' Home Journal* completed and returned an "Intimacy Today" survey questionnaire (Shaver, Pullis, & Olds, 1980). The second study was an in-home interview survey of 108 married couples living in the metropolitan area of Sydney, Australia (Antill, 1983). The results of each of these studies are reviewed in turn, followed by a discussion of their relevance to Ickes' (1981) theory of sex-role influences in dyadic interaction.

Shaver, Pullis, and Olds (1980)

From the more than 30,000 readers who responded to the 55-item Intimacy Questionnaire published in the November 1979 issue of the *Ladies' Home Journal*, Shaver, Pullis, and Olds (1980) selected a random sample of 2,100 female respondents for purposes of data analysis. Among the data these women provided were (1) assessments of their own and their husbands' or male partners' sex-role orientations (as rated on Spence, Helmreich, & Stapp's "Personal Attributes Questionnaire"; Spence et al., 1975) and (2) self-ratings of satisfaction with various aspects of their lives and their intimate relationships.

The results of the survey, although not reported in as much fine-grained detail as a professional audience might wish, are nonetheless informative about the kinds of satisfactions and dissatisfactions expressed by women in relationships of varying sex-role composition. A strong theme pervading these data is the pronounced dissatisfaction of traditionally feminine women who were married to or living with partners whom they perceived as traditionally masculine men. Compared with women in the entire sample, the women in these "masculine man–feminine woman" dyads were significantly *more* likely to report such stress symptoms as feeling fat, tiring easily, feeling sad or depressed, feeling worthless, feeling shy, and feeling that "you just can't go on" (p. 23). In addition, on all measures of general happiness or satisfaction with their lives, these women were significantly *less* likely to report (1) being satisfied with life as a whole, (2) feeling responsible for the way things turn out, (3) feeling control over the important events in their lives, and (4) expecting to be happy in the future.

The dissatisfaction of these women was further evidenced in their ratings of the quality of their relationships. Feminine women whose partners were perceived as masculine men were significantly less likely than women in the total sample to rate either their love relationships or their sex lives as satisfactory. These women were also the most likely to report feeling "underloved," i.e., to say that they loved their male partners more than they were loved in return. After summarizing these findings, the authors of the survey concluded that "the traditional couple, a feminine woman married to a masculine man, suffers considerably from the one-sidedness of each partner" (p. 43). Only the women's suffering in these relationships is documented, however, since ratings of the male partners' happiness and satisfaction were not obtained.

In contrast to the pervasive dissatisfaction expressed by the women in the "masculine man–feminine woman" dyads, the women in dyads in which one or both partners were androgynous tended to be quite satisfied with the quality of their lives and their intimate relationships. In particular, androgynous women paired with androgynous men not only reported relatively low stress symptoms but also reported considerable success in communicating and solving problems with their partners. In addition, they reported high levels of (1) satisfaction with their lives as a whole, (2) responsibility for their outcomes, (3) control over important life events, and (4) optimism about the future. Of more specific relevance to our theoretical concerns, their ratings of satisfaction with their sex lives and intimate relationships were also quite high.

Clearly, these patterns of data are consistent with the predictions derived from Ickes' (1981) theory. On the other hand, the data are frustratingly incomplete in that they only permit comparisons across different dyad types of the *women's* happiness and satisfaction. They tell us nothing about the reactions of the *men* with whom these women were paired. For this reason, the data do not permit tests of many of the predictions suggested by Hypotheses 5b, 6b, and 7b.

It is interesting to note, however, that despite the limitation just discussed, it is possible to examine Hypothesis 5b in an *indirect* manner by comparing the level of satisfaction expressed by women in sex-role-stereotyped (masculine man–feminine woman) dyads with that expressed by women in sex-role-*reversed* (feminine man-masculine woman) dyads. Although such sex-role-reversed combinations are statistically rare, they are theoretically informative in that the logic of Hypothesis 5b suggests that the "masculine" women in these "feminine man–masculine woman" dyads should be more satisifed with their relationships than should the "feminine" women in the traditional "masculine man–feminine woman" dyads. The reason for this prediction is, of course, that although an interdependent integration of instrumental and expressive capabilities may fail to occur in *both* dyad types, the resulting low level of interactional involvement could still be sufficient to satisfy a "masculine" woman's low expressive needs while failing to satisfy the high expressive needs of a traditionally "feminine" woman.

This reasoning appears to find support in the data reported by Shaver et al. (1980). Women in sex-role-reversed dyads (and "masculine" women in general) were more likely to report being satisfied with their lives and with their intimate relationships than were women in stereotypically sex-typed dyads (and "feminine" women in general). Although the results for the life-satisfaction measures may be due in part to the greater capacity of masculine women to independently obtain rewards through the use of their instrumental capabilities, the results for the relationship-satisfaction measures can be theoretically explained in terms of the lesser need of masculine women for relationships providing high levels of interactional involvement.

In addition to documenting the various findings just reviewed, the Shaver et al. (1980) survey also provided considerable data about the feelings of women in dyads in which one or both partners are undifferentiated. In general, the levels of satisfaction expressed by women in these dyad types were relatively low, a finding that is compatible with Ickes' (1981) theory, although not explicitly predicted by it (see pp. 105–106). A more detailed review of the data concerning dyads in which one or both members are undifferentiated is, unfortunately, beyond the scope of this chapter.

In the midst of all these results that are consistent with Ickes' (1981) theory, at least one finding emerged in the Shaver et al. (1980) data that cannot be readily derived from the theoretical postulates reviewed above. This theoretically anomalous finding is represented by a pattern of data indicating that women are generally satisfied with relationships in which their male partners are feminine sex-typed (i.e., sex-role-reversed). Although the logic of the theory could be extended to predict this outcome for dyads in which the men are feminine sex-typed and the women are androgynous, some additional theoretical assumption(s) would be required before the theory could predict this outcome for dyad types in which the men are feminine sex-typed and the women are either masculine, feminine, or undifferentiated. More will be said later about this anomalous finding.

With the exception of the finding just discussed, the results of the Shaver et al. (1980) survey study are generally quite consistent with the predictions derived from Ickes' (1981) theory of sex-role influences in dyadic interactions. These survey data are important in demonstrating that the theory can be generalized beyond the experimentally engineered, short-term relationships of men and women in the laboratory to the naturally occurring and relatively long-term relationships of men and women in the "real world." They also are important in providing both direct and indirect tests of certain hypotheses (5b, 6b, and 7b) regarding satisfaction with these relationships—hypotheses that were not tested in the study by Ickes and Barnes (1978). On the other hand, these data (1) tell us nothing about the objective levels of interactional involvement in the various dyad types studied, (2) depend upon the women's perceptions of their male partners' sex-role orientations, and (3) convey only the women's feelings about the quality of these relationships. Fortunately, only the first of these three limitations applies to the survey data we consider next.

Antill (1983)

After recruiting potential subjects at various shopping centers in the metro-politan area of Sydney, Australia, Antill's research assistants conducted in-home interviews with 108 married couples. During these interviews, both spouses independently completed a questionnaire concerning "married life in Australia." The questionnaire included, among other items, the Bem Sex-Role Inventory (BSRI; Bem, 1974) and the Spanier Dyadic Adjustment Scale—a widely used measure of marital quality and marital satisfaction (Spanier, 1976). On the basis of the spouses' responses to these measures, Antill (1983) examined satisfaction with the marriage "as a function of both husbands' and wives' sex-role categories" (p. 146).

Although Antill interpreted his results in terms of the similarity ("birds of a feather") versus complementarity ("opposites attract") distinction, they can be reinterpreted in terms of Ickes' (1981) theoretical model. The major findings of Antill's study are presented in Table 8-2, in which the mean satisfaction scores for each dyad type are based on the *summed* scores of the husbands and wives within these dyads.

In most respects, the patterns of means in Table 8-2 are consistent both with the results of the Shaver et al. (1980) survey and with the predictions of Ickes' theory. As the theory predicts, and as Shaver et al. found, marital satisfaction was (1) relatively high in dyads in which both husband and wife were androgynous ($M = 245.6$) and (2) relatively low in sex-role-stereotyped dyads composed of masculine male and a feminine female ($M = 218.9$). According to Antill (1983), "The difference between the two groups is significant,

Table 8-2. Mean Couple Happiness Scores for Each Combination of Husband and Wife Sex Roles

		Wife			
Husband	M	A	U	F	*M*
M	229.6 (5)	221.2 (5)	209.3 (11)	218.9 (13)	217.7 (34)
A	209.6 (10)	245.6 (10)	221.6 (5)	243.6 (7)	230.2 (32)
U	168.5 (2)	213.3 (7)	217.7 (10)	226.4 (7)	215.1 (26)
F	245.0 (2)	236.5 (2)	229.8 (4)	250.9 (8)	243.1 (16)
M	214.3 (19)	230.3 (24)	216.9 (30)	232.7 (35)	224.5 (108)

Note. Adapted from "Sex role complementarity versus similarity in married couples" by J. K. Antill, *Journal of Personality and Social Psychology*, 1983, *45*, 145–155. M = masculine; A = androgynous; U = undifferentiated; F = feminine. Numbers in parentheses are the sample *n*s for each dyad type.

$t(21) = 3.20, p < .01$" (p. 150). In addition, (3) satisfaction was generally low in dyads in which one or both partners were undifferentiated, a finding that again replicates Shaver et al.'s (1980) results and is suggested, although not explicitly predicted, by Ickes' (1981) theory (see p. 120).

Unfortunately, the ns for each combination were generally too small to permit statistically strong comparisons of the husbands' versus the wives' satisfaction within the various dyad types. For this reason, it is not too surprising that none of the matched t-tests for these comparisons was significant (Antill, personal communication). However, for the two specific cases in which the theory predicts differences in the satisfaction of husbands versus wives, the means were ordered as predicted. In sex-role stereotyped relationships, involving masculine husbands and feminine wives, the wives had lower satisfaction scores ($M = 108.2$) than their husbands ($M = 110.8$); however, in sex-role-reversed relationships, involving feminine husbands and masculine wives, the husbands had lower satisfaction scores ($M = 118.5$) than their wives ($M = 126.5$). This ordering of the two sets of means makes sense if it is assumed that (1) the levels of interactional involvement in these two dyad types are low (i.e., an interdependent integration of instrumental and expressive capabilities does *not* occur) and (2) only the masculine-sex-typed members of these dyads are satisfied with a low level of interactional involvement.

The neat match between theory and data was again disrupted, however, by the same "anomalous" finding reported by Shaver et al. (1980): the consistently high levels of satisfaction expressed by women—regardless of their own sex-role orientation—who were married to sex-role-reversed, feminine sex-typed men (see Table 8-2, fourth row of means).

Obviously, the clear-cut replication of this finding suggests that it can no longer be regarded as a mere anomaly: It appears to be a stable and replicable phenomenon. In attempting to explain this phenomenon, we can probably rule out the possibility that satisfaction is invariably high in all dyad types in which one or both of the partners are sex-role-reversed. As the first column of means in Table 8-2 reveals, there is considerable variability in (and generally low levels of) satisfaction for those dyad types in which the woman is sex-role-reversed (i.e., masculine). Thus, the presence of sex-role-reversed dyad members per se does not appear to guarantee a satisfying relationship.

A simpler and more compelling explanation is the one proposed by Antill (1983), that marital happiness or satisfaction is directly related to the *femininity* of one's partner. An examination of the marginal means in Table 8-2 led Antill to conclude that:

> Males appear to be happiest when paired with androgynous and feminine females (both high-femininity groups) and relatively less happy when paired with masculine and undifferentiated females (both low-femininity groups). . . . As with the males, females also appear to be happier when paired with androgynous and feminine partners and relatively less happy when paired with masculine and undifferentiated partners [p. 149]. . . . The present study has provided evidence for the overwhelming importance of femininity in married relationships. Androgynous partners were only an asset in terms of

happiness in that such individuals by definition are high on femininity. (p. 152)[2]

This conclusion—that "happiness is a feminine marriage partner"—was further substantiated in Antill's data when the marital satisfaction scores of husbands and wives were correlated with their partners' scores on the masculinity and femininity subscales of the BSRI. The zero-order correlation between the husbands' satisfaction and their wives' masculinity was only .05 (*ns*), whereas the correlation between the husbands' satisfaction and their wives' femininity was .28 ($p < .005$). Similarly, the zero-order correlation between the wives' satisfaction and their husbands' masculinity was only .03 (*ns*), whereas the correlation between the wives' satisfaction and their husbands' femininity was .31 ($p < .001$). Moreover, as Antill notes later in his paper:

> As if to emphasize the point that femininity is critical to marital happiness, the overall happiness of both husband and wife was even more highly related to their spouse's femininity as seen by themselves. Thus, the husband's happiness is correlated ($r = .48$, $p < .001$) with his assessment of his wife's femininity. . . . Similarly, the wife's happiness is correlated with her assessment of her husband's femininity ($r = .61, p < .001$). (p. 154) (see Footnote 2)

On the basis of correlations as strong as these, one is indeed tempted to conclude that "happiness is a feminine marriage partner," or, more prosaically, that "satisfaction in marital relationships is directly related to the degree to which one's partner is perceived as nurturant and emotionally supportive (i.e., as having those attributes measured by the femininity subscale of the BSRI)."

One should not be tempted to generalize this conclusion, however, to all dyadic interactions. In the more casual and short-term interactions of same-sex (male-male and female-female) dyads studied in the laboratory by Ickes et al. (1979), ratings of satisfaction with the interactions did *not* vary directly with the partners' femininity. On the contrary, as the data in Table 8-3 indicate, satisfaction ratings were high when both partners were masculine males (Table 8-3, first column of means), but were relatively low when both partners were feminine females (Table 8-3, fourth column of means).

These data are clearly inconsistent with a general rule stating that one's satisfaction with a dyadic relationship is directly related to the actual or perceived femininity (i.e., emotional supportiveness) of one's partner. They *are* consistent, however, with the predictions derived from Ickes' (1981) theory. In accordance with Postulates I and II of the theory, the interactions of dyads composed of two masculine males or two feminine females (the ST-ST dyad types) were both characterized by low levels of interactional involvement (see Ickes et al., 1979, Table 2). However, the masculine males in the first dyad type

---

[2]Copyright (1983) by the American Psychological Association. Reprinted by permission of the publisher and author.

Table 8-3. Interactions of Sex Composition and Sex-Role Composition: Means by Dyad Type

Dependent Measure	Male-male dyads			Female-female dyads			Interaction $F(2, 54)$
	ST-ST	ST-A	A-A	ST-ST	ST-A	A-A	
Awkward, forced, and strained	2.3	6.1	4.7	4.9	5.2	4.3	3.21*
Smooth, natural, and relaxed	9.9	6.8	8.2	6.6	7.0	8.4	4.29*
Perceived rapport with other	7.8	5.8	7.6	5.6	7.7	8.3	4.66*
Overall satisfaction with interaction	15.4$_a$	6.5$_c$	11.0$_{abc}$	7.3$_c$	9.5$_{bc}$	12.4$_{ab}$	5.54**

Note. From "Sex and sex-role influences in same-sex dyads" by W. Ickes, B. Schermer, and J. Steeno, *Social Psychology Quarterly*, 1979, *42*, 373–385. Copyright 1979 by the American Sociological Association. Reprinted by permission.
For a given measure, means not sharing a subscript in common are significantly different beyond the .05 level by two-tailed *t*-test for independent groups.
*$p < .05$.
**$p < .01$.

were highly satisfied with their interactions (presumably because their expressive needs were low), whereas the feminine females in the second dyad type were relatively unsatisfied (presumably because their expressive needs were high and were therefore frustrated). This pattern of results obtained for dyads composed of two feminine females (i.e., relatively low interactional involvement and relatively low satisfaction ratings) is clearly a reliable one; it was later replicated by Lamke and Bell (1981).

A dilemma thus becomes apparent. On the one hand, Ickes' (1981) theory cannot account for the no-longer-anomalous satisfaction ratings of the women who were paired with feminine sex-typed men in the Shaver et al. (1980) and Antill (1983) survey studies. On the other hand, Antill's "femininity hypothesis" cannot account for either the behavioral data or the self-reported satisfaction data in the laboratory studies by Ickes et al. (1979) and by Lamke and Bell (1981). Although Ickes' (1981) theory is able to account for nearly all of the results obtained in the various studies of sex-role influences in dyadic interactions that we have reviewed in this chapter, an attempt to reconcile the theory with Antill's "femininity hypothesis" seems to be warranted in light of the survey studies' results. For this reason, the following theoretical reconciliation is proposed.

Proposed Theoretical Resolution

The proposed theoretical resolution is quite simple. It is based on the explicit recognition that what is satisfying in intimate relationships such as marriage or cohabitation may not be satisfying in the less-intimate relationships between strangers, acquaintances, or casual friends. Specifically, the resolution takes the form of modifying Ickes' (1981) theory to incorporate Antill's (1983) "femininity hypothesis" into Postulate IV as follows:

> IV. In addition to determining the level of interactional involvement in the dyadic interaction (an *interpersonal* outcome), the sex-role orientations of the dyad members help determine the subjective reaction of each dyad member to the dyadic relationship (a *personal* outcome). In intimate relationships (i.e., those defined in terms of strong, mutual expectations that one's interaction partner will provide a consistently high level of nurturance and emotional support), the degree of satisfaction that dyad members experience regarding their relationship will vary directly with the degree to which they perceive their partners to be nurturant and emotionally responsive and supportive (i.e., high in femininity).
>
> In nonintimate relationships (i.e., those *not* defined in terms of strong, mutual expectations that one's interaction partner will provide a consistently high level of nurturance and emotional support), the degree of satisfaction that dyad members experience regarding their relationship will depend on the degree to which the level of interactional involvement in the relationship is consistent with their own dispositions to be *expressive* (i.e., high in femininity). Thus, (1) individuals with *masculine* orientations, having relatively little capability and motivation to be expressive, should be satisfied with relatively low levels of interactional involvement, whereas (2) individuals with *feminine* or *androgynous* orientations, having a relatively greater capability and motivation to be expressive, should be satisfied only with relatively high levels of interactional involvement.

This theoretical resolution, which reconciles Antill's (1983) "femininity hypothesis" to Ickes' (1981) theory, has a number of general implications that are worth noting. First, it requires the theory to take explicit account of the *types of relationship* involved. As Clark (Chap. 5 of this volume) has pointed out, type-of-relationship is an important moderating variable in determining whether other variables will contribute to the compatibility or incompatibility of a relationship. However, this variable has been neglected in much of the theory and research to date.

Second, incorporating this type-of-relationship variable into the theory enables us to suggest two different *rules* by which dyad members determine their level of satisfaction with intimate versus nonintimate relationships. In intimate relationships, the operative rule seems to be: "The more my partner cares about me, is nurturant, emotionally supportive, and responsive, etc. (i.e., displays stereotypically feminine patterns of behavior), the more satisfied I am with the relationship." On the other hand, the operative rule in nonintimate relationships appears to be: "The better the match between the level of interactional involvement in the relationship and my own disposition to be expressive (e.g., to share my feelings and be responsive to my partner's feelings), the more satisfied I am with the relationship." The distinction between these two rules may help explain why, for example, a masculine sex-typed man could be satisified with the relatively unemotional, low-involvement relationship he has with his "macho" fishing buddy, and yet be dissatisfied if he has the same type of relationship with his wife.

Third, in distinguishing between these two rules, the theory suggests some useful insights about the different *expectations, obligations,* and *desires* that dyad members may have with respect to their intimate versus nonintimate relationships. Although the intimate/nonintimate distinction employed here is not intended as equivalent to the communal/exchange distinction proposed by Clark (this volume, chap. 5; Clark & Mills, 1979; Mills & Clark, 1982), it is nonetheless likely that there is considerable overlap between intimate and communal relationships. Thus, intimate–communal relationships "are characterized by members' *obligations* and, usually, by their *desire* to be emotionally responsive to each other's needs" (Clark, Chap. 5, italics added), as well as by members' *expectations* that this will be the case. In contrast, the expectations, obligations, and desires that dyad members have regarding their nonintimate relationships should reflect a much weaker emphasis on emotional responsiveness to each other's needs. The empirical documentation of the hypothesized differences in the expectations, obligations, and desires associated with the two relationship types is already well-advanced, as Chapter 5 of this volume clearly illustrates.

Fourth, in distinguishing between these two rules, the theory suggests some useful insights about the kinds of *attributions* that dyad members may make to account for conflict and dissatisfaction in their intimate versus nonintimate relationships. Specifically, if satisfaction in intimate relationships is directly related to the degree to which one's partner is perceived as providing traditionally "feminine" inputs to the relationship, then conflict and dissatisfaction in the relationship should likely be attributed to the partner's failure to provide such inputs. In contrast, if satisfaction in nonintimate relationships varies according to the match between one's own expressive needs (i.e., "femininity") and the level of interactional involvement that the relationship provides, then conflict and dissatisfaction should likely be attributed to the relationship's failure (i.e., to the failure of the unique "interaction of personalities") to provide an optimal match. Thus, *partner attributions* may predominate in members' explanations regarding conflict and dissatisfaction in their intimate relationships ("He/she doesn't seem to care about me, provide emotional support, etc."), whereas *relationship* (i.e., "unique interaction") *attributions* may predominate in members' explanations regarding conflict and dissatisfaction in their nonintimate relationships ("We just don't 'hit it off' together, aren't a good match, etc.").

Fifth, it is important to note that the modification of the theory proposed above affects only its predictions regarding the dyad members' *subjective reactions* to their interaction (i.e., their individual or personal outcomes). It leaves unchanged the theory's predictions regarding the level of *interactional involvement* that will characteristically occur in their relationship (i.e., their dyadic or interpersonal outcomes). The most obvious theoretical implication of this distinction is that the type-of-relationship variable primarily moderates the influence of sex-role orientations on dyad members' feelings about their relationship; it does little or nothing to moderate the influence of members' sex-role orientations on their level of interactional involvement. Some of the more subtle, less-obvious implications of this and other distinctions just made are explored below.

Further Implications for Theory and Research

In addition to the general implications discussed above, the reconciliation of Antill's (1983) "femininity hypothesis" to Ickes' (1981) theory suggests a number of more subtle and specific insights regarding the processes by which men's and women's sex-role orientations affect the compatibility of their relationships. In this final section of the chapter, we will consider an expanded scenario depicting hypothetical events in the imagined relationship of our traditional, sex-role-stereotyped couple, Mike Manley and Felicia Femme. This scenario will be used to suggest and illustrate some of the dynamic processes that may underlie and potentially explain the dissatisfaction expressed by the members (particularly the female members) of dyads in which a stereotypically masculine man is paired with a stereotypically feminine woman. Although all of these hypothesized processes are consistent with Ickes' (1981) theory, they follow from the theory in only an intuitive and heuristic sense, and should not be regarded as logical derivations.

The Sex-Role-Stereotyped Couple Revisited

In the earliest stage of their relationship, Mike Manley and Felicia Femme were strongly attracted to each other. Mike's strongly masculine sex-role orientation imposed a clear-cut masculine "style" on his features, his dress, and his expressive behavior that Felicia found to be physically, as well as sexually, attractive. By the same token, the impact of Felicia's clear-cut feminine style on her looks and behavior had a similar effect on Mike (cf. Lippa, 1978; Ickes & Barnes, 1978, p. 679).

More important, however, Felicia recognized and admired in Mike those stereotypically masculine, "instrumental," take-charge, make-things-happen traits and abilities that she generally lacked. Here was someone who was highly active and instrumental—someone who could make decisions, take effective action, earn a good living, and provide well for the *physical needs* of herself and her children—all of the things she doubted she could do on her own. At the same time, Mike recognized and admired in Felicia those stereotypically feminine, "expressive," emotionally responsive and supportive traits and abilities that he generally lacked. Here was someone who was highly responsive and expressive—someone who could nurture him, bolster his ego, radiate approval, and provide well for the *emotional needs* of himself and his children—all of the things he doubted he could do on his own.

In their courtship and early marriage, everything seemed perfect. Each of them benefited, as expected, from the complementary qualities that the other possessed and that had, in fact, attracted them to each other. Moreover, because they were still under the spell of their "limerent" feelings (Tennov, 1979; Shaver & Hazan, this volume, Chap. 7), the *expectations* that Mike and Felicia had developed about their mutual *obligation* and *desire* for high levels of emotional responsiveness in intimate relationships motivated them to meet these expectations in their behavior. This "limerent motivation" guaranteed that—for a while, at least—their emotional needs in the relationship would be mutually satisfied.

As time passed, however, the "limerent" fire that had fueled their emotional investments in each other began to die down. Although Mike did not notice much difference in Felicia's emotional responsiveness to him (consistent with her high level of feminine expressiveness), Felicia gradually became aware of a marked reduction in Mike's capacity and willingness to meet her emotional needs. And, as the decades-old habits associated with Mike's "high-masculine-assertive but low-feminine-expressive" nature gradually reasserted themselves, Felicia's emotional needs became increasingly frustrated. Mike's ambition and drive to achieve became increasingly evident, and although he provided well for Felicia's and the children's physical needs through his instrumental activity, he increasingly seemed to be married to his work, not to her.

Having more than satisfied his low expressive needs with all of the instrumental talking he had to do with others at work during the day, Mike often came home at night tired and uncommunicative. Felicia, her expressive needs starved from a day spent at home alone without human contact [according to Shaver et al.'s (1980) survey data, feminine sex-typed wives are the least likely to work outside the home], routinely tried to engage him in conversation, but without much success. Mike insisted that she stop "nagging him" and said that he just wanted to be left alone to read the newspaper, watch television, and so forth, "in peace." During these times that they were both at home, the housework and child care were left pretty much up to Felicia. After all, she was the nurturant and feminine one, not Mike. Moreover, he was usually so wrapped up in his own thoughts about his plans and goals at work that he was generally oblivious to what went on around him at home anyway.

In response to Mike's self-absorption, Felicia would often bide her time until they went to bed, only to meet with the greatest frustration of all: Even their sex life was becoming emotionally impoverished. For Mike, sex was an increasingly efficient, goal-oriented drive to reach orgasm; for Felicia, it was an increasingly passive and emotionally barren act. For Mike, sex was something to be hurried through so he could turn over and go to sleep—his thoughts already back on the work he would do tomorrow. For Felicia, sex was something empty and unfulfilling—something that lacked the laughter and shared intimacy of the extended foreplay and afterplay she had so much enjoyed in the early stages of their relationship.

Despite her unhappiness, it was a long time before Felicia had the courage to file for divorce. Her lack of instrumentality, and the resulting fear that she was not up to the pressures of working to support herself and her children, led her to spend many unhappy years in a relationship that failed to meet her emotional needs. Mike was actually a bit surprised when he was served with the divorce papers. Although he had heard Felicia's "gripes" again and again over the years, he had generally discounted them because, from his standpoint, the relationship was fine. He got all the intimacy and emotional support *he* needed, and the sex was okay, so what was this divorce all about? He knew that Felicia blamed him for the break-up of their marriage, but he was not exactly sure why. Perhaps he would never know why. As Senator Proxmire once said, you just can't analyze love.

Hypotheses for Future Research

Senator Proxmire's sentiments notwithstanding, attempts to analyze the love that develops and fades in intimate relationships are of major practical, as well as theoretical, importance. If there is any truth in the senator's claim that the public wants love to remain "a mystery," there is probably little, if any, truth in the corollary claim that the people in our society also want the causes of divorce or its effects on both parents and children to remain a mystery. Yet we cannot fully understand how love fades without understanding how it develops. And we cannot answer the question of why some relationships fail without simultaneously learning why others succeed.

As additional small steps toward this understanding, the following specific hypotheses are proposed. Some of them follow directly from the theoretical resolution proposed earlier in this chapter; others are more loosely and intuitively derived from Ickes' (1981) theory. Some may prove to be true steps and others false steps, but all are potentially falsifiable and are therefore of scientific value:

> *Hypothesis A*: Women whose husbands or male partners are either undifferentiated or masculine sex-typed should be more sexually and emotionally frustrated than women whose husbands or partners are androgynous or feminine sex-typed. These differences, which may not be apparent in the earliest stages of the relationship, should become increasingly evident as the relationship continues. (Shaver et al.'s [1980] survey data provide strong support for the first of these propositions; the second remains to be tested.)
>
> *Hypothesis B*: Androgynous or feminine sex-typed women whose husbands or male partners are either undifferentiated or masculine sex-typed should be more sexually and emotionally frustrated than their husbands are. Conversely, androgynous or feminine sex-typed men whose wives or female partners are either undifferentiated or masculine sex-typed should be more sexually and emotionally frustrated than their wives are. (These predictions, which can be derived *both* from Ickes's [1981] original theory *and* from Antill's [1983] "femininity hypothesis," have not yet received a strong empirical test.) As in Hypothesis A, these differences are expected to increase over time.
>
> *Hypothesis C*: Fear of not being able to work and "make it on their own" should be a greater deterrent to separation or divorce for feminine sex-typed women than for androgynous or masculine sex-typed women. (Shaver et al.'s data offer some hints that this may be true, not only for feminine sex-typed women, but for undifferentiated women as well.) By the same token, fear of not

being able to work and "make it on their own" should be a greater deterrent to separation or divorce for feminine sex-typed men than for androgynous or masculine sex-typed men. (These predictions remain to be tested.)

Hypothesis D: If separation or divorce does occur, and if the relationship was an intimate one, androgynous and feminine sex-typed women whose husbands or male partners are either undifferentiated or masculine sex-typed should be likely to attribute the "cause" of the breakup to their partners' failure to provide appropriate emotional inputs to the relationship (e.g., show concern, "love" them enough, be emotionally responsive and supportive). The same prediction should apply to the separation or divorce attributions of androgynous or feminine sex-typed men whose wives or female partners are either undifferentiated or masculine sex-typed. The *partners'* attributions in both of these cases should be more variable, less likely to locate the "cause" of the breakup in the other person, and less likely to focus specifically on emotional inputs to the relationship. (These predictions remain to be tested.)

These hypotheses are only a few of many that could be derived from the theory and data reviewed in this chapter. Obviously, they are not intended to be exhaustive. Instead, they should be regarded as illustrative of just some of the many ways in which individuals' sex-role orientations can affect the compatibility or incompatibility of their relationships.

Acknowledgments. The author would like to thank Phillip Shaver for his helpful comments on an earlier draft of this chapter. He would also like to thank Phillip Shaver, Cathy Pullis, Debra Olds, and the publishers of the *Ladies' Home Journal* for allowing several of the findings from their November 1979 "Intimacy Today" survey study to be reported here. Appreciation is expressed as well to John Antill for providing additional data to supplement the findings reported in his 1983 journal article.

References

Antill, J. K. (1983). Sex role complementarity versus similarity in married couples. *Journal of Personality and Social Psychology, 45,* 145–155.

Bakan, D. (1966). *The duality of human existence.* Chicago: Rand McNally.

Bales, R. F. (1955). Adaptive and integrative changes as sources of strain in social systems. In A. P. Hare, E. F. Borgatta, & R. F. Bales (Eds.), *Small groups: Studies in social interaction.* New York: Knopf.

Bales, R. F. (1958). Task roles and social roles in problem-solving groups. In E. E. Maccoby, T. M. Newcomb, & E. L. Hartley (Eds.), *Readings in social psychology* (3rd ed.). New York: Holt, Rinehart & Winston.

Bem, S. L. (1974). The measurement of psychological androgyny. *Journal of Consulting and Clinical Psychology, 45,* 196–205.

Block, J. H. (1973). Conceptions of sex roles: Some cross-cultural and longitudinal perspectives. *American Psychologist, 28,* 512–526.

Clark, M. S., & Mills, J. (1979). Interpersonal attraction in exchange and communal relationships. *Journal of Personality and Social Psychology, 37,* 12–24.

Deaux, K. (1976). *The behavior of women and men.* Monterey, CA: Brooks/Cole.

Ickes, W. (1981). Sex-role influences in dyadic interaction: A theoretical model. In C.

Mayo & N. Henley (Eds.), *Gender and nonverbal behavior*. New York: Springer-Verlag.

Ickes, W. (1982). A basic paradigm for the study of personality, roles and social behavior. In W. Ickes & E. S. Knowles (Eds.), *Personality, roles and social behavior*. New York: Springer-Verlag.

Ickes, W. (1983). A basic paradigm for the study of unstructured dyadic interaction. In H. T. Reis (Ed.), *Naturalistic Approaches to Studying Social Interaction*. New Directions for Methodology of Social and Behavioral Science, no. 15. San Francisco: Jossey-Bass.

Ickes, W., & Barnes, R. D. (1978). Boys and girls together—and alienated: On enacting stereotyped sex roles in mixed-sex dyads. *Journal of Personality and Social Psychology, 36*, 669–683.

Ickes, W., Schermer, B., & Steeno, J. (1979). Sex and sex-role influences in same-sex dyads. *Social Psychology Quarterly, 42*, 373–385.

Kaplan, A., & Sedney, M. A. (1980). *Psychology and sex roles: An androgynous perspective*. Boston: Little, Brown & Company.

Lamke, L., & Bell, N. (1981). *Sex-role orientation and relationship development in same-sex dyads*. Unpublished manuscript, Arizona State University, Tempe, AZ.

Lippa, R. (1978). The naive perception of masculinity-femininity on the basis of expressive cues. *Journal of Research in Personality, 12*, 1–14.

Mills, J., & Clark, M. S. (1982). Exchange and communal relationships. In L. Wheeler (Ed.), *Review of personality and social psychology* (Vol. 3). Beverly Hills, CA: Sage, 1982.

Parsons, T., & Bales, R. F. (1955). *Family, socialization, and interaction processes*. New York: Free Press of Glencoe.

Sampson, E. E. (1977). Psychology and the American ideal. *Journal of Personality and Social Psychology, 35*, 767–782.

Shaver, P., Pullis, C., & Olds, D. (1980). Report on the LHJ "Intimacy Today" Survey. Private research report to the *Ladies' Home Journal*.

Spanier, G. B. (1976). Measuring dyadic adjustment: New scales assessing the quality of marriage and similar dyads. *Journal of Marriage and the Family, 38*, 15–28.

Spence, J. T., & Helmreich, R. (1978). *Masculinity and femininity: Their psychological dimensions, correlates, and antecedents*. Austin, TX: University of Texas Press.

Spence, J. T., Helmreich, R., & Stapp, J. (1975). Ratings of self and peers on sex-role attributes and their relation to self-esteem and conceptions of masculinity and femininity. *Journal of Personality and Social Psychology, 32*, 29–39.

Tennov, D. (1979). *Love and limerence: The experience of being in love*. New York: Stein & Day.

Chapter 9

The Role of the Self in the Initiation and Course of Social Interaction

Harry T. Reis

The notion that people select their friends is perhaps trite. No one would doubt that individuals have a say in deciding which acquaintances will become friends and which will not. Often this process may be portrayed as something akin to a beauty contest: Individuals acquire a certain asset value contingent upon the socially desirable characteristics they possess, and this value determines their access to rewarding social relations. If such an account were correct, then friendship, social activity, and satisfaction should reveal markedly skewed distributions, with those enjoying an abundance of desirable traits being most rewarded.

An alternative to the above model might view the process as a random lottery. In this view, people are brought into proximity by a variety of factors, many of which are essentially random, or at least not under their direct control. They then become friends, simply because of the opportunities that proximity offers.

Neither of these views is accurate. The choice of acquaintances and the development of friendship is a complex process characterized by systematic differences in social inference, recursive patterns of influence and reaction, and progressive assessments of rewards and alternatives. At every stage of the process, the nature of the interaction is greatly affected by the psychological makeup of the participants. Most, if not all, of these factors tend to operate without the actors' conscious awareness, and the process is difficult to perceive in action because relevant covariation information is not readily accessible. For one thing, we are involved both as actor and target, thereby making discrimination of the simultaneous influence sources difficult. For another, because many psychological aspects of the self are not obvious, the causal factors underlying friendship formation are not likely to be disclosed by observation. Instead, what is generally more apparent is the variety of interactions in which we participate, and the range of others with whom we socialize. Consequently, the systematic patterns that would highlight people's roles as active constructors of their social lives are usually obscure.

My goal in this chapter is to discuss the different ways in which the self is responsible for constructing the social world in which it participates. I will first separate the phenomena into three general categories of influence: the opportunity to meet, possibilities for continuity, and recursive influence. These categories will then be integrated by application to two general cases: loneliness and physical attractiveness.

Before beginning, it may be useful to discuss the relationship of a self-oriented perspective to the theme of this volume, compatibility and incompatibility. For a long time, lay and psychological viewpoints were dominated by the doctrine of static matching. According to this doctrine, people possess varying degrees of an assortment of traits and values, and these are either aligned compatibly in a dyad or not. An extreme version of this hypothesis is utilized by "computer matching" services, in which an ideal partner is presumably identified by the specification of an appropriate set of descriptors. Although the static matching model may be oversimplified, it does recognize the role of both individuals' personal characteristics in affecting the interaction that results. However, the model assumes a static, rather than a transactional, process: Personal traits are enacted similarly, from one interaction to another, regardless of the partner's response.

More recently, the dynamic aspects of interpersonal relations have been emphasized in studies of expectancy-confirmation processes (Darley & Fazio, 1980). Herein one partner's response is shaped and channeled by the expectancy-derived stimulus of the other's actions. Although attention to the manner in which interactants influence each other's responses is an important step forward, this view seems somewhat oversimplified in that the personal characteristics of the reactor are lost. That is, partners are seen as mostly malleable, reacting to the behavior of the actor independent of their own needs, values, and expectations.

Analyses of compatibility and incompatibility must take both of these perspectives into account. If compatibility is based on the relationship's stability, integrative functioning, and the level of satisfaction experienced by its members (see the Introduction to this volume), the emphasis must be on how interaction forges a different set of behaviors than two individuals would have produced had they been acting alone or with a different partner (Kelley, 1979). However, the starting point for this analysis must be the individuals themselves, in two respects: the needs and values they bring to the interaction, and the tendencies with which they act on, and react to, each other. From this perspective, compatibility would be seen not so much as an alignment of needs and values, but rather in terms of the ability to co-act with another person in creating social events that are satisfying to both partners. This is a matter of flexibility, implicating the socially directive aspects of the self in two ways: in determining the behaviors that are personally rewarding, and in allowing oneself to be responsive to a partner's outcomes.

Three Sources of the Impact of the Self

Opportunity to Meet

Obviously, if two people never meet, they have virtually no opportunity to discover whether they could be compatible with each other. Factors that direct social encounters thereby play a major role in social relations, at least in defining the limits of what is possible. There are two steps involved in this process. First, aspects of the self must alter the probability that two randomly selected individuals will come into contact. Second, their meeting must make an ongoing relationship more likely. We will examine the first of these steps in this section.

On an intuitive level it seems apparent that the probability of meeting is affected by personal characteristics. Skills and intelligence bear upon the educational settings and the careers that people pursue. Attitudes and interests predispose people to participate in a wide variety of vocational, recreational, religious, and professional activities (Fishbein & Ajzen, 1975). Personality traits also have an impact on behavior: High-risk-takers are presumably more likely than low-risk-takers to join a parachuting club, for example, whereas persons low in self-confidence are more likely than those high in self-confidence to enroll in an assertiveness-training group. In a more empirical vein, Snyder and Ickes (in press) recently reviewed a large literature indicating that personality factors affect the choice of social situations.

Once two individuals engage in the same activity or put themselves in the same setting, the likelihood is increased that they will come into contact with each other and hence become acquainted. This simple principle may in part be responsible for the observed similarity in values and traits that close friends and lovers show. That is, since contact is funneled toward similar others by behavioral choices, there are fewer possibilities for attraction among dissimilar persons. This general constraint notwithstanding, random events may still play a significant role. Bandura (1982) provides some evocative examples of how chance encounters can alter life paths. He illustrates his argument with a case that is probably familiar to all: a serendipitous meeting with a stranger or casual acquaintance that blossoms into full-fledged romance. Although the same two individuals might never have met again, that single encounter led to further interaction and a deeper relationship.

Although a first encounter may be random, the factors that bring people to its site are generally not. The role of random social contact is reminiscent of the classic "Westgate" study by Festinger, Schachter, and Back (1950). These researchers found that the probability of friendship increased as the physical distance between residences decreased. The only meaningful function served by physical proximity was to increase the likelihood of contact. In a related study, Segal (1974) demonstrated that 45% of a group of 52 police trainees asked to nominate a close friend selected someone who was immediately adjacent in alphabetical ordering. Because most of this group's activities were conducted alphabetically, and assuming that alphabetical rank is not related to attitudes or traits, it seems safe to infer that random contact led to friendship. There are many other studies of the effects of propinquity on the development of relationships, all pointing to similar conclusions.

Although these examples would seem to argue for the role of chance, it must be remembered that random pairing occurs within the context of activity-centered similarity. The residents of Westgate were all married veterans returning to school; Segal's subjects were all police trainees. They therefore possessed the initial similarities likely to make interaction both probable and rewarding. After all, propinquity increases the probability of friendship by providing opportunities for people to reward one another. Such opportunities would fail if there was not a psychological basis for their potential to be actualized. Thus, even when the undeniable role of serendipity is considered, the self plays an essential role by determining the environments in which people participate, and hence the partners to whom they might be exposed. How these partners are selected, once initial exposure has occurred, is discussed in the following section.

Possibilities for Continuity

After two individuals have come into contact, psychological aspects of the self play a critical role in determining whether interaction will be initiated, and whether a relationship will subsequently develop. In this section we will discuss the influence of an actor's actions or feelings on friendship formation. Factors that rely upon systems of mutual influence will be considered in the following section. Because there are psychological differences in the processes of approach and continuity in relationships, these processes will be considered separately.

Initiation. The decision to approach another individual, whether conscious or unconscious, depends upon the resolution of two sets of countervalent forces: driving and restraining (Lewin, 1951). Driving forces are factors indicating that the other is a desirable partner, or in other words, someone with whom interaction appears likely to be rewarding. These tendencies are countered by restraining forces—assessments of the likelihood that such rewards will actually be received, or in other words, the probability of being accepted by the other. The equilibrium that results from these opposing tendencies determines the strength of self-directed motives to seek interaction with the other. If driving forces outweigh restraining forces, the individual anticipates that the other will be attracted to oneself much as one is attracted to the other, and that an exchange of liking and rewards may be expected. Berscheid (in press) has recently used this single principle of anticipated reciprocal liking to summarize research on the numerous factors that affect attraction in initial encounters.

The desirability of the other is typically inferred from social cues, in that usable data are often minimal and limited to what is available visually or through public knowledge and mutual acquaintances. Many characteristics make a partner desirable. One of the most potent variables in initial attraction is physical attractiveness. A large number of positive traits are generally ascribed to physically attractive people, frequently by virtue of stereotypic inferences that may or may not be accurate (Berscheid & Walster, 1974; Sorell & Nowak, 1981). Although some negative traits may also be associated with attractiveness (see, for example, Dermer & Thiel, 1975), the overwhelming positivity of this stereotype, when coupled with the aesthetic value of beauty itself, makes attractive persons highly desired interaction partners (Berscheid & Walster, 1974). Despite the predominance of physical attractiveness as a topic for empirical studies, cues about many other attracting factors are usually apparent in initial encounters: status, gregariousness, intelligence, vitality, wealth, height, and so on. More in-depth information may also be available from communications with third parties.

The social desirability of these traits at times seems ubiquitous (witness the content of most classified "personal ads"). Nevertheless, there are individual differences in preferences, with some factors showing small variation around a culturally shared level (e.g., attractiveness, friendliness), and others displaying large variability (e.g., wealth, leisure activities). That variations in these preferences may be informative about the personality and value structure of the person is central to the theories of Kelly (1955). To Kelly, the manner in which people interpret their environment is a direct reflection of choices based on personal needs, experiences, and other idiosyncratic—but highly systematic—factors. Kelly designed what he called the Rep Test specifically to identify these personal constructs. The test works by isolating the specific dimensions that perceivers use to compare and contrast different acquaintances. Individual differences in attitudes, abilities, and activity preferences also influence attraction by virtue of the importance of similarity between two interaction partners. A large body of evidence attests to the pervasive impact of similarity in social relations (Berscheid, in press). Analyses of the underlying mechanisms by which similarity affects attraction often focus on self-derived factors. For example, Wheeler (1974) has noted that selective affiliation with similar others is one realization of social-comparison processes. In a somewhat related vein, Swann (1983) has argued that social partners are chosen on the basis of the perceived likelihood that they will verify our self-conceptions. Buss (in press) applies this point specifically to marriage, in his inference that the similarity of spouses' activities arises from the creation of a social environment that reinforces individual predispositions. Thus, attraction to others is based on both social desirability and similarity, but in both instances potential benefit to the self is central.

Attracting forces are balanced by estimates of the probability of acceptance. A number of laboratory studies, such as that of Huston (1973), indicate that subjects are less likely to initiate interaction when they perceive rejection to be likely. In a more naturalistic mode, Reis, Wheeler, Spiegel, Kernis, Nezlek, and Perri (1982) found that fear of rejection by the opposite sex was inversely related to the frequency of interaction, as well as to the quality of those interactions that did occur. Anticipated acceptance and rejection depend in part upon the principle of reciprocity of reward, a central tenet of most social-exchange theories. Perhaps the most explicit version of this notion is to be found in Walster, Berscheid, and Walster's (1973) propositions about equity theory. This theory predicts—and is supported by available evidence to confirm—that dyadic relationships in which one partner receives more rewards than the other, relative to their respective inputs, are unstable and likely to be terminated. However, crucial to our current concerns, the mechanism for this breakup is not clear. That is, does the overrewarded partner seek to end the relationship because he or she feels guilty and anticipates rejection? It is also plausible that termination is induced by the underrewarded partner, with the net effect being the same for both.

In some instances, fear of rejection is one aspect of low self-esteem. Recently, empirical attention has been drawn to the process in which an overly negative assessment of the self, and hence of one's acceptability, leads to social withdrawal or unsatisfying interaction. Brockner (1983) has proposed a model of the self-perpetuating nature of low self-esteem. Although his analysis derives primarily from studies of task performance, it is consistent with many investigations of social relations as well. There are three stages to his model. First, people with low self-esteem have poorer expectations of how they will perform. Combined with a lower assessment of one's acceptability, this would lead to shunning interaction (Leary, 1982) or perhaps to seeking less desirable partners. Second, persons with low self-esteem tend to become more self-focused during the task, thus hampering their performance. Self-focus appears to hinder social performance as well (Schlenker & Leary, in press) and would seem to interfere with the capacity to enjoy social contact, since self-awareness is usually negative and inhibits spontaneity and responsiveness. Finally, Brockner (1983) notes that persons with low self-esteem typically evaluate their performance as poorer, especially when standards are ambiguous (as social standards usually are) and tend to attribute their failures to dispositional causes. These same cognitive patterns also have been shown to characterize depressed and lonely individuals (Hansson, Jones, & Carpenter, 1984; Lewinsohn, Mischel, Chaplin, & Barton, 1980).

The importance of fear of rejection is also borne out by two other paradigmatic studies. Kiesler and Baral (1970) demonstrated that men whose self-esteem was situationally elevated were more likely to approach an attractive female. In an ingenious study, Bernstein, Stephenson, Snyder, and Wicklund (1983) gave men the opportunity to approach an attractive woman. In one condition, subjects had no plausible justification for this approach, save the desire to affiliate. In another condition, subjects had available a reasonable and public explanation that made it unlikely that the woman would perceive their social intent, thereby diminishing the probability of rejection. This manipulation increased the percentage of men who did approach the woman from 25% to 75% in one study, and from 33% to 72% in a replication.

Before proceeding, it might be noted that fear of rejection can also restrain attempts to alter the nature of existing relationships. The importance of this point is emphasized by the observation that most social relations are not formally initiated, at least in the premeditated and conscious sense that this term connotes. Rather, people tend to find themselves in the presence of others through chance encounters, task requirements, and other relatively impersonal circumstances. Some decision, often enacted without awareness, is then needed to change the interaction to one with a more social nature. These acts can be conceptualized as initiations of a *social* relationship, just as approaches involving strangers are. The primary difference is that, in the former case, the interactants already have more information about each other. Psychological factors relevant to initiation can thereby inhibit or altogether block the development of deeper connections out of an existing acquaintance, just as they affect initial contacts. For example, fear of rejection might restrain attempts to change a professional or platonic friendship into a romantic involvement. A poignant example of this phenomenon occurs in the story of Cyrano de Bergerac and Roxane. Although lifelong close friends, Cyrano fears to reveal his love for the beautiful Roxane, saying:

> And tell me how much hope remains for me
> with this protuberance!
> Oh I have no more
> Illusions! . . . My friend, I have my bitter days,
> knowing myself so ugly, so alone.

Instead, he surreptitiously composes heart-stirring love letters for the beautiful but simple-minded Christian, whom Roxane loves not for his pretty face, as Cyrano assumes, but for the eloquence and depth of feeling displayed in his (Cyrano's!) letters. It is only many years later, after Christian has died and Roxane has entered a convent, that, as Cyrano lies dying, his secret is revealed. Roxane speaks:

> Why were you silent for so many years,
> All the while, every night and every day,
> He gave me nothing—You knew that—you knew
> Here, in this letter lying on my breast,
> Your tears—You knew they were your tears—
> . . . I never loved but one man in my life,
> And I have lost him—twice . . .

Development. The processes that guide the development of a relationship beyond initial attraction are decidedly more complex, mostly because of increasing interdependence: The rewards that each partner receives become

---

dependent upon the actions of both. (This mutual influence is the subject of the following section.) Individual attraction is still relevant, however. The same general reward processes that determine initial attraction are also important in maintaining later attraction. Following Berscheid's (in press) framework, these processes can be summarized as follows: (1) Individuals will continue to be attracted to others who possess traits they perceive to be desirable; (2) similarity of interests and traits will be helpful because it frequently underlies anticipated reward and shared activities; and (3) attraction will be greatest to those perceived as likely to reciprocate liking.

Even though the processes may be the same, the content may differ. For one thing, the characteristics perceived to be desirable are likely to change somewhat. Attitudes toward family may increase in impact over time, for example. A second difference is that judgments about rewards in established relationships are more likely to be based on experienced levels of satisfaction, rather than on expectations rooted in social inference. Such assessments are likely to be held with greater confidence and should also be more stable, due to the increased data base. Despite these differences, and despite the partners' greater reliance on each other for interaction and reward, the general processes that predict attraction, satisfaction, and stability—that is, compatibility—are similar in the initial and developmental stages of the relationship. In both stages, they rely heavily on the self.

A brief example may make this point clearer. As Gilligan (1982) and Peplau and Gordon (in press) point out, when compared with women, men are found to be relatively more fearful of intimacy in a close heterosexual relationship. In the later stages of a relationship, this difference is likely to lead both partners to perceive their needs as dissimilar and their outcomes as not being reciprocated. The failure of some men to be emotionally intimate is one of the most common complaints of females in marital discord (see Chap. 8 of this volume). Yet the achievement of intimacy is generally considered one of the touchstones of relationship development (Erikson, 1950; Levinger & Snoek, 1972). As such, the resolution of these dispositional differences is a major factor in compatibility and incompatibility. Gender and sex-role differences in intimacy clearly belong to the psychological self, in that they derive from deeply rooted needs and socialization experiences. Consequently, one of the key dimensions of long-term compatibility in a heterosexual romantic dyad is rooted in the self.

Just as in the case of initiation, behavior in well-established relationships is also affected by ego-protective strategies. The work of Tesser and his colleagues (summarized in Tesser, 1983) indicates that although we want our friends to perform well, too much achievement by similar others may threaten our self-esteem. Consequently, people prefer that close friends do well on tasks irrelevant to their sense of self, allowing them to "bask in reflected glory" (Cialdini, Borden, Thorne, Walker, Freeman, & Sloan, 1976), but to do less well than themselves on tasks that are central to their own self-concepts. The interplay of these three parameters (closeness to other, relevance to the self-concept, and level of performance) has been supported in a number of varied studies. For example, Tesser and Smith (1980) found that college students were less helpful to friends than to strangers when the task was highly relevant to their self-concept. Even more relevant is a study of friendship nominations among 5th and 6th grade students (Tesser, Campbell & Smith, 1983). When asked to name their close friends, the majority of children nominated classmates whose performance was superior to their own on irrelevant tasks, but somewhat poorer than their own on relevant activities.

Interactive Influence

To borrow an analogy from statistics, the reward model presented above implies that relationship satisfaction is a function of two main effects—that is, those terms representing the level of satisfaction that each of the two partners produces independently. However, in a factorial analysis of variance, significant main effects do not constrain the interaction to be nonsignificant, and this is true in social relations as well. In both cases, the interaction effect refers to the extent to which the behavior of one independent variable (or one partner in a dyad) depends upon the other independent variable (or partner). This dependence provides dyadic social behavior with much of its flexibility and complexity (as in the analysis of variance), and no doubt most of the delight (unlike the analysis of variance!). Researchers have investigated interactive influences in two ways. The first research tradition has stressed problems of interdependence, in which the coordination of two actors' behaviors produces a unique outcome. The second, more recent approach emphasizes shaping processes, in which one actor's behavior serves as a stimulus for the response of the other.

Interdependence. In their painstaking analysis of interdependence, Kelley and Thibaut (1978) make it plain that the specialness of social relations arises from the manner in which each participant modifies his or her behavior in order to take the other's outcomes into account. They describe three general patterns of interdependence, each of which is present in most interactions to some extent: reflexive control (in which outcomes depend exclusively on one's own actions), fate control (in which outcomes depend exclusively on the other's actions), and behavior control (in which outcomes depend on both partners' actions). Some degree of behavior control is typically the rule in social relations, and it illustrates well the interactive basis of compatibility. For example, there may be no intrinsic advantage to preferring hockey or chamber music for recreation. However, a dyad whose members have shared tastes is likely to be more satisfying than one whose members are mismatched. Ickes and Barnes (1977) give an empirical demonstration of this phenomenon in the realm of personality variables. In their study, two unacquainted strangers were unobtrusively observed during a 5-min waiting period. Pairs in which the subjects were mismatched on the trait of self-monitoring experienced longer silences and greater self-consciousness than pairs in which both subjects were high or low on this trait.

Kelley and Thibaut's (1978) analysis of interdependence has an additional dynamic component. To them, interdependence exists at two levels: in "the given matrix," which describes the outcomes that actors would accrue if they considered only their own perspective, and in the "dispositional matrix," which describes the actors' stable traits and their attitudes toward each other. The ultimate course of a single interaction depends upon how these dispositional tendencies motivate the actors to transform the given matrix—in other words, how actors modify their personal feelings to take the other's outcomes into account. Coordination provides the fabric of the relationship, in that feelings about the relationship depend upon both the fit of the partners' given matrices *and* the extent to which their transformational tendencies are responsive to each other's needs. For example, even if one partner preferred hockey and the other chamber music, an empathic transformational tendency would allow both to feel rewarded in sharing the other's activity choice. In contrast, a self-interested orientation would lead to separate behaviors, or, in the case of turn-taking, to a lack of enjoyment in the activity.

Although this analysis of interdependence focuses on the operating characteristics of the dyad, it also reveals the controlling functions of the self. The starting point is the given matrix, or the personal value an individual would place on certain activities. These values are rooted in the self, although the resulting outcomes depend on the specific mesh of the values held by both partners. The dispositional matrix refers to the partners' characteristic responses to each other's needs, outcomes, and behavior. These responses include such interpersonal attitudes as empathy, egocentrism, self-denial, and competition, as well as the feelings engendered by having a partner whose social behavior reflects one or another of these styles. Interpersonal orientations also arise from the self, presumably from a synthesis of the person's psychological needs and past experiences. The combination of the given and dispositional matrices determines compatibility.

An example may clarify these processes. Imagine a marriage in which both partners are self-centered, perhaps as a consequence of each having had a "spoiled" childhood. This trait is clearly an aspect of the self, in that it describes a tendency to approach the environment in an egocentric manner. Assuming a couple's interest in similar activities, their life together might be fairly stable and rewarding for both. With a divergence in interests, however, the partners would not be able to share mutually satisfying interaction, nor would they be able to engage in preferred activities with their spouse. As a result, their relationship would probably be unsatisfying and unstable. However, compatibility would depend far less on the preference for similar activities if both partners were more empathic. In this instance, each partner would feel gratified by the other's satisfaction, and the individualized rewards from the given matrix would matter less.

Recursive influence. A special case of interdependence occurs when the response of each partner is modified by the prior behavior of the other. This pattern is recursive, in the sense that each actor's behavior is stimulated by, and also serves to stimulate, the behavior of the other. Multiple steps then characterize larger interaction sequences. Kelley (1983) describes these cycles as option-consequence lists. Essentially, his notion is that each action a dyad enacts not only determines the members' rewards for that event, but also presents them with new outcome possibilities for subsequent behavior. In this way, interdependence also includes a degree of control over the temporal course of events.

A good example of this process is the affect reciprocity displayed by married couples. Gottman (1979), among others, has identified reciprocity sequences as long as six steps. Positive affect expressed by one spouse is generally returned by the other spouse, in turn leading to continued positive affect from the first spouse, and so on. On the other hand, negative affect seems to be reciprocated only in distressed couples, often leading to escalation of the negativity. Members of a nondistressed couple are more likely to respond to negative affect with a neutral comment. Thus, the expression of negative affect is likely to activate a different interaction sequence in a distressed couple than in a nondistressed pair.

Recent empirical studies of expectancy-confirmation processes can also be examined in terms of recursive influence. A prototypical example is presented by Snyder, Tanke, and Berscheid (1977). In their study, men were led to believe that their partner in an anonymous phone conversation was either an attractive or an unattractive woman. The women did not actually differ as suggested, nor were they aware of this manipulation. When the women's portions of the conversations were rated independently, those whose male partners believed them to be attractive came across more positively than those whose partners believed them to be unattractive. Apparently, the callers' expectations led them to be friendlier to ostensibly attractive women than to ostensibly unattractive ones, and these behaviors in turn induced the women to reciprocate in kind. Other instances of such self-fulfilling prophecies in social circumstances are cited by Darley and Fazio (1980).

The general process of expectancy confirmation indicates a potent effect of the self on interaction sequences, in that expectations may come to fruition largely because the actor believes them and therefore generates behaviors likely to elicit confirming responses. Although little empirical attention has been directed to the source of these expectations, they presumably arise from the same personal origins as any other predictions: past experience, individual needs, and cultural stereotypes. Expectancy confirmation satisfies the initial requirement for a recursive process because the originating person's action varies the cues to which the partner responds, altering the interaction sequence that follows. However, most analyses of this process seem to assume that the partner is essentially malleable, responding freely and unrestrainedly to the actor's expectations. There are three reasons to question this assumption. First, interaction partners undoubtedly have expectations of their own that may also trigger complementary or competing self-fulfilling prophecies. Second, people often attempt to compensate for an unfavorable expectation in the hope of averting an unpleasant interaction (Ickes, Patterson, Rajecki, & Tanford,

1982). Third, although individuals are often flexible in expressing social traits, there nonetheless are important cross-situational consistencies (Epstein, 1979). Thus, an expectation might not elicit behavioral confirmation when it is too discrepant with the actual behavioral predispositions or skills of the target. Otherwise, we would never be able to learn that first impressions can be wrong.

This is not to deny the impact of expectancy-confirmation processes. Particularly in the instance of stereotypic knowledge, they constitute potent shaping forces, as suggested by the earlier discussion of factors that affect meeting and continuity possibilities. More research is needed to identify the conditions under which these processes are more or less likely to modify social behavior in ways that extend beyond simple interdependence predictions. As a step in this direction, the following delimiting conditions are proposed:

1. *Discrepancy size.* Targets probably have a latitude of acceptance for each of their trait domains. These affect the extent to which targets are able and willing to vary their trait-relevant behavior. The central tendency and width of these latitudes differ from one trait domain to another, and from person to person. An expectation of behavior too discrepant from the target's traits is likely not to be confirmed and may even produce negative effects such as reactance.

2. *Ambiguity.* The more ambiguous the trait in question, the more likely it is that subtle influence will elicit it. Traits that are clearly manifested or about which physical reality is apparent are less likely to be altered.

3. *Awareness.* Aspects of the self about which a target is aware are likely to be resistant to shaping. For example, someone who knows that she dislikes cocktail parties is less likely to be induced to see their merits than someone unaware of her feelings.

4. *Personal investment.* The more central a given value or trait to a target's self-concept, the less responsive it will be to subtle recursive manipulation. A person for whom distrust is a core aspect of personality will be less likely to respond to a stranger's expectation of trust than will someone for whom distrust is a more peripheral aspect of the self. In this regard, the resistance of depressed and lonely persons to intervention by well-meaning friends seems noteworthy.

Self-Expression: General Comments

In the preceding discussion, the self has been described as influencing social conduct through three types of forces: *personal effects*, in which the traits and values of persons influence their responses to the social environment; *dyadic effects*, in which outcomes are based on the coordination of two partner's personal effects; and *recursive influence*, in which each actor's behavior alters the stimuli to which the other responds. A fundamental question that might be posed at this juncture is "Why would the self want to express itself in social interaction?" or "What functions are fulfilled by this type of self-expression?" Because the functional approach has been applied most profitably to the study of attitude formation, I will extrapolate from analyses such as those of Katz (1960) and McGuire (1969). These authors discuss four nonexclusive functions: instrumentality, knowledge, expression, and ego-defense.

The notion of *instrumentality* suggests that social relations help propel people toward the attainment of desired goals. Some of these goals are inherently social. For example, proponents of the social-needs approach argue that people have various needs that can only be fulfilled within social relationships. Weiss (1974) presents six such needs: attachment, social integration, opportunity for nurturance, reassurance of worth, reliable alliance, and obtaining guidance. It is to be emphasized that the status of these activities as goals does not depend on their origin. They may have an evolutionary-biological source, or they may be founded in socialization. Regardless, goals that require varied forms of social contact for realization exist. Social relations are also useful for achieving nonsocial aims. Social psychology has a long tradition of studying how group membership facilitates locomotion toward desired goals (Cartwright & Zander, 1968). Furthermore, research cited earlier supports the relevance of shared activity preferences for the choice of spouses and close friends.

A second function of the self that social relations help satisfy is the need for *knowledge* about the environment. Such knowledge enables us to understand events in a manner that makes them interpretable, and hence more predictable and controllable. Information is often transmitted socially, both by direct communication of data describing physical reality, and through social-comparison processes regarding events or qualities that are more ambiguous. An interesting complexity is added by virtue of the consideration that much of the environment about which knowledge is sought is social as well. Thus, social interaction serves as a source of both answers and questions. An interesting example of this duality is provided by the Orvis, Kelley, and Butler (1976) and Harvey, Wells, and Alvarez (1978) studies of attribution processes within married couples. Their data demonstrate how attributions help couples define the conditions under which particular behaviors are either prescribed or prohibited. In addition to helping couples understand their relationship, these attributions facilitate the development of a deeper relationship, about which, in turn, further insight will be desired.

The third function of social relations is *expression*. Social relationships allow individuals to express their identity and unique characteristics to others, thereby establishing a social sense of self. To some extent, this is a self-presentation process, but it is important to remember that self-presentation involves not only external projection, but personal identity as well (Cooley, 1902). The types of partners one chooses reflect one's values and ideals. Furthermore, because social partners help determine the nature and quality of one's activities, specific choices will affect the expression of self more generally.

Ego defense is the final function that interpersonal relations may satisfy. Many self-esteem protecting motives have been posited in social psychology, all of them relevant to social functioning. These defenses help channel perception and interaction so as to protect the person from events that threaten the self-concept. The work cited earlier on fear of rejection is a good example of this function. By avoiding contact altogether, the potential denigration of rejection is averted, leaving self-esteem unaffected. Ego-defensive functions operate for other aspects of the self as well. Fear of intimacy, for instance, would be well-served by an emphasis on superficial relationships, coupled with self-serving rationalizations for terminating any relationships that approach deeper levels of involvement.

Two Examples of the Impact of the Self on the Course of Social Conduct

To this point, the impact of the self has been examined piecemeal, in terms of distinct processes. One of the dynamic aspects of the self, however, is that it functions as an integrated whole. By way of exemplifying the processes described above, integrated accounts will be presented for two prototypical examples: loneliness and physical attractiveness. The discussion will emphasize the manner in which the self shapes and governs the reaction to the social environment.

Loneliness

Loneliness is an aversive emotional state in which the discrepancy between a person's desired and achieved levels of social contact produces unpleasant emotions and negative self-perceptions (Peplau & Perlman, 1982). Most lay accounts of loneliness begin with external factors, dealing with the absence or inadequacy of friends or with circumstantial restrictions on socializing (Rubenstein & Shaver, 1982). Nevertheless, social psychological investigations have focused primarily on the person.

A number of recent studies have examined lonely people's cognitions about themselves. With regard to attributions, for example, these studies indicate that lonely people exhibit the classic "learned helplessness" attribution pattern: Social failures are attributed to a lack of ability, whereas successes are attributed to external circumstances (e.g., Anderson, 1980; Furman, Shaver, & Buhrmester, 1984). Regardless of whether these self-attributions are veridical, they may have self-fulfilling consequences: Such attributions tend to produce lower expectations and poorer coping in subsequent similar situations (Anderson, 1980; Goetz & Dweck, 1980). The importance of attributions in this process is further substantiated in a study by Brodt and Zimbardo (1981). Using a standard misattribution paradigm, they found that when anxiety could be attributed to an external factor, the social performance of shy females improved considerably.

This attributional difference is part of a more general pattern of negative self-perception by the lonely. Lonely people tend to see themselves negatively on a wide variety of self-esteem and competence measures (Peplau, Miceli, & Morasch, 1982). Even if these assessments are incorrect, they may nonetheless have self-defeating (and self-perpetuating) effects. Horowitz, French, and Anderson (1982) describe how self-perceptions of incompetence inhibit social contact. Expectations of social failure can be used as a reason for avoiding contact, or for not trying hard (self-handicapping). This pattern may become reified, so that the lonely person uses his or her status as lonely and social incompetent as a justification for continued isolation and the lack of active coping strategies. Of course, such behavior is self-defeating. The absence of interaction precludes the development of meaningful friendships, the primary factor in avoiding loneliness (Wheeler, Reis, & Nezlek, 1983). It is also likely to perpetuate deficiencies in social skill, since experience in interactions is a primary source of such skills. Finally, isolation may reinforce the self-perception of social incompetence and perhaps further stigmatize the person as a "loner." Although the self might protect itself from fear of rejection by isolation, this behavior makes matters worse in the long run.

Although some studies suggest that the problem is more a matter of negativity of self-perception than of unfavorable evaluations by others (Lewinsohn et al. 1980; Wittenberg & Reis, 1984), it is nevertheless important to note that lonely people do tend to be deficient in a variety of social skills. Jones (1982) reviewed a number of studies indicating that the lonely are more cynical and rejecting in their assessments of others, and appear to lack many of the skills necessary to initiate and maintain social relations (e.g., initiation, disclosure, sociability). These inadequacies have a number of consequences for interdependence. Most central is the implication that lonely people are not likely to be rewarding social partners. Relatively poor skills, combined with a negative view of self and others, would make a lonely person a most unsatisfying partner. Lonely people particularly seem unable to focus attention on their partners, paying greater notice to themselves instead (Jones, Hobbs, & Hockenbury, 1982). This may not be surprising, given that social anxiety, a negative self-image, and a state of relative deprivation are all likely to heighten self-consciousness. However, using Kelley's (1979) terminology, such an extreme self-focus tends to make the transformational tendencies that reward other people improbable. Inter-action with lonely people is therefore less likely to produce rewards for their partners and will also tend to yield interdependence patterns that are not mutually satisfying. This analysis implies that lonely people will generally be incompatible with each other as well as with nonlonely people, for, although interaction would eliminate their isolation, they are still less likely to attend to each other's needs and interests.

To summarize, the motivating properties of the self create two behavioral tendencies that distinguish the lonely from the nonlonely. First, they engender negative or competence-denying cognitions about the self that are likely to perpetuate themselves. Second, they foster and then help to maintain social-skill deficits that make lonely persons less desirable interaction partners. Thera-peutic interventions could be designed to take into account how the various functions of the self are (pathologically) fulfilled in lonely people. A model program might focus on the inability to give or receive rewards in social interaction, and the ego defenses that preserve this state. The notion that the self may help perpetuate the state of loneliness suggests that programs attending solely to skills training are likely to be ineffective, since they do not deal with the ego processes that instigate and defend a negative self-perception. In fact, social success induced by a training program may well be attributed to that program, thereby reinforcing the attributional pattern of helplessness described earlier.

Physical Attractiveness

One of the most disquieting facts about social attraction is the powerful and pervasive impact that physical appearance has. Despite the "undemocratic" nature of this variable (Aronson, 1969), an impressive body of research has shown it to be an important, if not *the* most important, factor in social preference. This advantage seems to apply throughout the entire life span, from early infancy to old age (see Sorell & Nowak's, 1981, excellent review of developmental patterns). Furthermore, although many commentators have speculated that the preference for physically attractive others should be limited to initial encounters, research demonstrates that the effect is sustained over time (e.g., Mathes, 1975; Reis, Nezlek, & Wheeler, 1980).

It would appear, then, that the social relations of attractive and unattractive persons are significantly different. Two of the functions of the self listed earlier, instrumentality and ego defense, seem most relevant to these differences. Some of the instrumental functions can be conceptualized as "gatekeeper effects." As Aristotle once noted, "Beauty is a greater recommendation than any letter of introduction." Attractive people get more attention upon initial observation, and are perceived to be more desirable social partners in general (Berscheid, in press). Because first encounters set the stage for later interaction, attractiveness confers an important initial advantage. Part of this benefit stems from a halo effect, whereby the attractive person is perceived as having other socially desirable attributes as well. In addition, due to the asset value of attractiveness, association with an attractive other enhances one's own social desirability (Kernis & Wheeler, 1981; Sigall & Landy, 1973) and thus motivates continued interaction. Further, because attractive persons control more valuable assets, they have more opportunities to reinforce others, and presumably have more choice over the selection of partners.

These benefits would be of limited utility if the impact of attractiveness were restricted to status-by-association and the aesthetic merits of beauty. Studies of the traits inferred to attractive persons indicate that they are generally perceived to possess a wide variety of positive social characteristics, such as sociability and sensitivity (e.g., Dion, Berscheid, & Walster, 1972). Whether or not these inferences are correct, the mere expectancy of a positive interaction is likely to lead to its confirmation. In the Snyder et al. (1977) study described earlier, telephone conversations involving males who were told that their female targets were attractive were rated more positively on a variety of dimensions than were conversations in which the target was supposedly unattractive. Andersen and Bem (1981) found a similar effect with female callers and male targets. Two studies my colleagues and I have conducted produced related results. Using self-reports of ongoing interaction, Reis et al. (1980, 1982) showed that attractive persons of both sexes participated in interactions that were experienced as more intimate and pleasant. Because attractive people engage in more enjoyable interactions, the implication is that they control the distribution of relatively more rewards, by virtue of their choice of partners.

Whether attractive people actually possess the traits stereotypically ascribed to them is not clear. Nevertheless, the available evidence indicates that attractive individuals perceive themselves more positively, are perceived more positively by others, and socialize in a more favorable manner. However, all but one of the available studies of which we are aware used one of three methods self-reports, responses to hypothetical stimulus persons, or measures based on interactions in which the partners were aware of the subject's attractiveness. Self-reports of attractive people may be swayed by a history of being treated as desirable. Hypothetical responses are informative regarding social perception, but not necessarily regarding actual behavior. Interactions in which attractiveness is apparent may become more enjoyable by virtue of the partner's actions. Thus, our knowledge about the effect of beauty on social skills is limited. The one exception is Goldman and Lewis's (1977) study, in which attractive subjects were rated as more skillful in anonymous conversations with partners blind to their looks. However, the experimenters with whom they interacted were aware of their attractiveness.

This reservation notwithstanding, self-perception differences are indicative of the role that attractiveness plays in forming ego-defensive motives, which then affect subsequent social behavior. With regard to such motives, there appear to be some interesting gender differences in the correlates of beauty. Attractive men enjoy greater self-confidence, sociability, and assertiveness, and less fear of rejection (e.g., Krebs & Adinolfi, 1975; Reis et al., 1982). Among females, the pattern is less uniformly favorable. Although attractive women perceive themselves as more likable, as having greater control of their lives (Adams, 1979), and as higher in self-esteem (e.g., Lerner & Karabenick, 1974), they are also less assertive, less likely to initiate interaction with men, and less trusting of men (Reis et al., 1982) than other women are. The impact of attractiveness on women's assertiveness and initiation seems reasonable, given that greater social desirability makes one the target of another person's initiation more often. Lessened trust also seems plausible, given cultural beliefs about being treated as a "sex object."

In this manner, a lifetime's experience of attractiveness may produce different ego-defensive mechanisms for men and women. Earlier, the social ramifications of fear of rejection and lack of self-confidence were discussed. To the extent that these factors inhibit the pursuit of satisfying social relations, unattractive men are at a clear disadvantage. Beauty has many advantages for females, but the drawbacks are noteworthy. A relative lack of trust in men might inhibit the development of an intimate friendship. Also, to the extent that stereotypic beliefs about the asset value of beauty are salient, a female perceiving herself as pretty might attribute male interest to her looks rather than to other, more intrinsically gratifying personal characteristics. Thus, it might be harder to alter an attractive woman's self-concept with social feedback. Further, if attractive women rely on their appearance to foster social participation, then aging, with the inevitable loss of youthful beauty, may have more negative consequences for their self-concepts and social behavior. Males are less likely to experience this loss, since their attractiveness is less strongly correlated with age, and their social relations seem to be less consciously rooted in the value of appearance.

Compatibility: The Interdependence of Two Selves

In the major part of this discussion, I have focused on the impact of an individual self on interaction patterns. Yet compatibility and incompatibility occur beyond the individual, at the dyadic level. By way of concluding, it might prove useful to comment on how two individuals come to interact in a manner that is gratifying for both. Although behavior in an ongoing relationship might best be examined at the level of the dyad, motivation and satisfaction ultimately reside in the individual members. Two closely related partners may influence each other substantially, resulting in complex patterns of interdependence at the behavioral, affective, and cognitive levels. (Kenny's [in press] recent mathematical model of social relations acknowledges this complexity in that each score has three components: two representing the general behavioral tendencies of each participant, and one representing their unique relationship with each other.) However, the motivation to act and the subjective evaluation of outcomes takes place within the individual.

Compatibility can therefore be regarded as the extent to which the relationship helps both partners fulfill their own needs. These needs can be grouped according to the four functions of the self presented earlier. Instrumental needs are those that pertain to goal attainment, and many of the goals are themselves particular types of social relations (e.g., companionship, intimacy, provisions for a family). Berscheid (in press), for example, makes a compelling case for the affective value of being liked by a significant other. In addition to interpersonal goals, attainment of other sorts of goals in the context of interaction is also important. Buss's (in press) study indicates that activity-related aims can be fulfilled more readily when couples share a social environment. On a more elementary level, if a relationship interferes with valued nonsocial goals, then it would have a negative effect on the person's outcomes. This suggests the importance of interdependence, and in particular, of transformational tendencies. As discussed earlier, these tendencies refer to the manner in which the other's outcomes are taken into account. When both members of a dyad evaluate a situation similarly, conflict is unlikely. Only when they individually disagree would their tendencies to consider the other's point of view matter. Because this is probably the typical case in ongoing relationships, the manner in which couples systematically integrate both perspectives is a major determinant of compatibility. Kelley (1979) notes this central role in arguing that feelings about a partner's transformations may be a more potent reward than the resulting behavior itself. For example, a wife might feel rewarded more by her husband's thoughtfulness in forgoing his preferences and taking the vacation she fancies than she does by the vacation itself.

Dyadic interaction also helps fulfill the knowledge function of the self. Social comparison is one motive for selective affiliation, and, by and large, people prefer others who validate their point of view (Berscheid & Walster, 1974). Moreover, dyadic functioning is enhanced if both individuals perceive reality similarly, since many activities require consensual decisions (e.g., child-rearing practices, time allocation among work, family, and leisure).

Expressive functions of the self are also active in social relations. A person's activities and opinions express his or her unique characteristics and experiences, and it is easier for such expression to occur in tandem with a partner. Perhaps the most obvious implication for compatibility of this factor is its role in allowing friendship to develop out of initial encounters, solely by bringing people with similar interests together. As noted earlier, similarity is traditionally one of the best predictors of reciprocity of liking. Furthermore, the choice of a friend is often one of the most telling reflections of an individual. This is the case because social relations comprise the greater part of people's goal-directed behavior. Consequently, we generally assume—though often in too linear or simplistic a fashion, and with far too little data—that people's selections of friends reveal their inner needs and values. As the old saw goes, "You can tell a lot about a person from the company she keeps."

Finally, the operation of ego-defensive needs also influences harmony in ongoing interaction. Compatibility here will be determined by whether a relationship is consistent with the ego-defensive tendencies of both partners. The element of interdependence arises from each person simultaneously serving as self and as stimulus for the other. If the threat produced by one exceeds the other's capacity to cope, then tension and a lack of satisfaction are likely to result. For example, a casual acquaintance between two people, one fearing intimacy and the other fearing loneliness, is not likely to develop into a deeper, compatible relationship. Compatibility of defenses may also affect initial encounters. If attractive women expect to be approached, and unattractive men fear rejection, then this dyadic combination is not likely to be initiated. Thus, in terms of the ego-defensive functions of the self, compatibility depends on the interplay of two individual tendencies.

Much of what is known about compatibility boils down to two simple considerations: whether two people like each other, and whether they like the way they spend time together. But, of course, therein lies the complexity. The processes described above are numerous, and they apply to a long list of specific traits, attitudes, and behaviors. Their operation is often covert and subtle, but nonetheless powerful. They evolve on the basis of development, experience, and enlightenment. As intricate a subject as the functioning of the self is in a single individual, the interdependence of two persons offers a geometrically expanded set of possibilities. If nothing else, that should make this topic compatible with researchers seeking phenomena to study for years to come.

References

Adams, G. R. (1979). *Beautiful is good: A test of the "kernel of truth" hypothesis.* Unpublished manuscript, Utah State University.

Andersen, S. M., & Bem, S. L. (1981). Sex typing and androgyny in dyadic interaction: Individual differences in responsiveness to physical attractiveness. *Journal of Personality and Social Psychology, 41,* 74–86.

Anderson, C. A. (1980). *Motivational and performance deficits as a function of attributional style.* Unpublished doctoral dissertation, Stanford University.

Aronson, E. (1969). Some antecedents of interpersonal attraction. In W. J. Arnold & D. Levine (Eds.), *Nebraska Symposium on Motivation.* Lincoln, NB: University of Nebraska Press.

Bandura, A. (1982). The psychology of chance encounters and life paths. *American Psychologist, 37,* 747–755.

Bernstein, W. M., Stephenson, B. O., Snyder, M. L., & Wicklund, R. A. (1983). Causal ambiguity and heterosexual affiliation. *Journal of Experimental Social Psychology, 19,* 78–92.

Berscheid, E. (in press). Interpersonal attraction. In G. Lindzey & E. Aronson (Eds.), *Handbook of social psychology.* Reading, MA: Addison-Wesley.

Berscheid, E., & Walster, E. (1974). Physical attractiveness. In L. Berkowitz (Ed.), *Advances in experimental social psychology* (Vol. 7). New York: Academic Press.

Brockner, J. (1983). Low self-esteem and behavioral plasticity: Some implications. In L. Wheeler & P. Shaver (Eds.), *Review of personality and social psychology.* Beverly Hills, CA: Sage.

Brodt, S. E., & Zimbardo, P. G. (1981). Modifying shyness-related social behavior through symptom misattribution. *Journal of Personality and Social Psychology, 41,* 437–449.

Buss, D. M. (in press). Toward a psychology of person-environment (PE) correlation: The role of spouse selection. *Journal of Personality and Social Psychology.*

Cartwright, D., & Zander, A. (1968). *Group dynamics: Research and theory.* New York: Harper & Row.

Cialdini, R. B., Borden, R. J., Thorne, A., Walker, M. R., Freeman, S., & Sloan, L. R. (1976). Basking in reflected glory: Three (football) field studies. *Journal of Personality and Social Psychology, 34,* 366–375.

Cooley, C. H. (1902). *Human nature and the social order.* New York: Harper & Row.

Darley, J. M., & Fazio, R. H. (1980). Expectancy confirmation processes arising in the social interaction sequence. *American Psychologist, 35,* 867–881.

Dermer, M., & Thiel, D. L. (1975). When beauty may fail. *Journal of Personality and Social Psychology, 31,* 1168–1176.

Dion, K. K., Berscheid, E., & Walster, E. (1972). What is beautiful is good. *Journal of Personality and Social Psychology, 24,* 285–290.

Epstein, S. (1979). The stability of behavior: I. On predicting most of the people much of the time. *Journal of Personality and Social Psychology, 37,* 1097–1126.

Erikson, E. (1950). *Childhood and society*. New York: W. W. Norton.

Festinger, L., Schachter, S., & Back, K. (1950). *Social pressures in informal groups: A study of human factors in housing*. Stanford, CA: Stanford University Press.

Fishbein, M., & Ajzen, I. (1975). *Belief, attitude, intention and behavior: An introduction to theory and research*. Reading, MA: Addison-Wesley.

Furman, W., Shaver, P., & Buhrmester, D. (1984). *Social needs, loneliness, and attributional style*. Unpublished manuscript, University of Denver.

Gilligan, C. (1982). *In a different voice*. Cambridge, MA: Harvard University Press.

Goetz, T. E., & Dweck, C. S. (1980). Learned helplessness in social situations. *Journal of Personality and Social Psychology*, *39*, 246–255.

Goldman, W., & Lewis, P. (1977). Beautiful is good: Evidence that the physically attractive are more socially skillful. *Journal of Experimental Social Psychology*, *13*, 125–130.

Gottman, J. M. (1979). *Marital interaction: Experimental investigations*. New York: Academic Press.

Hansson, R. O., Jones, W. H., & Carpenter, B. N. (1984). Relational competence and social support. In P. Shaver (Ed.), *Review of Personality and Social Psychology*. Beverly Hills, CA.: Sage.

Harvey, J. H., Wells, G. L., & Alvarez, M. D. (1978). Attribution in the context of conflict and separation in close relationships. In J. H. Harvey, W. Ickes, & R. F. Kidd (Eds.), *New directions in attribution research*. Hillsdale, NJ: Erlbaum.

Horowitz, L. M., French, R., & Anderson, C. A. (1982). The prototype of a lonely person. In L. A. Peplau & D. Perlman (Eds.) *Loneliness: A sourcebook of current theory, research and therapy*. New York: John Wiley.

Huston, T. L. (1973). Ambiguity of acceptance, social desirability, and dating choice. *Journal of Experimental Social Psychology*, *9*, 32–42.

Ickes, W., & Barnes, R. D. (1977). The role of sex and self-monitoring in unstructural dyadic interactions. *Journal of Personality and Social Psychology*, *35*, 315–330.

Ickes, W., Patterson, M. L., Rajecki, D. W., & Tanford, S. (1982). Behavioral and cognitive consequences of reciprocal versus compensatory responses to preinteraction expectancies. *Social Cognition*, *1*, 160–190.

Jones, W. H. (1982). Loneliness and social behavior. In L. A. Peplau & D. Perlman (Eds.), *Loneliness: A sourcebook of current theory, research and therapy*. New York: Wiley.

Jones, W. H., Hobbs, S. A., & Hockenbury, D. (1982). Loneliness and social skill deficits. *Journal of Personality and Social Psychology*, *42*, 682–689.

Katz, D. (1960). The functional approach to the study of attitude. *Public Opinion Quarterly*, *24*, 163–204.

Kelley, H. H. (1979). *Personal relationships: Their structures and processes*. Hillsdale, NJ: Erlbaum.

Kelley, H. H. (1983). *Option-consequence lists as descriptions of social interdependence*. Unpublished manuscript, University of California, Los Angeles.

Kelley, H. H., & Thibaut, J. W. (1978). *Interpersonal relations: A theory of interdependence*. New York: Wiley.

Kelly, G. A. (1955). *A theory of personality*. New York: W. W. Norton.

Kenny, D. A. (in press). The social relations model for dyadic data structures. In L. Berkowitz (Ed.), *Advances in experimental social psychology*. New York: Academic Press.

Kernis, M. H., & Wheeler, L. (1981). Beautiful friends and ugly strangers: Radiation and contrast effects in perceptions of same-sex pairs. *Personality and Social Psychology Bulletin*, *7*, 617–620.

Kiesler, S. B., & Baral, R. L. (1970). The search for a romantic partner: The effects of self-esteem and physical attractiveness on romantic behavior. In K. L. Gergen & D. Marlowe (Eds.), *Personality and social behavior*, Reading, MA: Addison-Wesley.

Krebs, D., & Adinolfi, A. A. (1975). Physical attractiveness, social relations, and personality style. *Journal of Personality and Social Psychology, 31*, 245–253.

Leary, M. R. (1982). Social anxiety. In L. Wheeler (Ed.), *Review of personality and social psychology*. Beverly Hills, CA: Sage.

Lerner, R. M., & Karabenick, S. (1974). Physical attractiveness, body attitudes, and self-concept in late adolescents. *Journal of Youth and Adolescence, 3*, 307–316.

Levinger, G., & Snoek, J. D. (1972). *Attraction in relationship: A new look at interpersonal attraction*. Morristown, NJ: General Learning Press.

Lewin, K. (1951). *Field theory in social science*. New York: Harper & Row.

Lewinsohn, P. M., Mischel, W., Chaplin, W., & Barton, R. (1980). Social competence and depression: The role of illusory self-perceptions. *Journal of Abnormal Psychology, 89*, 203–212.

Mathes, E. W. (1975). The effects of physical attractiveness and anxiety on heterosexual attraction over a series of five encounters. *Journal of Marriage and the Family, 37*, 769–781.

McGuire, W. J. (1969). The nature of attitudes and attitude change. In G. Lindzey & E. Aronson (Eds.), *Handbook of social psychology (2nd Ed.)*. Reading, MA: Addison-Wesley.

Orvis, B. R., Kelley, H. H., & Butler, D. (1976). Attributional conflict in young couples. In J. H. Harvey, W. Ickes, & R. F. Kidd (Eds.), *New directions in attribution research*. Hillsdale, NJ: Erlbaum.

Peplau, L. A., & Gordon, S. L. (in press). Women and men in love: Sex differences in close heterosexual relationships. In V. E. O'Leary, R. K. Unger, & B. S. Wallston (Eds.), *Women, gender and social psychology*. Hillsdale, NJ: Erlbaum.

Peplau, L. A., Miceli, M., & Morasch, B. (1982). Loneliness and self-evaluation. In A. Peplau & D. Perlman (Eds.), *Loneliness: A sourcebook of research and therapy*. New York: Wiley.

Peplau, L. A., & Perlman, D. (Eds.), (1982). *Loneliness: A sourcebook of current theory, research, and therapy*. New York: Wiley.

Reis, H. T., Nezlek, J., & Wheeler, L. (1980). Physical attractiveness in social interaction. *Journal of Personality and Social Psychology, 38*, 604–617.

Reis, H. T., Wheeler, L., Spiegel, N., Kernis, M. H., Nezlek, J., & Perri, M. (1982). Physical attractiveness in social interaction: II. Why does appearance affect social experience. *Journal of Personality and Social Psychology, 43*, 979–996.

Rostand, E. (1981). *Cyrano de Bergerac* (B. Hooker, Trans.). New York: Bantam.

Rubenstein, C. M., & Shaver, P. (1982). The experience of loneliness. In L. A. Peplau & D. Perlman (Eds.), *Loneliness: A sourcebook of current theory, research and therapy*. New York: Wiley.

Schlenker, B. R., & Leary, M. R. (in press). Social anxiety and self-presentation: A conceptualization and model. *Psychological Bulletin*.

Segal, M. W. (1974). Alphabet and attraction: An unobtrusive measure of the effect of propinquity in a field setting. *Journal of Personality and Social Psychology, 30*, 654–657.

Sigall, H., & Landy, D. (1973). Radiating beauty: The effects of having a physically attractive partner on person perception. *Journal of Personality and Social Psychology, 28*, 218–224.

Snyder, M., & Ickes, W. (in press). Personality and social behavior. In G. Lindzey & E. Aronson (Eds), *Handbook of social psychology*. New York: Random House.

Snyder, M., Tanke, E. D., & Berscheid, E. (1977). Social perception and interpersonal behavior: On the self-fulfilling nature of social stereotypes. *Journal of Personality and Social Psychology, 35*, 656–666.

Sorell, G. T., & Nowak, C. A. (1981). The role of physical attractiveness as a contributor to individual development. In R. Lerner (Ed.), *Individuals as producers of their environment*. New York: Academic Press.

Swann, W. B., Jr. (1983). Self-verification: Bringing social reality into harmony with the self. In J. Suls & A. G. Greenwald (Eds.), *Social psychological perspectives on the self*. Hillsdale, NJ: Erlbaum.

Tesser, A. (1983). *Self-evaluation maintenance processes: Implications for relationships and development*. Unpublished manuscript, University of Georgia.

Tesser, A., Campbell, J., & Smith, M. (1983). *Friendship choice and performance: Self-evaluation maintenance in childhood*. Unpublished manuscript, University of Georgia.

Tesser, A., & Smith, J. (1980). Some effects of friendship and task relevance on helping: You don't always help the one you like. *Journal of Experimental Social Psychology, 16*, 582–590.

Walster, E., Berscheid, E., & Walster, G. W. (1973). New directions in equity research. *Journal of Personality and Social Psychology, 25*, 151–176.

Weiss, R. S. (1974). The provisions of social relationships. In Z. Rubin (Ed.), *Doing unto others*. Englewood Cliffs, NJ: Prentice Hall.

Wheeler, L. (1974). Social comparison and selective affiliation. In T. L. Huston (Ed.), *Foundations of interpersonal attraction*. New York: Academic Press.

Wheeler, L., Reis, H. T., & Nezlek, J. (1983). Loneliness, social interaction, and sex roles. *Journal of Personality and Social Psychology, 45*, 943–953.

Wittenberg, M. T., & Reis, H. T. (1984). Loneliness and social perception in a naturalistic environment. Unpublished manuscript, University of Rochester.

Chapter 10

Marital Compatibility and Mutual Identity Confirmation

Roger M. Knudson

The present chapter focuses upon marital compatibility and the ongoing process of mutual identity confirmation between spouses. The perspective to be developed is rooted fundamentally in the assumption that persons are at all times actively engaged in constructing and maintaining a definition of reality within which they orient themselves and which guides their conduct. Such a definition of reality includes not only a perspective on the "external world," but equally importantly includes a definition of the individual's self or identity. Furthermore, the definition specifies the individual's place in this world so that identity and the overall framework of meaning within which the person attempts to make sense of life are always highly interrelated (Berger & Berger, 1983; Berger & Luckmann, 1966).

Marriage, from this perspective, begins when two individuals, each with a separate definition of reality, attempt to develop a new, shared, "consensually valid" definition of each other, the relationship between them, and the place of their relationship in the broader network of relationships within which they live. The process of forming and maintaining a marriage may thus be thought of as an ongoing negotiation between representatives of two separate realities regarding the exact nature or "reality" of the marriage. Compatibility may then, in turn, be understood in terms of the degree to which, at any given point in time, the parties to this negotiation have achieved and can sustain a shared construction of reality.

The perspective is supported by a wide range of evidence, both experimental and clinical, that will be reviewed below. In addition, as we shall see, the perspective leads to a number of as-yet-unresolved questions about how compatibility is achieved and maintained. It is important from the outset, however, to elaborate a number of additional assumptions that are made throughout the following discussion.

1. A first assumption is that, in constructing reality, people are fundamentally motivated to construe their experience as predictable, consistent, and meaningful. From this perspective, the self may be understood to be those

reality-structuring processes of the individual by means of which predictability, consistency, and meaning are strived for. Such a view of persons is developed by a wide range of theorists including Mead (1934), Fingarette (1963), Perry (1970), and Loevinger (1976), and is well represented in the seminal work of Kegan (1982). It is important to emphasize the *process* nature of the self in this conception. The separation of nouns from verbs in English predisposes us to a view in which nouns "are" things that may act or be acted upon but are separable from action. It is only with conscious effort that we are able to maintain a conception of self as a process rather than as a static thing. As Kegan (1982) puts it, however, ". . . what a human organism organizes is meaning. Thus it is not that a person makes meaning, as much as that the activity of being a person is the activity of meaning-making" (p. 11). Loevinger (1976) expresses this same key idea as follows: "The striving to make experience meaningful is . . . not something that a thing called *ego* does; the striving for meaning is what ego is" (p. 61). Or, in the felicitous language of Gregory Bateson: " 'I' is a verb."

2. A second assumption deserving elaboration is that the self is a social phenomenon in that, rather than being established once and for all, identity depends in an ongoing way upon validating confirmation by the world. In a recent study, Csikszentmihalyi and Rochberg-Halton (1981) document some of the crucial ways that physical objects found in the home play a role in this ongoing process of self-confirmation. Much more widely examined, however, is the role of other persons, particularly the few truly significant others in an individual's life, in providing this confirmation. As Berger and his colleagues (Berger & Kelner, 1964; Berger & Luckmann, 1966) argue, the principal means by which the individual's world view is sustained are the presence, the actions, and particularly the speech of significant others.

Berger and Kelner (1964) assert the following proposition:

> In everyday life . . . it is proper to view the individual's relationship with his significant others as an ongoing conversation. As the latter occurs, it validates over and over the fundamental definitions of reality once entered into, not, of course, so much by explicit articulation, but precisely by taking the definitions silently for granted and conversing about all conceivable matters on this taken-for-granted basis. Through the same conversation the individual is also made capable of adjusting to changing and new social contexts in his biography. In a very fundamental sense it can be said that one converses one's way through life.
>   If we concede these points, we can now state a general sociological proposition: The plausibility and stability of the world, as socially defined, is dependent upon the strength and continuity of significant relationships in which conversations about this world can be continually carried on. Or to put it a little differently: The reality of the world is sustained through conversation with significant others. (pp. 4–5)

It follows as an immediate corollary to this assumption that marriage will be for most persons one of the most significant, if indeed not *the* most significant, conversations through which two individuals maintain, as well as change and develop, their definition of self and world.

3. A third assumption is that marital compatibility should also be perceived as an ongoing process. In conceiving of marriage as reality/identity sustaining conversation, it should be recognized that two separate claims regarding the identity of self and others are simultaneously being proffered. Neither spouse unilaterally defines the relationship. Rather, each spouse's proffered definition remains contingent upon confirmation by the response of the other. Thus, as has been emphasized by Bateson (1972) and others strongly influenced by him (e.g., Haley, 1963; Lederer & Jackson, 1968; Watzlawick, Beavin, & Jackson, 1967), communication involves an *ongoing negotiation* of the definition of the interactants' relationship. In a marriage, then, it is via this negotiation that the competing, and often conflicting, claims made by these two individual definitions of reality must in some way be coordinated. Since the degree of such coordination may vary with changing circumstances as well as with change or development in one or both of the spouses, compatibility is assumed to be changeable rather than fixed. It is not a quality that inheres in a given relationship from first meeting " 'til death do us part."

Interpersonal-Interactionist Approaches

One major area of investigation lending empirical support to the conception of marriage as a mutual identity-confirming conversation is frequently labeled the "interpersonal" or "interactionist" approach to personality. Research in this area not only has documented that individuals are powerfully motivated to maintain a consistent definition of self, but also has provided extensive evidence bearing on the processes by which such consistency is maintained.

A classic formulation is provided by Secord and Backman's (1961, 1965) "interpersonal approach" to personality. Secord and Backman have developed an elaborate calculus of behavioral stability and change involving as components:

1. An aspect of the person's self-concept.
2. The person's perceptions of the person's own behavior related to that aspect of the self-concept.
3. The person's perception of relevant aspects of the other.

In this model, the person seeks to achieve congruency. This state is said to exist when the person *perceives* that the behaviors of both self and other imply a definition of self congruent with the relevant aspects of the person's self-concept. Secord and Backman suggest that stable, patterned relations result from congruency since individuals tend to repeat interactions characterized by congruency and also develop positive feelings toward others with whom they have congruent interactions, this effect serving in turn to perpetuate the relationship.

Swensen (1973) proposes the following process:

> Ordinarily in an interaction, if two people are reasonably mature and if the
> anxiety level is not so high that perception of the other is distorted, the attitude
> and behavior of each toward the other changes. This change is generally in the
> direction of consensual validation. That is, each corrects the view the other has
> of him, until, assuming the relationship becomes intimate, each develops a view
> of the other that is in reasonable harmony with the other's view of himself.
> (p. 44)

Consistent with this model, interpersonal interaction may be viewed as the
sending and receiving of messages at two fundamentally different levels. One
such level is the *content* level, referring to the information conveyed. In addition
to the content, however, there is also a *relationship* level of communication,
which indicates to the recipient how the sender intends the message to be taken.
Relationship level messages are thus *metacommunications* (communications
about content level communications) and are the means by which each
interactant attempts to define the nature of the relationship. As Watzlawick et
al. (1967) put it:

> . . . on a relationship level people do not communicate about facts outside their
> relationship, but offer each other definitions of the relationship and, by
> implication, of themselves. . . . [To] take an arbitrary starting point, person P
> may offer the other, O, a definition of self. P may do this in one or another of
> many possible ways, but whatever and however he may communicate on a
> content level, the prototype of his metacommunication will be "This is how I
> see myself." (p. 83)

Watzlawick et al. add in a footnote that a more complete statement of this
message would be, "This is how I see myself in relation to you in this
situation."

Such a message may be termed a *direct perspective* perception. This is only
one of several levels of perspective involved in "negotiations" concerning how
the relationship is to be defined. There are also *meta-perspective* perceptions
(i.e., the perceptions one person has of the other's direct perspective views).
Continuing the illustration from above, P's response to O would include the
meta-perspective assertion, "This is how I see you seeing me." More complex
yet, *meta-meta-perspective* perceptions may also be involved. For example, O
replies to P, "This is how I see you seeing me seeing you" (Laing, Phillipson, &
Lee, 1966; Watzlawick et al., 1967, p. 90). Each level of perspective is also
associated with a "target" of perception, which in a marital relationship is either
self or spouse. For example, the direct perspective perception stated above
focuses on self (i.e., "This is how I see *myself* in relation to you"). There is a
corresponding direct perspective perception focused on the spouse (i.e., "This is
how I see *you* in relation to me").

With each party to an interaction attempting to define the relationship in
terms of these multilevel perceptions of self and other, one assumes that the
various messages must be in reasonable agreement with one another in order for
the interaction to continue smoothly. P, for example, must communicate to O

that he (P) sees O much as O sees herself. Carson (1969) asserts that such "self-confirming or relationship-confirming interpersonal responses are the coin of the realm" (p. 173) in the development and maintenance of interpersonal relations; and it is the repeated exchange of these communications that eventuates in the recurrent interaction sequences which come to characterize a relationship.

When incongruency (nonconfirmation of identity) is experienced, the Secord and Backman model suggests that efforts to restore congruency will be brought into play. Least likely, perhaps, is that the person's self-concept will change. Instead, Secord and Backman identify five categories of congruency-restoring (and congruency-sustaining) processes:

1. *Cognitive restructuring.* Self may misperceive Other's behavior so as to achieve congruency with aspects of his behavior and self-concept. He may also misinterpret his own behavior so as to achieve maximum congruency with an aspect of his self-concept and his perception of Other.

2. *Selective evaluation.* Self maximizes congruency by evaluating more favorably those interpersonal system components that are congruent; he minimizes incongruence by devaluating those components that are incongruent.

3. *Selective interaction.* Self maximizes engagement in congruent patterns of interpersonal behavior by selecting and interacting with those Others whose behavior requires a minimum change from previously congruent interpersonal situations in which Self has engaged.

4. *Evocation of congruent responses.* Self maintains congruency by developing techniques that evoke congruent responses from other persons.

5. *Congruency by comparison.* When Other confronts Self with an incongruent evaluation, Self may accept the evaluation but minimize the effect of incongruency by attributing the trait to significant others. Thus, its presence in himself is lessened by comparison: he has no more of it or no less of it than other people (1965, p. 97).

Nowhere is the empirical support for the interpersonal-interactionist perspective more comprehensively detailed than in a review by Snyder and Ickes (in press). On the basis of the evidence marshalled in this review, it seems safe to conclude that, in broad outline, the perspective now rests on firm empirical foundations. For each of the congruency-maintaining processes suggested by Secord and Backman (1965), Snyder and Ickes cite several studies demonstrating that such processes are operative in persons' interactions with others. On the basis of this accumulated body of evidence, they conclude that "individuals construct for themselves social worlds that are suited to expressing, maintaining, and acting upon their conceptions of self, their social attitudes, and their characteristic dispositions."

Once this general conclusion is granted, however, we may immediately identify a number of thorny issues for which neither the research to date nor the theoretical model provides any clear guidance. Snyder and Ickes themselves point up one such unresolved issue when they note: "There has been relatively little theoretical work that attempts to specify the conditions in which certain aspects of the self-concept will become salient at the expense of others." This is no small concern. One section of their review of the literature, by way of illustrating just what a puzzle is lurking here, focuses on characteristic dispositions of the self and choice of situations. The conclusion to the section is—not surprisingly in light of the more general conclusion above—that "individuals appear to gravitate actively toward social situations that will foster and encourage the behavioral expression of their own characteristic dispositions and interpersonal orientations." Thus, for example, there have been empirical demonstrations that extraverts seek out "extraverted situations that provide opportunities to engage in extraverted behaviors" (Snyder & Ickes, in press). Similar findings obtain for sensation-seekers choosing sensation-providing situations, authoritarians choosing authoritarian settings, individuals with an internal locus of control gravitating toward situations in which outcomes are determined by skill, and those with an external locus of control choosing situations in which outcomes are more dependent upon chance. In addition, the authors cite studies of situation choice as a function of arousal-seeking, need for achievement, neuroticism, repression-sensitization, self-monitoring, sex-role orientation, social skills, and success/failure orientation.

With this welter of traits "competing" as it were for situational confirmation, the complexity of specifying which disposition or set of dispositions will be most salient becomes apparent. The possibility of selecting a spouse who consistently provides confirmation for some single disposition seems plausible enough. Indeed, for example, there have been demonstrations that individuals high on arousal/stimulation-seeking do in fact select spouses who are themselves high on sensation-seeking (Farley & Davis, 1977; Farley & Bloomquist Mueller, 1978). Attempts to move beyond a single trait, however, as in the literature examining the "complementary needs hypothesis" (Winch, 1958), have failed thus far to provide positive results (Fishbein & Thalen, 1981; Murstein, 1976; Tharp, 1963). We will return to the issue of complementary needs in the following section, but at this juncture let us simply note that we can currently say virtually nothing with confidence about which aspects of the self it will be most important for a spouse to confirm in which situations in order to promote compatibility.

This one issue hardly exhausts, however, the sources of complexity in the ongoing exchange of self and other definitions in the marital conversation. We may ask not only which features of the self most pressingly demand confirmation, but *which self* is most salient. Here again Snyder and Ickes' (in press) review is instructive. Recognizing the widely made distinction between the current self and the individual's ideal self, the authors suggest that individuals may in certain circumstances seek out responses from others that are incongruent with the current self but consistent with the ideal self, thus perhaps promoting change in the former in the direction of the latter. Their examples of such circumstances are along the lines of therapy or education and do not include marriage, but it is a commonplace to observe marriages in which one (or both) spouses idealizes the other and has a clear expectation of being "improved," i.e., changed in the direction of the ideal self, via the relationship.

Not only do individuals sometimes tolerate situations incongruent with the current self in order to change the self, but also they may enter or remain in such situations in order to change the situation or to change other persons. Snyder and Ickes provide as examples such individuals as missionaries, proselytizers, social workers, and revolutionaries who "may have to commit themselves to months or even years of patient work in a situation they abhor in order to effect the intended changes" (Snyder & Ickes, in press). Again they fail, at least apparently, to recognize the aptness of this as a description of not a few marriages! It is a truism that marital partners often have a conception of the "ideal other" which is projected onto the spouse and to which the spouse is expected increasingly to conform.

Beyond these issues of "which disposition" and "which self" there is an even more tangled web of complexities, the "knots" in the Laingian "spiral of reciprocal perspectives" (Laing, 1961, 1971; Laing et al. 1966; Knudson, Sommers, & Golding, 1980). There are, as already noted above, several levels of interpersonal construal: direct, meta, and meta meta. Comparisons within and between these various levels of interpersonal perception of self and other generate a number of different types of congruency/incongruency of perception.

To give some illustration of the complexity here, consider first, for example, the husband's direct perspective perception of self ("I see myself as very independent"). A comparison of this perception with the wife's direct perspective view of the husband ("I see him as very independent") generates an index of *agreement* about the husband. Comparing one person's direct perspective with the other's meta perspective provides an index of *understanding*. Thus the husband's view of himself ("I see myself as independent") might be compared with the wife's meta-perspective view of her husband's self view ("I think he sees himself as quite independent"). Both agreement and understanding are thus *interpersonal* measures based on comparing the husband's perceptions with those of the wife. There is a third set of such interpersonal comparisons, called *realization of understanding*, which involves comparing one person's meta perspective to the other's meta-meta perspective. Continuing the example from above, the wife's meta view ("He sees himself as independent") may be compared with the husband's meta-meta view of himself ("My wife thinks I see myself as somewhat dependent"). In this illustration, then, the husband and wife agree about the husband and the wife understands the husband's view of himself, but the husband fails to realize that he is understood.

In addition to the interpersonal contrasts, there is also a set of *intrapersonal* comparisons. These include indexes of *feeling agreed with* which result from comparing one's own direct and meta-perspective perceptions ("I see myself as independent and I think my wife sees me as independent"). They also include indexes of *feeling understood*, comparing one's own direct perspective of self with one's meta-meta perspective of self ("I see myself as independent, but I think my wife thinks that I see myself as somewhat dependent"). Here the husband feels agreed with, he thinks his wife sees him as he sees himself, yet he does not feel understood, thinking that she does not correctly perceive how he sees himself.

As this example illustrates, not only are there a large number of comparisons, but in addition to being congruent or incongruent, some of these perceptions may be either correct or incorrect. In the example above, the wife understands the husband's view of self, yet the husband fails to realize that he is understood and so feels incorrectly misunderstood. Similarly, one might feel agreed with in the absence of actual agreement or presume understanding exists when in fact there is none.

Given this complex, interlocking network of perspectives, we may return to the matter of obtaining self-confirmatory responses with yet another set of queries. When we speak of the self being confirmed, does this imply only agreement or are understanding and realization of understanding also involved? Furthermore, are intrapersonal comparisons more important than interpersonal ones? Clearly one may feel agreed with either correctly or incorrectly depending upon whether the other actually agrees. The Secord and Backman model appears to emphasize the intrapersonal feeling of agreement, but has less to say about the connection between this feeling and the actual interpersonal state of affairs. Secord and Backman (1965) and Carson (1969) argue that it is the "evocation of congruent responses," the process of actually inducing the other to behave in ways that confirm the self, which appears to be most adaptive for establishing stable congruence.

There do not appear to be clear data to support this claim, however, particularly in the case of long-term relationships such as marriage. Shrauger and Schoeneman (1979), in a review of more than 60 studies, found that perceived agreement between self-concept and how others were believed to see the self was consistently high in most studies, whereas actual interpersonal agreement tended to be lower. As an alternative to evoking congruent responses, couples may develop relationships in which certain "hot" issues known to be potentially conflict-producing are consistently, even rigidly, avoided. Goffman (1959) refers to such an arrangement as a "veneer of consensus" and describes its process as follows:

> . . . there is usually a kind of division of definitional labor. Each participant is allowed to establish the official tentative ruling regarding matters which are vital to him but not immediately important to others. . . . In exchange for this courtesy he remains silent or noncommittal on matters important to others but not immediately important to him. We have then a kind of interactional *modus vivendi*. Together the participants contribute to a single over-all definition of the situation which involves not so much a real agreement as to what exists but rather a real agreement as to whose claims concerning what issues will be temporarily honored. (pp. 9–10)

In sum, however much support the interpersonal-interactionist literature provides for the conception of marriage as a mutual identity-confirmation process, it clearly leads to a set of very complex issues that have at best only begun to be investigated empirically. Moreover, the research reviewed in the interpersonal-interactionist area takes, in general, a relatively narrow focus. In the extreme, marital identity confirmation is studied in terms of single dispositions. This falls considerably short of examining the processes by which two individuals (attempt to) mutually sustain their respective *identities as a whole*. The latter sort of investigation would depend upon first having a scheme for describing each spouse's construction of self and reality *as a whole* and then exploring the "goodness of fit" between different such constructions. It is to some approaches to such description of the individual's overall organization of experience that we turn in the next section.

The Development of the Self

As a potentially powerful supplement to the interpersonal-interactionist literature, we turn now to recently emerging theories of self (or ego) development in the structural-developmental tradition. After many years of intertwined theory building and measurement construction, Loevinger and her colleagues (Loevinger, 1966, 1976; Loevinger & Wessler, 1970; Loevinger, Wessler, & Redmore, 1970) published a detailed description of a set of qualitatively distinct stages in the development of the self, as well as a technique for their measurement. There is a clear logic to the sequence of stages, and each stage has an inner logic of its own as well. A considerable body of research has been generated employing Loevinger's measure, including a set of studies that lend substantial support to its construct validity (Hauser, 1976; Holt, 1980; Loevinger, 1979). Loevinger's account is powerfully complemented by the more recent work of Kegan (1982, 1983). Kegan emphasizes the development of ego in terms of subject-object relations and gives particular attention to the process of transition between stages (Loevinger & Knoll, 1983). Together the two theories provide us with a richly detailed account of a series of levels of self-development, each of which represents a qualitatively distinct construction of reality.

In both Loevinger's and Kegan's models, the development of the self is characterized by both increasing differentiation and increasing integration of one's framework of meaning. As Kegan puts it, "Any stable organismic organization . . . is a kind of 'evolutionary truce' maintaining the current extent of *differentiation from* and *integration with* the whole. Thus every equilibrated level of adaptation represents a kind of temporary compromise between the move toward differentiation and the move toward integration; every developmental era is a new solution to this universal tension." Even more important for our purposes, he adds, "What is being kept dynamically stable . . . is the present distinction between self and other" (Kegan, 1982, p. 413). Thus each stage, as a new construction of reality, constitutes not simply a new relationship of self to other, but a qualitatively new definition of one's conception of self-in-relation-to-other.

Since many readers may be unfamiliar with the work of either Loevinger or Kegan, a digression seems necessary at this point to provide a brief description of the stages of development in these two models. The account given below of these stages is necessarily oversimplified, but it should add some substance to the subsequent discussion of how such stage conceptualizations might be applied.

The earliest period of self-development is labeled by Kegan "Incorporative" and corresponds to Loevinger's I-1 stage, the latter being divided into "presocial" and "symbiotic" phases. The initial task in this stage, given that the infant has no self at birth, is to construct a stable outer world separate from the self—as Kegan puts it, "having [a world] to relate to rather than be embedded in" (1982, p. 79). In the earlier, presocial phase, no distinction is made between animate and inanimate objects. This is followed by the symbiotic phase, in which the child distinguishes the mothering other from other objects but makes no differentiation between the self and the mothering other.

The transition from the I-1 stage to the second stage occurs approximately at the time that language use is acquired. Kegan characterizes such transitions as a process of "emergence from embeddedness" (differentiation). In this process, what was subject ("self") becomes object ("other") from the emerging perspective of the new subject. This requires the formation of a new subject-object relation (integration). In addition, however, there is a kind of repudiation of the former subject. That is, in order to construct a new self, what was previously "me" must become part of the "not-me" (Kegan, 1982, pp. 81–82). We will return to this point in what follows.

At the second stage, Loevinger's I-2, or "Impulsive Stage," and Kegan's "Impulsive Balance," a new construction emerges in which impulses are the predominant factor. In Kegan's useful way of putting it, the transition is from "I *am* my reflexes" to "I am impulses/perceptions; while I *have* my reflexes" (Kegan, p. 79). In other words, a new structure of personal organization has evolved which coordinates or mediates the reflexes, while the individual is now egocentrically preoccupied with satisfying bodily needs. The individual at this stage is concrete, oriented to the present, and essentially passive in the sense that others are viewed mainly as a source of supplies. Others are thus "good" if they are "nice to me," but "bad" if they are "mean to me." The significance of rules is not recognized and impulse control is thus dependent upon external constraint. Indeed, as Kegan points out, nonexpression of the impulses constitutes a threat to the self, which at this stage *is* the impulses.

Loevinger's I-Delta (I-Δ), or "Self Protective Stage," corresponds to Kegan's "Imperial Balance." Loevinger's discussion of the stage tends to emphasize the opportunistic and hedonistic nature of the individual. The individual now understands that there are rules, but the main rule appears to be "don't get caught." Morality is thus purely expedient; getting caught defines an act as wrong. There is an increased ability to delay gratification as the child learns to anticipate short-term rewards and punishments. Constraint has thus moved from the external to the internal, but the control is fragile and used to obtain satisfaction of one's own immediate needs or to avoid punishment. From this perspective, Loevinger suggests, life is viewed as a zero sum game: For someone to win, someone else must lose. Hence one must be "self protective," and one's relationships will be exploitative and manipulative.

Kegan gives relative emphasis here to the emergence of a self conceptualized in terms of roles. Again, what was self has now become other: "I *have* my impulses; I am my roles." The self at this level is able to do its own praising, but remains dependent upon feedback confirming that it is correct. While there is a private world for the individual at this stage, the balance is called "imperial" by Kegan because there is as yet no shared reality.

At the "Conformist Stage" (I3) in Loevinger's system, Kegan's "Interpersonal Balance," the self is identified with the group. One therefore conforms to the rules simply because they are the rules of the group, from whom the self seeks acceptance and approval. Rather than fearing punishment, as in the previous stage, the individual now fears disapproval and shame for violating the norms. As Kegan (1982) puts it, "There is no self independent of the context of 'other people liking' " (p. 96). Since the welfare of the self is identified with that of the group, the individual values niceness, helpfulness, and is concerned with appearance, status, and reputation. Continuing with Kegan's description, at this stage "I have my impulses, but I *am* my relationships." One consequence is that at this stage intimacy is not yet possible. One cannot share one's self in relationship with another since there is no self independent of the relationship.

Loevinger suggests that the transition from I3 to I4, the "Self-Aware Transitional Level" (I3/4), is the probable modal level for adults in this society. She further suggests that since it is apparently a stable position for adult character, it should be regarded as transitional only in a theoretical sense. At this level, the individual has to some extent differentiated a self from the group, but the individual has not yet replaced the group standards with self-evaluated ones. There is an increase is self-awareness, though this is still expressed in banal terms. Alternative possibilities in situations are recognized in a beginning way as is an understanding of psychological causation. Loevinger suggests that at this level, while the perception of individual differences is more differentiated than at the Conformist Stage, where differences in terms of traits are generally not perceived, one tends to conceptualize individual differences largely in terms of "pseudotraits" such as norms, virtues, or moods.

The next stage is Loevinger's "Conscientious Stage" (I4), Kegan's "Institutional Balance." At this stage the individual is guided by self-chosen, self-evaluated inner rules rather than those of the group. There is at this stage a sense of self-as-self. The individual can say "I have my relationships" rather than "I am my relationships." At this stage, Kegan suggests, "I am my career" (or "I am my ideology, my institution"). The person at this stage is marked by a new capacity for independence and aspires to achievement defined now in terms of self-chosen standards. The inner life is more richly differentiated and the capacity for self-criticism emerges. Correspondingly, feelings and motives, rather than actions, become the terms in which relationships are experienced. Others too are perceived as differing along many trait dimensions rather than only in broad stereotypes. Interpersonal mutuality is possible at this stage, and

Loevinger characterizes the individual at this stage as "his brother's keeper," someone who feels a strong sense of responsibility for others. Significantly, emotional conflict is recognized at this stage as internal. As Kegan points out, however, since the self at this stage has evolved as a set of organizing structures for the regulation of such conflict, inner conflict is not tolerable at this stage. Thus the person at this stage is preoccupied with thoughts of duty, obligation, and performance, and must be vigilant in regard to feelings, particularly the affiliative and erotic, which might upset the smooth operation of the institution that the self is.

Loevinger terms the next stage the "Autonomous Stage (I5), Kegan the "Interindividual Balance." This stage is distinguished by the individual's capacity to both acknowledge and cope with inner conflict as well as by respect for the autonomy of others, the latter's individual differences now being not only perceived but valued. There is a recognition, moreover, of the ways in which autonomy is limited and the consequent inevitability of mutual interdependence in relationships. The capacity for intimacy emerges at this level, since the person now has a self ("I have a self or selves" at I5 vs. "I am my self" at I4) to share with another.

Finally, Loevinger identifies a highest stage, the "Integrated Stage" (I6), which is of mainly theoretical interest since persons at this stage are very rarely found.

To the extent that an individual's characteristic functioning may be located in one of these stages, the question we may then return to is how compatible that individual's construction of reality might be with that of another person. Are individuals at a given stage generally compatible only with others at that same stage or is there a range of stages within which a potentially compatible other might be found?

A number of intriguing and potentially researchable questions follow immediately from this way of framing the general compatibility issue. The literature discussed above concerning interpersonal perception in marriage—for example, that including Laing's complex accounts of levels of reciprocal perspective taking—has proceeded without attention to the developmental capacity of either spouse for meaningful perspective taking. The theoretical models of Loevinger and Kegan suggest that individuals at different stages will differ not only in terms of their ability to take the perspective of the other, but also in terms of their access to their own experience and consequent ability to articulate their own perspective to the other. Thus, for example, prior to asking whether an individual's meta-level or meta-meta-level perceptions are accurate or inaccurate, we would ask whether the individual had the capacity to take a meta- or meta-meta-level perspective on self or other.

As another example, one might well return to Secord and Backman's list of congruence-maintaining processes to explore their relationship to stage of development. Here the issues would include not merely whether individuals at a given developmental stage characteristically employ certain of these congruence-maintaining processes, but also the more complex question of how two individuals coordinate their separate efforts to maintain congruency.

To elaborate briefly only one final example of how taking developmental level into account may permit the recasting of old questions, we might again consider that hoary standby of the marital literature, the complementary-needs hypothesis.

The theory of complementary needs (Winch, 1958) states that persons choose partners whose needs complement their own pattern of needs. The theory has generated considerable research even though reviewers have repeatedly concluded that no clear-cut support of complementarity has yet been produced (Fishbein & Thalen, 1981; Murstein, 1976; Tharp, 1963). A recurrent criticism has been that no rationale has ever been provided for stating which needs will be complementary. On the face of it, it is implausible that all couples in a large group study will evidence complementarity on exactly the same needs. Recently, Meissner (1978), in his overview of the current psychoanalytic perspective on marriage, has suggested that the "complementary needs" hypothesis should be revised to take into account the developmental level of the members of the dyad.

The models of self-development detailed by Loevinger and Kegan appear especially promising candidates for such research since they permit us to predict what the salient needs at each developmental stage will be. While space does not permit a complete account of the predicted relationships between needs for all possible pairings of levels of self-development in marriage partners, a brief sketch of what the theory suggests for two such pairings follows: First consider the union of two persons at what Loevinger calls the Conformist stage (I3), Kegan's "Interpersonal Balance." This relationship is then contrasted with a marriage of two individuals at the Conscientious Stage (I4), Kegan's "Institutional Balance."

For an I3–I3 couple, the theory suggests that the crucial concern is with a sense of belonging. Thus we would expect to find these couples exhibiting highly similar levels of those needs that pertain to group membership and group stability. In terms of Murray's (1938) list of needs, we might expect such couples to evidence complementarity for such needs as Affiliation, Defendance, Impulsivity, Change, Cognitive Structure, and Sentience. We might also expect that at this stage conformity to sex-role stereotypes would produce highly negative correlations for Aggression and Nurturance, with husbands high on Aggression but low on Nurturance and vice versa for the wives.

For the I4–I4 couple, an entirely different set of predictions follows from the theory. Here the leading concerns include achievement of long-term goals and ideals, duty, responsibility for others, and greater mutuality in relationships. Thus we would expect complementarity for such Murray needs as Achievement, Endurance, Social Recognition, Dominance, Autonomy, and Understanding. In contrast to the I3–I3 couples, we might now expect positive correlations for Aggression and Nurturance.

(Parenthetically, my students and I now have data which suggest that when engaged couples are grouped by developmental level, clear and theoretically consistent patterns of need complementarity do emerge. The number of couples studied for many of the possible pairings of level of development is as yet quite small, so the findings remain merely suggestive at this point.)

In addition to their potential for guiding our understanding of how well any two individuals' constructions of reality might mesh with each other, the structural-developmental theories also raise important questions about the processes of growth in a marriage. As already noted, Kegan's analysis of the process of transition from one stage to the next suggests that the emergence of a new self requires in a sense a rejection of the old self. One says in effect, "I am a new person, a new 'me.'" By implication, "I am no longer the person I used to be; I am *not* the old 'me.'" However, since self and context as viewed in these models are never genuinely separable, to reject the old me is also to reject the context in relation to which the old me was constructed. The critical issue for marital compatibility is that one's spouse is a major part of that context. Thus, in order to develop, the individual rejects both "old me" and spouse, and the question that arises is how the marriage may survive such periods of transition. How, that is, may the marriage endure the separation from the old pattern of relationship until such time as a reintegration—the establishment of a new pattern of relating—is achieved?

Empirical investigation of these last questions has not, to my knowledge, even begun. The question of what holds a marriage together during periods of individual growth by one or both of the spouses, however, leads us to ask whether there may be an even broader context within which to view the spouses' attempts to construct a mutually compatible reality. We turn to one such broader context in the final section of this chapter.

A Brief Glance at Mutual Reality Maintenance in Transgenerational Perspective

Promising as we believe the avenues for research just suggested are for developing our understanding of the mutual identity-confirmation processes in marriage, there is one additional body of literature that deserves attention. This is the ever-more-rapidly-expanding family therapy literature. In this predominantly clinically oriented literature, it has been a commonplace assumption for decades that marriage represents an attempt to join together not merely two individuals' constructions of reality but in fact *two families'* constructions. This is quite consistent with our initial assumption of the self as a social process if one recognizes that the others upon whom one's definition of self depends most crucially for confirmation prior to marriage are generally the members of one's family of origin. At the same time, the importance of this perspective often seems to be obscured by an overemphasis on processes of differentiation from the family of origin and a corresponding deemphasis or even failure to recognize the accompanying processes of (re)integration with the family of origin. From many accounts, one might conclude that the respective families of origin of two spouses are relevant to understanding the marriage only to the extent that one or both spouses has failed to satisfactorily differentiate from (individuate, separate from, leave behind) the family.

An alternative perspective, suggested perhaps most strongly by "transgenerational" approaches to marital and family therapy such as those of Boszormenyi-Nagy (Boszormenyi-Nagy, 1972, 1974, 1979; Boszormenyi-Nagy & Spark, 1973; Boszormenyi-Nagy & Krasner, 1980; Boszormenyi-Nagy & Ulrich, 1980), Framo (1982), and Stierlin (1977, 1981; Stierlin, Rucker-Embden, Wetzel, & Wirsching, 1980), is that the separate realities being negotiated through a couple's marriage are in ongoing ways *family* constructions of reality. Particularly instructive in this regard, we believe, is the suggestion by Boszormenyi-Nagy (e.g., Boszormenyi-Nagy & Ulrich, 1980) that beyond the personal and the transactional dimensions of analysis, there is a dimension of *ethical* connectedness of individuals to their family of origin. This dimension of relationship has been discussed by Boszormenyi-Nagy in terms of the "transgenerational ledger of entitlements" and by Stierlin in terms of the closely related concept of "delegation" and the important distinction between "missions" and roles. Each of these concepts is briefly discussed in the following.

From the perspective of Boszormenyi-Nagy, the family is an *ongoing* social system that is held together in a fundamental, dynamic way by a ledger of transgenerational accountability (Boszormenyi-Nagy, 1974). This ledger is based on the existentially given fact that issues of mutual obligation and entitlement exist in every relationship. As Karpel and Strauss (1983) point out, these issues are the source of the most basic questions that members of a family may address to one another: "Can I count on you? Can I trust you? Will you be fair to me? Will I get what I deserve from you? Will you stand by me? Will I be fair to you? Will I give you what you deserve?" (Karpel & Strauss, 1983, p. 30). The "principle of equitability" asserts further that each individual is entitled to have his or her interests considered in a way that is fair from a multilateral perspective in which each person considers not only self-interests but the interests of all others as well (Boszormenyi-Nagy & Ulrich, 1980, p. 160).

In effect, for each member of the family, the ledger is a regularly updated record of both the benefits and the injuries given and received for which the individual remains personally accountable. At the level of the family as a whole, the intergenerational ledger sums these individual accounts of entitlement and indebtedness and so reflects the long-term relative balance of fairness between and among members of the family. It thus indexes the trustworthiness of the family relationships. Trustworthiness is never a static quality but is the product of ongoing efforts to repay obligations and acknowledge the legitimate claims of others. As Boszormenyi-Nagy puts it:

Genuine trustworthinerss cannot be imposed by either forcible oppression or by manipulative skill. It has to be deserved or merited on the basis of a multilateral input or investment on the part of all partners. The balance of relational fairness depends on a relatively symmetrical investment of trust in caring mutuality. (1979, p. 4)

The ledger, as described by Boszormenyi-Nagy and Ulrich (1980), represents the convergence of two processes: legacies and the accumulation of merits.

Legacies (from the latin *lex*: low and *ligare*: to bind) are the specific set of expectations and obligations imposed upon the individual by virtue of his or her unique position in the family constellation. While some may be only between parent and child, many will derive from accounts that have been unsettled over several generations. Particularly when the family ledger contains such obligations unfulfilled across the generations, there is the potential for exploitation of individual family members. The second process contributing to the ledger is the accumulation by the individual of merit, which is earned via contributing to the other's welfare, acknowledging the claims of the other, and fulfilling obligations. This too is a relational balance factor which Boszormenyi-Nagy emphasizes is not contained in any single individual's mind, but is determined by the equity of the give-and-take between persons.

While many of the implications of this approach to understanding families cannot be pursued here, one set of implications is especially important for our purposes. These implications follow from the delegation principle which Stierlin (1977) links to the legacies construct.

Delegation, Stierlin (1977) points out, derives from the Latin *delagare*, which had two related meanings: (1) to send out and (2) to entrust with a mission. Thus Stierlin distinguishes incisively between the process of role socialization by the family and the process of *mission delegation*. The distinction is well expressed, Stierlin further suggests, in the contrast between "I play a role" implying "I am an actor performing a part" versus "I fulfill a mission" with its implication of both obligation and commitment (Stierlin, 1977, p. 276).

It is the delegation process, far more than the role-socialization process, that is rooted in the family's efforts to settle accounts and (re)establish balance of the ledger. A mission thus carries an ethical imperative that role performance does not.

The idea that marriage is a union not of two individuals but of the representatives from two families takes on new meaning in light of the distinction between role and mission. Of course, agreement or disagreement over appropriate role performance is certainly an ingredient in marital compatibility. The concept of family-delegated mission(s) suggests, however, another level of analysis, a level at which each spouse will be required to share in the other's *lifelong ethical responsibility* to contribute to the balance of the family of origin's ledgers. There are, we may note, three ledgers that become intertwined in the marriage: the ledger from the husband's family of origin, the ledger from the wife's family of origin, and the newly created ledger reflecting the emerging balances of entitlement and indebtedness between the husband and wife in their own marriage and between them as parents and their children as the latter are born and grow up. This network of multilateral obligations constitutes what Boszormenyi-Nagy has termed "the deep ethical context" (1979, p. 4) of family relationships. Trustworthiness at this level constitutes the most basic resource of family relationships; its absence, Boszormenyi-Nagy asserts, constitutes "the primary pathogenic condition of human life" (1979, p. 4).

Compatibility between spouses, then, may be seen as most deeply rooted at this level in the ethical dynamics of the relationship. Crucially important is the issue of how to equitably deal with competing equally valid claims. As three-generational families become commonplace and increased life expectancies lead to a growing number of four-generational families, such issues become increasingly complex. Likewise, in the growing numbers of second marriages, the obligations that remain after divorce as well as those created by remarriage are not only complex but often seemingly mutually contradictory. Yet it is upon the couple's ability to establish and maintain, with each other and with the members of their families, ethically valid solutions to these sorts of dilemmas that the compatibility of their marriage will be founded. Whatever form the new reality created by a couple should take, unless it establishes an order experienced as trustworthy by all those who participate in it, it is unlikely to endure, much less provide the relational resources for growth and self-fulfillment which all of us look to our marriages to provide.

References

Bateson, G. (1972). *Steps to an ecology of mind.* San Francisco: Chandler.

Berger, B., & Berger, P. (1983). *The war over the family.* Garden City, NY: Doubleday/Anchor.

Berger, P., & Kellner, H. (1964). Marriage and the construction of reality. *Diogenes, 46,* 1–24.

Berger, P., & Luckmann, T. (1966). *The social construction of reality.* Garden City, NY: Doubleday/Anchor.

Boszormenyi-Nagy, I. (1972). Loyalty implications of the transference model in psychotherapy. *Archives of General Psychiatry, 27,* 374–380.

Boszormenyi-Nagy, I. (1974). Ethical and practical implications of intergenerational family therapy. *Psychotherapy and Psychosomatics, 24,* 261–268.

Boszormenyi-Nagy, I. (1979). Contextual therapy: Therapeutic leverages in mobilizing trust. In *The American family.* Philadelphia: Smith, Kline, and French Company.

Boszormenyi-Nagy, I., & Krasner, B. R. (1980). Trust-based therapy: A contextual approach. *American Journal of Psychiatry, 137,* 767–775.

Boszormenyi-Nagy, I., & Spark, G. (1973). *Invisible loyalties: Reciprocity in intergenerational family therapy.* New York: Harper & Row.

Boszormenyi-Nagy, I., & Ulrich, D. (1980). Contextual family therapy. In A. S. Gurman & D. P. Kniskern (Eds.), *Handbook of family therapy.* New York: Brunner/Mazel.

Carson, R. C. (1969). *Interaction concepts of personality.* Chicago: Aldine.

Csikszentmihalyi, M., & Rochberg-Halton, E. (1981). *The meanings of things: Domestic symbols and self.* Cambridge: Cambridge University Press.

Farley, F. H., & Bloomquist Mueller, C. (1978). Arousal, personality, and assortative mating in marriage: Generalizability and cross-cultural factors. *Journal of Sex and Marital Therapy, 4,* 50–53.

Farley, F. H., & Davis, S. A. (1977). Arousal, personality, and assortative mating in marriage. *Journal of Sex and Marital Therapy, 3,* 122–127.

Fingarette, H. (1963). *The self in transformation: Psychoanalysis, philosophy, and the life of the spirit.* New York: Basic Books.

Fishbein, M. D., & Thalen, M. H. (1981). Psychological factors in mate selection and marital satisfaction: A review. *JSAS Catalog of Selected Documents in Psychology, 9,* 84.

Framo, J. L. (1982). *Explorations in marital and family therapy: Selected papers of James L. Framo.* New York: Springer-Verlag.

Goffman, E. (1959). *The presentation of self in everyday life.* Garden City, NY: Doubleday/Anchor.

Haley, J. (1963). *Strategies of psychotherapy.* New York: Grune and Stratton.

Hauser, S. T. (1976). Loevinger's model and measure of ego development: A critical review. *Psychological Bulletin, 83,* 928–955.

Holt, R. P. (1980). Loevinger's measure of ego development: Reliability and national norms for male and female short forms. *Journal of Personality and Social Psychology, 39,* 909–920.

Karpel, M. A., & Strauss, E. S. (1983). *Family evaluation.* New York: Gardner Press.

Kegan, R. (1982). *The evolving self.* Cambridge, MA: Harvard University Press.

Kegan, R. (1983). A neo-Piagetian approach to object relations. In B. Lee & G. G. Noam (Eds.), *Developmental approaches to the self.* New York: Plenum.

Knudson, R. M., Somers, A., & Golding, S. L. (1980). Interpersonal perception and mode of resolution in marital conflict. *Journal of Personality and Social Psychology, 38,* 751–763.

Laing, R. D. (1961). *Self and others.* London: Tavistock.

Laing, R. D. (1971). *Knots.* New York: Pantheon.

Laing, R. D., Phillipson, H., & Lee, A. R. (1966). *Interpersonal perception: A theory and a method of research.* New York: Springer-Verlag.

Lederer, W. J., & Jackson, D. D. (1968). *Mirages of marriage.* New York: Norton.

Loevinger, J. (1966). The meaning and measurement of ego development. *American Psychologist, 21,* 195–206.

Loevinger, J. (1976). *Ego development.* San Francisco: Jossey-Bass.

Loevinger, J. (1979). Construct validity of the sentence completion test of ego development. *Applied Psychological Measurement, 3,* 281–311.

Loevinger, J., & Knoll, E. (1983). Personality: Stages, traits, and the self. *Annual Review of Psychology, 34,* 195–222.

Loevinger, J., & Wessler, R. (1970). *Measuring ego development* (Vol. 1). San Francisco: Jossey-Bass.

Loevinger, J., Wessler, R., & Redmore, C. (1970). *Measuring ego development* (Vol. 2). San Francisco: Jossey-Bass.

Mead, G. H. (1934). *Mind, self, and society.* Chicago: University of Chicago Press.

Meissner, W. W. (1978). The conceptualization of marriage and family dynamics from a psychoanalytic perspective. In T. J. Paolino & B. S. McCrady (Eds.), *Marriage and marital therapy from three perspectives: Psychoanalytic, behavioral, and systems theory.* New York: Brunner/Mazel.

Murray, H. A. (1938). *Explorations in personality.* New York: Oxford.

Murstein, B. I. (1976). *Who will marry whom? Theories and research in marital choice.* New York: Springer Publishing Company.

Perry, W. (1970). *Intellectual and ethical development in the college years.* New York: Holt, Rinehart and Winston.

Secord, P. F., & Backman, C. W. (1961). Personality theory and the problem of stability and change in individual behavior: An interpersonal approach. *Psychological Review, 68*, 21–32.

Secord, P. F., & Backman, C. W. (1965). An interpersonal approach to personality. In B. A. Maher (Ed.), *Progress in experimental personality research* (Vol. 2). New York: Academic Press.

Shrauger, J. S., & Schoeneman, T. J. (1979). Symbolic interactionist view of self-concept: Through the looking glass darkly. *Psychological Bulletin, 86*, 549–573.

Snyder, M., & Ickes, W. (in press). Personality and social behavior. In G. Lindzey & E. Aronson (Eds.), *Handbook of social psychology* (3rd ed.). Boston: Addison-Wesley.

Stierlin, H. (1977). *Psychoanalysis and family therapy.* New York: Aronson.

Stierlin, H. (1981). *Separating parents and adolescents: Individuation in the family.* New York: Aronson.

Stierlin, H., Rucker-Embden, I., Wetzel, N., & Wirsching, M. (1980). *The first interview with the family.* New York: Brunner/Mazel.

Swensen, C. H. (1973). *Introduction to interpersonal relations.* Glenview, IL: Scott, Foresman.

Tharp, R. G. (1963). Psychological patterning on marriage. *Psychological Bulletin, 60*, 97–117.

Watzlawick, P., Beavin, J. H., & Jackson, D. D. (1967). *Pragmatics of human communication.* New York: Norton.

Winch, R. F. (1958). *Mate selection: A study of complementary needs.* New York: Harper and Brothers.

Chapter 11

Cognitive Interdependence in Close Relationships

Daniel M. Wegner, Toni Giuliano, and Paula T. Hertel

This chapter is concerned with the thinking processes of the intimate dyad. So, although we will focus from time to time on the thinking processes of the individual—as they influence and are influenced by the relationship with another person—our prime interest is in thinking as it occurs at the *dyadic* level. This may be dangerous territory for inquiry. After all, this topic resembles one that has, for many years now, represented something of a "black hole" in the social sciences—the study of the group mind. For good reasons, the early practice of drawing an analogy between the mind of the individual and the cognitive operations of the group has long been avoided, and references to the group mind in contemporary literature have dwindled to a smattering of wisecracks.

Why, then, would we want to examine cognitive interdependence in close relationships? Quite simply, we believe that much could be learned about intimacy in this enterprise, and that a treatment of this topic, enlightened by the errors of past analyses, is now possible. The debate on the group mind has receded into history sufficiently that its major points can be appreciated, and at the same time, we find new realms of theoretical sophistication in psychology regarding the operation of the individual mind. With this background, we believe it is possible to frame a notion somewhat akin to the "group mind"—and to use it to conceptualize how people in close relationships may depend on each other for acquiring, remembering, and generating knowledge.

Interdependent Cognition

Interdependence is the hallmark of intimacy. Although we are all interdependent to a certain degree, people in close relationships lead lives that are intertwined to the extreme. Certainly, the behaviors they enact, the emotions they feel, and the goals they pursue are woven in an intricate web (Davis, 1973; Kelley, Berscheid, Christensen, Harvey, Huston, Levinger, McClintock,

Peplau, & Peterson, 1983). But on hearing even the simplest conversation between intimates, it becomes remarkably apparent that their thoughts, too, are interconnected. Together, they think about things in ways they would not alone. The idea that is central in our analysis of such cognitive interdependence is what we term *transactive memory*. As will become evident, we find this concept more clearly definable and, ultimately, more useful than kindred concepts that populate the history of social psychology. As a preamble to our ideas on transactive memory, we discuss the group mind notion and its pitfalls. We then turn to a concern with the basic properties and processes of transactive memory.

A Brief History of the Group Mind

The analogy between the individual mind and the social system was extra-ordinarily popular among 19th-century social theorists. Traceable in large part to the philosophies of Hegel (1807/1910) and Rousseau (1767), the tendency to draw this analogy gave rise to a variety of related ideas—the group mind, for one, but also notions of "collective consciousness," the "*Volksgeist*," "collec-tive representations," the "mind of the crowd," and the "collective un-conscious." Trading on the analogy was serious business at the time, and few eyebrows were raised when Herbert Spencer (1876) even went so far as to compare different brain structures to the different houses of the British Parliament.

This line of theorizing was represented in various ways in subsequent writings in sociology (e.g., Durkheim, 1915), psychology (e.g., Wundt, 1910/1916), and psychoanalysis (e.g., Jung, 1922), and formed a major theoretical rallying point for the young science of social psychology (e.g., LeBon, 1903; McDougall, 1920; Ross, 1908). In each case, some variation on the "group mind" was used as a characterization of a property of the group. Principally, this idea was used to capture *within-group similarity*; a group contains individuals with similar attitudes, similar understandings of the world, shared language, and otherwise seemingly unitary outlooks. Also, the group mind could represent *social agency*; the group seemed to behave and think as a unit, an agent that could have dealings with other agents, reflect on itself, change its mind, and in many other ways resemble an individual. Finally, the group mind provided a way of appreciating the Gestalt or *configural* properties of groups; the group's actions might not be reducible to those of particular individuals, and the idea of the group mind offered theorists a repository for these emergent, irreducible events.

The problem in all of this, it should come as no surprise, was that the group mind did not have a group body. Thus, there was the immediate question of where these properties of the group mind resided (see, e.g., MacIver, 1921). The more critical feature of this problem, however, was that the group mind had no voice. How would one ask the group mind a question? Would one ask the leader? In this case, the group mind is a useless concept, for its workings should be entirely observable in the leader's reports. Would one take a vote? In this case, the group mind concept is again valueless, for it becomes less exact than the vote itself. Would one simply observe the group? This solution was suggested by Sir Frederic Bartlett (1932), who argued that to catch the group mind at work (at least as this mind was being conceptualized by theorists at the time), one would need to observe its voiceless embodiment—the group as a whole—and find the group doing something collectively that had not been suggested or preordained by any of its individual members. Obviously, at this point the idea of the group mind loses touch with reality. For the group mind's thought to be observed in this way, a group action specifically *not* associated with any observable means of communication would be necessary.

Unfortunately, most of the proponents of the concept of a group mind eventually reached just this impasse. Many commentators, Bartlett included, pointed out that a group mind could be explained by the overlap of individual minds entering and leaving the group over time. The continuity and homogeneity of the group's outlook could merely be a matter of the continuous communication of group attitudes, knowledge, and customs to new members. This kind of explanation seemed entirely too common and uninteresting to group mind theorists, though, because it seemed to challenge the supposition that the group mind should be different from the minds of group members. Without this difference, of course, the group mind becomes but a superfluous addendum to the analysis of individual minds. So, in the pursuit of some unique, emergent quality of group mental life, theorists began turning to obscure avenues of explanation. Jung (1922) and Pareto (1935) sought the origins of the group mind in genetics, a topic so little understood that it could be safely adduced, along with occasional references to the supernatural, as an explanation of like-mindedness among group members. Even McDougall (1920) briefly entertained the hypothesis that telepathic communication formed the foundation of group mental life. With magic as its last recourse, the group mind concept slipped ignominiously into the history of social psychology, and by its absence ordained the study of the individual as the prime focus of the field (cf. Allport, 1968; Knowles, 1982).

Is there anything in the idea worth preserving? Along with the early theorists, we believe that an emphasis on the difference between group and individual mental processes is an indispensable part of the definition of each. At the same time, we believe that the early theorists made two critical errors in defining the group mind that must be rectified for the furtherance of any similar idea. First, we propose that identifying the group mind with the *similar mental processes and contents of group members* is an error. As will be seen, we believe that such similarity may be both a cause and a consequence of group mental operations— but it is *not* the defining quality of such operations themselves. Second, we suggest that sidestepping *communication processes among group members* in the analysis of group mental life is an error. We hope to show that such processes are the very center of group thought, and that far from cheapening or demystifying the unique properties of the group mind, these communication processes operate to *produce* the distinction between the group mind and the minds of individual members. This said, it is still the case that the "group mind" terminology is steeped, perhaps forever, in error and opprobrium. Thus, we abandon such traditional language at this point, hoping to establish a more verifiable (and falsifiable) analysis by means of the idea of transactive memory.

The Nature of Transactive Memory

Ordinarily, psychologists think of memory as an individual's store of knowledge, along with the processes whereby that knowledge is constructed, organized, and accessed. So, it is fair to say that we are studying "memory" when we are concerned with how knowledge gets into the person's mind, how it is arranged in the context of other knowledge when it gets there, and how it is retrieved for later use. At this broad level of definition, our conception of transactive memory is not much different from the notion of individual memory. With transactive memory, we are concerned with how knowledge enters the dyad, is organized within it, and is made available for subsequent use by it. This analogical leap is a reasonable one as long as we restrict ourselves to considering the *functional equivalence* of individual and transactive memory. Both kinds of memory can be characterized as systems that, according to general system theory (von Bertalanffy, 1968), may show rough parallels in their modes of operation. Our interest is in processes that occur when the transactive memory system is called upon to perform some function for the group—a function that the individual memory system might reasonably be called upon to perform for the person.

Transactive memory can be defined in terms of two components: (1) an organized store of knowledge that is contained entirely in the individual memory systems of the group members, and (2) a set of knowledge-relevant transactive processes that occur among group members. Stated more colloquially, we envision transactive memory to be a combination of individual minds and the communication among them. This definition recognizes explicitly that transactive memory must be understood as a name for the interplay of knowledge, and that this interplay, no matter how complex, is always capable of being analyzed in terms of communicative events that have individual sources and individual recipients. By this definition, then, the thought processes of transactive memory are completely observable. The various communications that pass between intimates are, in principle, observable by outside observers— just as each intimate can observe the communications of the other. Using this line of interpretation, we recognize that the observable interaction between individuals entails not only the transfer of knowledge, but the construction of a knowledge-acquiring, knowledge-holding, and knowledge-using system that is greater than the sum of its individual member systems.

Let us consider a simple example to bring these ideas down to earth. Suppose we are spending an evening with Rudy and Lulu, a couple married for several years. Lulu is in another room for the moment, and we happen to ask Rudy where they got the wonderful stuffed Canadian goose on the mantle. He says, "We were in British Columbia . . . ," and then bellows, "Lulu! What was the name of that place where we got the goose?" Lulu returns to the room to say that it was near Kelowna or Penticton—somewhere along Lake Okanogan. Rudy says, "Yes, in that area with all the fruit stands." Lulu finally makes the identification: Peachland. In all of this, the various ideas that Rudy and Lulu exchange lead them through their individual memories. In a process of interactive cueing, they move sequentially toward the retrieval of a memory trace, the existence of which is known to both of them. And it is just possible that, without each other, neither Rudy nor Lulu could have produced the item. This is not the only process of transactive memory. Although we will speak of interactive cueing again, it is just one of a variety of communication processes that operate on knowledge in the dyad. Transactive processes can occur during the intake of information by the dyad, they can occur after information is stored and so modify the stored information, and they can occur during retrieval.

The successful operation of these processes is dependent, however, on the formation of a transactive memory structure—an organizational scheme that connects the knowledge held by each individual to the knowledge held by the other. It is common in theorizing about the thoughts and memories of individuals to posit an organizational scheme that allows the person to connect thoughts with one another—retrieving one when the other is encountered, and so forth. In a dyad, this scheme is complicated somewhat by the fact that the individual memory stores are physically separated. Yet it is perfectly reasonable to say that one partner may know, at least to a degree, what is in the other's memory. Thus, one's memory is "connected" to the other's, and it is possible to consider how information is arranged in the dyadic system as a whole. A transactive memory structure thus can be said to reside in the memories of both individuals—when they are considered as a combined system.

We should point out here that transactive processes and structures are not exclusively the province of intimate dyads. We can envision these things occurring as well in pairs of people who have just met, or even in groups of people larger than the dyad. At the extreme, one might attribute these processes and organizational capacities to whole societies, and so make transactive memory into a synonym for *culture*. Our conceptualization stops short of these extensions for two reasons. First, we hesitate to extend these ideas to larger groups because the analysis quickly becomes unwieldy; our framework for understanding transactive memory would need to expand geometrically as additional individuals were added to the system. Second, we refrain from applying this analysis to nonintimate relations for the simple reason that, in such dyads, there is not as much to be remembered. Close dyads share a wealth of information unique to the dyad, and use it to operate as a unit. More distant dyads, in turn, engage in transactive processes only infrequently—and in the case of a first and only encounter, do so only once. Such pairs will thus not have a very rich organizational scheme for information they hold. We find the notion of transactive memory most apt, in sum, for the analysis of cognitive interdependence in intimate dyads.

Our subsequent discussion of transactive memory in this chapter is fashioned to coincide with the process-structure distinction. We begin by considering the processes involved in the everyday operation of transactive memory. Here, we examine the phases of knowledge processing standardly recognized in cognitive psychology—encoding, storage, and retrieval—to determine how they occur in transactive memory. The second general section examines the nature of the organizational structure used for the storage of information in the dyad. The structure of stored information *across* the two individual memories will be examined, with a view toward determining how this organization impinges on the group's mental operations. The final section concentrates on the role of transactive memory, both process and structure, in the life of the dyad. We consider how such memory may contribute to compatibility or incompatibility in relationships, and how an individual's personal memory may be influenced by membership in a transactive system.

Transactive Memory Processes

Communication is the transfer of information. When communication takes place between people, we might say that information is transferred from one memory to another. However, when the dyadic group is conceptualized as having one memory system, interpersonal communication in the dyad comes to mean the transfer of information *within* memory. We believe that multiple transfers can occur as the dyad encodes information, as it holds information in storage, and as it retrieves information—and that such transfers can make each of these processes somewhat different from its counterpart occurring at the individual level.

Transactive Encoding

Obviously, dyads do not have their sense organs in common. The physical and social environment thus must be taken in by each person separately. Social theorists have repeatedly noted, though, that an individual's perceptions can be channeled in social ways. Many have observed, for example, that one partner might empathize with another and see the world from the other's "point of view." Alternatively, cognitive constructions of a "group perspective" may be developed by both partners that lend a certain commonality to their intake of information (see Wegner & Giuliano, 1982). These social influences on encoding, however, are best understood as effects on the individual. How does the *dyad* encode information?

When partners encounter some event and encode it privately in their individual memories, they may discuss it along the way. And though we might commonly think of such a discussion as a "rehash," a mere echo of the original perceived event, there is reason to think that it could be much more. After all, whereas experiencing an event can be accomplished quite passively, discussing an event requires active processing of the information—and the generation of ideas relevant to the event. Several demonstrations of an individual memory phenomenon called the "generation effect" indicate that people will often remember information they have generated better than information they have simply experienced (Johnson & Raye, 1981; Slamecka & Graf, 1978). So, for instance, one might remember the number 37 better if one had been presented with "$14 + 23 = ?$" than if one had merely been presented with "37." Partners who talk over an event, generating information along the way, might thus come to an encoded verbal representation of the event that supplants their original, individual encoding.

The influence of the generation effect could, of course, take many forms. Ordinarily, it should lead partners to remember their own contributions to dyadic discussions better than the contributions of their partners. This phenomenon has been observed in several studies (e.g., Ross & Sicoly, 1979). But the generation effect could also contribute to one's memory for group-generated information. When a couple observes some event—say, a wedding—they may develop somewhat disparate initial encodings. Each will understand that it was indeed a wedding; but only one may encode the fact that the father of the bride left the reception in a huff; the other might notice instead the odd, cardboard-like flavor of the wedding cake. Their whispered chat during all this could lead them to infer that the bride's father was upset by the strange cake. Because this interpretation was generated by the group, both partners will have thus encoded the group's understanding of the events. Their chat could thus revise history for the group, leaving both with stored memories of the father angry over a sorry cake.

Evidence from another domain of cognitive research leads to a similar point. One of the most powerful determinants of encoding in individual memory is the degree to which the incoming information is semantically elaborated (e.g., Anderson & Reder, 1979). To elaborate incoming information is simply to draw inferences from it and consider its meaning in relation to other information. This is precisely what happens in dyadic communications about events. Partners often talk about things they have experienced as individuals or as a group. They may speak about each other's behavior, about the behavior of others they both know, about the day's events, and so on. In such discussions, it is probable that those particular events or behaviors relevant to the dyad will be discussed at length. They will be tied to other items of knowledge and, in the process, will become more elaborately encoded—and thus more likely to be available for later retrieval.

To the extent that generative or elaborative processes are effortful, or require careful thinking, their effects could be strengthened yet further. Encoding processes that are effortful for the individual typically lead to enhanced memory (Tyler, Hertel, McCallum, & Ellis, 1979; Walker, Jones, & Mar, 1983). When a couple engages in an argument, cognitive effort may be required for each person to understand what the other is saying and for each to convey a personal point of view. Such effort on the part of both could also be necessary when one partner is merely trying to teach the other something. It is the shared experience of argument, decision-making, or careful analysis that will be remembered more readily when the communication is effortful. After all, couples more frequently remember their "talks" than their routine dinner conversations.

These transactive encoding processes could conceivably lead a dyad to understand events in highly idiosyncratic and private ways. Their discussions could go far afield, linking events to knowledge that, while strongly relevant to the dyad, is embedded primarily in the dyad's known history or anticipated future. The partners' memories of the encoded events themselves could be changed dramatically by the tenor of their discussions, sometimes to the point of losing touch with the initial realities the partners perceived. To some degree, such departures from originally encoded experience might be corrected by the partners' discussions of events with individuals outside the relationship; such outsiders would serve to introduce a perspective on events that is uninformed of the dyad's concerns, and that therefore might help to modify memory of the events. But many experiences are discussed only within the relationship, and these are thus destined to be encoded in ways that may make them more relevant to the dyad's concerns than to the realities from which they derived.

Transactive Storage and Modification

Once information gets into transactive memory, it is stored, perhaps later to be retrieved. One important concern regarding storage is the way in which the information is organized: Does one person have it, do both have it, or are there yet other possible arrangements? We take up these questions later when we explore the structure of transactive memory. At this point, we wish to dwell a bit on a different aspect of storage—its dynamic properties. One of the most intriguing lessons of cognitive research on individual information storage is that there is no guarantee that information will be retrieved from storage in the same form in which it was originally encoded. Knowledge apparently can be modified, even as it resides in memory.

Studies of individual memory by Loftus and her colleagues (e.g., Loftus, Miller, & Burns, 1978) have shown that memory for previously perceived events can be influenced by subsequent events. Subjects who saw slides of an auto accident, for instance, and who were then asked questions containing erroneous implications about perceptual details of the accident, later falsely recognized slides depicting the implied details. Research by Hertel (1982) indicates that such modifications can also occur in an individual's memories for his or her cognitive and affective reactions to events. Information obtained well after an event can lead one to remember differently one's reaction to the event. Errors such as these may occur because information encountered subsequent to an event is integrated into one's stored representation of the event.

A straightforward extrapolation of these phenomena would suggest that similar modifications should occur in a dyad's memory. When the couple encodes an initial event and then witnesses subsequent events relevant to it, both partners may be subject to parallel individual memory modification, and their shared memory representation might thus be modified. We believe, though, that memory modification in the dyad could be quite a bit more complicated (and interesting) because of iterative effects that occur in the course of dyadic communication. Suppose, for instance, that a female partner is surprised at a remark made by her neighbor. The neighbor called over the fence to say that "Your dog is doing a fine job of fertilizing my lawn." The male partner may have originally observed the surprise reaction, but later saw the neighbor kick the dog. Still later he might consequently misrecall that the female partner had reacted with anger to the neighbor's remark. And quite conceivably, she could come to agree with her mate's report of her anger. Through a chain of communications, both partners may modify their memory of prior events, making this memory consistent with subsequent information that the dyad has obtained.

In a broader sense, the modification of transactive memory may be an inevitable part of communication. This is because internally represented thoughts may need to be modified by the individual to make them communicable. In studies of the social transmission of information, for example, Bartlett (1932) found that sending a story through a chain of people has certain predictable effects on the nature of the story. It usually becomes a simplified, short-hand account that resolves or drops any inconsistencies that were present in the original version. A transmitted story thus resembles the protocols people give when they recall information after storing it for a long time. Communicating information between people, like storing it within one person over time, yields pared-down, "schematic" representations of the information. Of course, something like this could occur merely through sloppiness in communication. But such social degeneration of information could also be the result of modifications that one individual makes in information for the purpose of transmitting it to another. The simple fact that communicated information must be put into words, for example, requires that it be discrete as opposed to continuous (Freyd, 1983). The speaker's injunction to make things understandable to a listener, in turn, may strip away inconsistencies and irrelevancies (cf. Zajonc, 1960).

These simplification processes, in combination with the aforementioned modifiability of the individual's memory, produce a highly modifiable transactive memory. One might, for example, tell a partner about a childhood incident in which one was frightened by a duck. The experience itself could not be transmitted, of course, only the words. Even these would necessarily be brief, failing to cover the wealth of detail one originally encoded, and perhaps missing much of the context of the episode as well. Later on, one's partner might then recount this experience, probably in new words and with different emphases (e.g., "There's a duck, dear; run and hide!"). One could fail at this time to point out the difference between this version and one's original experience. One might even "play along," elaborating the memory by telling a story of a violent and deranged waterfowl. As a consequence of repeated interactions of this kind over time, both partners could end up sharing in memory a skeletal and decidedly incorrect version of the duck story that one had encoded quite veridically at the outset. The impact of social transmission that Bartlett observed might not need long chains of people passing rumor; it could develop through the repeated cycling of information between just two partners.

Transactive Retrieval

Retrieval is usually considered the final step of memory processing—the point at which the effectiveness of encoding and storage become known. Therefore, when a couple is called upon to retrieve information, their success will depend in large part on the nature of the transactive processes that have enabled them to encode and store the information. But even at this final step, further transactive processing may occur.

As we noted earlier, the couple might search their transactive memory in a sequential, interactive process; one partner retrieves an item of information relevant to the target item, the other uses this item as a cue for yet another item, and so on. Such interactive cueing is often observed when a couple has a shared "tip of the tongue" experience. In trying to remember the name of a film, for instance, one person might volunteer that "It begins with a B." The other might say, "Ooh, ooh, wait, wait," and then later mention that the film was a comedy with a Faustian theme. This image might help the first to recall that Dudley Moore's costar wore a red satin "devil" suit in part of the movie. Eventually, one or the other partner might finally hit on the name.

It is unclear whether this transactive process would usually result in more successful retrieval than would parallel individual retrieval attempts. It is fairly obvious, though, that interactive cueing of this kind could often lead to quite different retrieved information. Members of a close relationship could easily lead each other astray, along lines of inquiry that both recognize as reasonable—but which are better characterized as flights of fancy than actual recollections. At other times, however, they might have the opposite tendency, keeping each other "in line" as they pursue the target item. The predominant consequences of interactive cueing are presently unknown, for as far as we can discern, no research has been conducted to examine this process.

There is another aspect of dyadic retrieval, however, that has a somewhat more proximal empirical base. Cognitive psychologists have investigated the effects of the *context* of individual retrieval attempts, finding that people are better able to retrieve information in contexts that resemble the ones in which the information was encoded (Tulving & Thomson, 1973). In our view, this finding suggests that individuals who have encoded information in the presence of an intimate will subsequently retrieve the information more effectively if the intimate is present during retrieval. The intimate partner provides an important context for everything one encodes for the duration of the relationship. On hearing a tune and humming it with one's partner, on gossiping about friends with the partner, and even on watching TV with the partner, there is a special context for encoded information. Later retrieval should be facilitated when the partner is present. In short, the family that encodes together should retrieve together.

This phenomenon may be responsible for the ease with which past pains in relationships are brought to mind in the presence of the other. Similarly, joys shared in the past may be retrieved primarily when the other is present. Moments shared with other people—whether old flames, parents, or even fellow workers—should be relatively more difficult to retrieve in the presence of one's current intimate partner. In a way, the co-presence of partners produces in each a special mindset, a readiness to remember the information first encountered in the same group setting.

Transactive Memory Structures

To build a transactive memory is to acquire a set of communication processes whereby two minds can work as one. To a certain degree, then, any couple that shares a common culture and language has a rudimentary transactive memory. The couple possesses a common set of background assumptions (cf. Cicourel, 1974; Clark & Haviland, 1977; Grice, 1975; Lewis, 1969) that they share as well with everyone else in their neighborhood. Thus, they begin a relationship, even as strangers, with a certain sense that each knows something that the other knows. This basic sense, however, can grow in quite different directions as changes occur in the *organization* of the couple's transactive memory. For one, as intimates become acquainted, they can each come to understand that there are certain areas one knows that the other does not; this change is the *differentiation* of transactive structure. And also, as they become acquainted, they can develop a sharing of unique knowledge that moves beyond the basic sharing that occurs between strangers in a culture; this change is the *integration* of transactive structure. Both differentiation and integration are processes, of course, and so might be classed with the various transactive memory processes we have discussed thus far. Each can occur during encoding, storage, and retrieval phases of transactive knowledge processing. These processes, however, impinge most clearly on the location of information in transactive memory, and so are considered here as we address the topic of transactive structure.

Differentiated Structure

A person beginning a close relationship will enjoy a background of familiarity with certain things—family, friends, special interests and skills—to which the partner has never been privy. And while the partner may guess that the person has such realms of knowledge, and even make fairly good estimates of its nature and extensity, the partner does not really know for sure what exists in the person's individual store of knowledge. So, if the partner was having trouble, say, tying a knot, he or she would not be able to say with much confidence whether the person would be of any assistance in this enterprise. Knowing that the person had been involved in scouting as a child, however, could offer an important key. Such a fact about a person is not likely to be immediately evident, of course, and so must be acquired at some point for the partner to have any success in taking advantage of the person's expertise.

As each member of the pair becomes more cognizant of the specialties of the other, the dyad's memory as a whole grows in differentiation. To describe this feature of transactive memory more explicitly, it is useful to introduce distinctions regarding three kinds of information a person may hold in personal memory: higher-order information, lower-order information, and location information. One can think of *higher-order information* as the topic, theme, or gist of some set of items of *lower-order information*. So, for example, the term "fruit" can be considered higher-order information with respect to terms such as "apple," "orange," and "banana." By the same token, "what George said" can be regarded as higher-order information than the actual words he spoke. Distinctions like this one have been made frequently in cognitive psychology, sometimes using terms such as "schema" to refer to higher-order information. We include the distinction here to indicate simply that there are degrees of the specificity of knowledge represented in memory. *Location information*, in turn, is information as to where any piece of higher-order or lower-order information may be found. In a sense, it is an "address." When one knows that information on Kant's *Critique of pure reason* can be found in a library, in a philosopher friend's memory, or even in one's own memory, one has location information about Kant's *Critique*.

Communication in the dyad may lead to the transmission of any of the three types of information. Certainly, one might tell a partner of the existence of some higher-order knowledge (e.g., "Sam and Wanda were at the party") or some lower-order knowledge (e.g., "He said he was ashamed of her when she got drunk"). One would also convey location knowledge in saying these things, for one would immediately give away that these facts were available in one's own memory. It is possible, however, that one could convey location information with regard to higher-order knowledge without conveying the lower-order knowledge associated with it. Simply noting that "I heard what Sam and Wanda were talking about at the party," for example, would communicate to one's partner that one held both higher and lower orders of information in one's memory—but it would not reveal the nature of the lower-order information. In making such communications, one would contribute to the differentiation of the transactive memory structure.

A differentiated transactive structure, in this light, is one that contains mutual higher-order and location information, but reserves lower-order information for one or the other partner's memory alone. Knowledge of general topics is shared by both persons, and with the simultaneous sharing of location information, each person obtains a personal "directory" for knowledge held by the dyad. The individual in this system may have any amount of lower-order information. At the extreme, one person might hold *all* the lower-order information available to the dyad. This person could find anything that the dyad knows merely by accessing his or her own memory. The other partner, in turn, would have similar access—but would be required to access the *other's* memory, through communication, to obtain any item of lower-order information. More commonly, of course, couples develop differentiated structures in which each partner holds some proportion of the lower-order information accessible to the dyad.

The development of differentiated transactive memory is an important effect of the reciprocal self-disclosure that usually accompanies relationship formation. Couples typically begin a relationship by revealing information about themselves to each other; starting with fairly mundane surface information, they move on to exchange more private knowledge of themselves (cf. Altman & Taylor, 1973; Archer, 1980). And, when they are trading knowledge of their life goals, personality traits, emotional investments, or other personal qualities, they are also building the differentiation of their transactive memory. Each fact about the self that is revealed to the other lends the other a sense of one's expertise and experience. Thus, self-disclosure regularly transmits higher-order information. Sometimes, much lower-order information is conveyed as well—such as when one tells the other not only that one "likes Greek food," but also details one's recipes for several Greek dishes. More commonly, though, these lower-order details will not be communicated. The other will have sufficient access to them merely by knowing the higher-order information and the location information that is communicated "piggyback" with it. In the future, when the pair wants Greek food, the expert in this domain will be expected by both parties to supply the needed lower-order information.

The differentiated organization of knowledge in the dyad makes for an efficient transactive memory. For all those domains of knowledge that the group might need to know—but that neither individual must know alone—differentiated organization eases the work of one or the other partner. Lower-order information can be communicated on a "need to know" basis, as when the Greek gourmet can direct the cooking of a mutually prepared meal, noting ingredients and steps to the other as they are necessary. And the partner who does not know the details of knowledge in a particular domain can nevertheless be confident that the dyad will be effective. To a degree, couples may even undertake to manage their affairs such that transactive memory will be differentiated. They may decide, for instance, that one should have responsibility for the group's checkbook balancing, that the other should have the responsibility for knowing about a child's progress at school, and so on. In this way, they avoid wasting transactive memory space on duplication of lower-order information. Indeed, such efficiency may often be produced in a relationship by virtue of partners' prior adoption of the specialized knowledge responsibilities that accompany sex roles, occupational roles, and the like.

Differentiated structure may be efficient, but it also may lead to certain problems in information management in the relationship. For instance, as higher-order information and location information are shared, and the transactive memory thus becomes differentiated and increasingly capable of accessing unshared domains of lower-order information, we would expect an increase in the pair's confidence in their knowledge in general. Organization of information regularly leads individuals toward greater confidence that they know the information (see, e.g., Pratt, Luszcz, Mackenzie-Keating, & Manning, 1982). With differentiation, each person would become increasingly likely to believe that the group would be able to retrieve most any information—though the person might not have any access to the information in personal memory. The female who has specialized in knowledge linked most strongly with her stereotypic sex role, for instance, may enter a relationship with a male and experience an immediate surge in confidence that her dyad will be able to fix a leaky faucet, play poker, or otherwise employ knowledge domains usually associated with the male sex role. Such presumptions may often be unfounded.

Differentiated structure could also lead on occasion to confusions regarding one's own knowledge. The "feeling of knowing" (Hart, 1967) might very well arise not only for domains that one indeed knows, but also for domains of information known only by virtue of transactive memory. If one partner keeps track of phone numbers, for example, the other may never have experienced any difficulty in retrieving a needed number. All the other must do is ask. On encountering a setting in which the partner is not present, however, the other could fail to appreciate the absence of the usual information source—and so continue to assume that the phone numbers are immediately available. Such confusions should be particularly intrusive in the very settings that usually allow for transactions between partners. At home, in familiar recreational contexts, and the like, it seldom happens that one is stranded without the other. Thus, much lower-order information may be taken for granted. Only when one must be alone will these assumptions be examined, and the extent of one's personal hold on information be discovered.

It is perhaps fortunate that transactive memory is never entirely differentiated. A conversation between partners who share little or no lower-order information, for instance, could be tiresome indeed. They would chat about generalities, but because they held no lower-order information in common, they could never get into the details of their individual domains of knowledge. They could reiterate their personal qualities and interests, delving again into the process of reciprocal self-disclosure. But eventually, they would have little new to say to each other—every higher-order item of knowledge would already be shared, and conversations would deteriorate rapidly (e.g., one says "I know every batting average in the American League"; the other says "I know you do, dear"). Given the human tendency to converse primarily about the new (Grice,

1975), such conversations would probably not even occur. An entirely differentiated transactive memory cannot be all that characterizes the mental operations of the dyad.

Integrated Structure

Woody Allen's short story "The Whore of Mensa" comments satirically on an important counterpoint to differentiated memory in relationships—the tendency to share knowledge. The male protagonist in this story encounters an educated young woman who, for a price, is willing to come over and discuss any subject. The man laments his wife's inability to satisfy his yearnings for mentally stimulating conversation; the young woman, he learns, gives good Proust. He is enthralled and spends large sums on her.

People in close relationships are not satisfied with differentiated transactive knowledge. They commonly try to find higher-order topics that are shared, and then trade their lower-order information on these topics, often at length. The remarkable feature of such sharing is that it frequently leads to new knowledge for both partners. Imagine, for example, that a couple is leaving a party. At different times, they each talked to Tex. The male notes that Tex was depressed this evening; he stared at the floor and barely talked. The female says that Tex was not at all depressed; in fact, she saw him for quite a while early in the party and he seemed unusually frisky and friendly. The male recalls that Tex said he was thinking about separating from his wife. And in short order, the couple reaches a conclusion: Tex was flirting with the female and feeling embarrassed about it in the presence of the male. This conclusion represents new knowledge which, independent of its correctness, is a qualitative departure from the knowledge held by both partners alone. Together, they unveiled their individual sets of lower-order information on the higher-order topic of "Tex" and, in so doing, reached a new, integrated understanding of that topic.

The development of integrated transactive memory structures is analogous to the development of integrated individual memory structures (cf. Hayes-Roth & Thorndyke, 1979). As in the case of individuals, dyads are likely to establish integrated structures when they learn that they hold related information in two locations. In the dyad, however, these locations will be the two individual memories. The partners who both know about "Tex at the party," about "Proust," or about any other higher-order topic are likely to explore their respective sets of lower-order information through communication. Such communication may, at times, lead only to the realization that the partners have unknowingly shared identical sets of lower-order information; their discussion leads them to understand that they held duplicate knowledge prior to the interaction. But also at times, communication can reveal that each partner has a somewhat different set of lower-order items classed under the same higher-order topic. When this happens, their transactive memory is ripe for the development of an integrated structure. They can put together their views of the topic to develop a shared higher-order conception.

The development of integrated transactive structures has been investigated in various guises in social psychology. Studies of group decision making (e.g., Davis, 1980; Kerr, 1981) and "social combination" processes (e.g., Laughlin, 1980) have examined the means by which groups reach integrated understandings of topics on the basis of initially disparate individual understandings. As a rule, these lines of research have indicated that groups strive toward a unity of conceptualization, a general view held by all members. This is certainly consistent with our notion of integrated transactive structure. With the present analytical framework, however, it is possible to go one step further in understanding such processes.

We believe that the press toward integrated structure in transactive memory is responsible for the unique, emergent properties of group mental life. What the group-mind theorists were searching for can be found in the seemingly "magical" transformations that occur when disparate sets of information are combined into new ideas. One partner may bring one set of knowledge, the other may bring something different, and they then may experience some conflict. But in the healthy dyadic relationship, this conflict does not necessarily lead to the dissolution of the group. Rather, it energizes the integration process, leading the couple to seek some new conceptualization that will transform their conflict into agreement. The new formulation that is reached, however, does not just promote compromise between partners. It also makes the group think about something in a way that the individuals would not; the group's viewpoint becomes unique.

This press toward unique integrations in close dyads was the topic of research by Giuliano and Wegner (1983). Their experiment was planned to induce a cohesive group state in some heterosexual pairs but not in others, and to compare the interactions of such "close" and "distant" couples during dyadic problem-solving. The problems posed to these couples were designed to resemble a typical hurdle that dyads must overcome repeatedly in daily life: The couple encounters an opportunity to retrieve a single target item from transactive memory—when each member has already retrieved a candidate item from personal memory. This could happen, say, when a couple must decide on a restaurant to visit when each partner has already thought of a possibility. The hypothesis was that "distant" couples, when faced with disagreement, would opt for the personal choice of one or the other partner; "close" couples, in contrast, were expected to use such conflict as a stimulus to invent a new, group-generated possibility. Quite simply, unique integrations would evolve in the face of conflict—but only when the couple had been induced to feel "close."

For each experimental session, two or three male/female pairs were randomly formed from a group of people who did not know one another. Pairs were taken to a room, seated at adjacent chairs facing opposite directions, and given several yards of yarn neatly wrapped around a stick. Partners were instructed to wrap the yarn around the two of them, exchange places, and wrap the yarn back onto the stick—all of this in privacy, but without talking. This exercise was designed to induce cohesiveness between partners. Out of concern that initial negative impressions might hinder the effectiveness of the cohesiveness manipulation, the researchers had subjects anonymously rate their initial impressions of other group members immediately after everyone arrived for the session. Strong negative first impressions (prior to pairing) on the part of at least one partner led to the exclusion of three pairs from the analyses. This left a total of 16 couples to become wrapped up with each other.

The problems to be solved were patterned after TV's "Family Feud" game show. The problems consisted of 20 categories (e.g., a place to get pizza; bedtime for college students) and subjects were instructed to predict the response most commonly given by 100 undergraduates who had been polled for their opinions. In order to compare individual and group memory structures, subjects completed this questionnaire twice. They filled out the questionnaire for the first time individually, just prior to being paired for the cohesiveness manipulation. The questionnaire was filled out by pairs the second time. Half of the subjects filled out the questionnaire with their original (yarn) partners. For the other half, opposite-sex pairs were formed such that the problems were solved by partners who had not experienced the cohesiveness manipulation together. The couples were tape-recorded as they discussed the categories and tried to develop a single answer that was ostensibly to be scored for popularity against the responses of the polled undergraduates.

The typical procedure that the couples followed in selecting their final response started with each partner revealing his or her earlier response. Then, they could adopt one of several strategies for determining a dyadic response. When partners initially had a similar individual response (about 24% of the time), the dyadic response could be the same as their individual responses or it could be different. Not surprisingly, couples whose individual responses coincided chose that response for the dyad on 99% of their agreements. A much wider range of options was available when individual responses differed. In many cases, partners in this situation would simply decide on the individual response of one or the other. For questions calling for a qualitative response (e.g., naming a musical group), this often happened—producing a lop-sided compromise between partners. For questions of a quantitative nature (e.g., the average age that females marry for the first time), responses were often derived from the two individual responses as a true compromise between them. When the ages of 18 and 22 were given, for instance, 20 would be the dyad's response.

The final possible strategy when individual responses differed was to develop a dyadic response that resembled neither individual response. Such strategies were, of course, of special interest in this research. Rather than signifying some sort of compromise between individual responses, they represent unique integrations—choices that are unpredictable from individual responses. This happened for questions requiring either quantitative or qualitative responses. In the case of a qualitative item such as "Name a good candy bar," for instance, individual responses of Mars and Milky Way might yield a group response of

Snickers. In the case of a quantitative item such as "Average bedtime for college students," individual responses of 12:00 AM and 1:00 AM might produce a group response of 1:30 AM.

In the parlance of transactive memory, the couples in this study were placed in the position of having a differentiated transactive structure. Each time they discussed their initial personal responses, and so communicated lower-order information, they took the chance of discovering differentiation—different items of information coming from the different personal repositories of transactive memory. Their strategies for resolving these discrepancies could then be of two types: *compromise strategies*, which were derived from individual structures, or *integrative strategies*, which were independent of them. The first type includes group responses that originated with one or the other partner, as well as responses derived as midpoints between the two individual responses. Strategies independent of individual responses are integrative in nature and uniquely represent the dyad.

The results revealed that integrative responses were the strategy of choice when "close" couples had to resolve differences. The correlations between the overall number of initial differences of "close" partners and their use of integrative strategies revealed a significant relationship for both qualitative questions [$r(16) = .43$, $p < .05$] and quantitative questions [$r(16) = .54$, $p < .02$]. For "distant" partners, the corresponding correlations revealed no significant relationships [$r(16) = .18$, qualitative; $r(16) = .00$, quantitative]. For "close" couples, therefore, initial discrepancies resulted in increased attempts to unite the pair with unique, group-generated solutions. The use of these unique integrations was not promoted by the degree of initial discrepancy for previously unpaired subjects. These results support the idea of a transactive communication process in a close dyad that prompts integrative communication whenever discrepancies in lower-order information are revealed.

The tape-recordings of the problem-solving sessions showed that couples sometimes verbally prearranged their strategy. Several couples clearly set out a "turn-taking" strategy for resolving discrepancies—"We'll do yours this time and mine next." It is interesting that commentators on group conflict resolution have often argued that such turn-taking is a primary cooperative response to incompatible individual preferences (e.g., Kelley & Thibaut, 1978). The present results suggest that this is *not* the strategy of choice in close dyads. Close couples faced with differentiated knowledge structures often do not verbalize their integrative strategy, but it seems to be pursued with a certain automaticity and urgency. Asked to "Name a magazine," for example, a couple produced individual responses of *People* and *Newsweek*—and instead of discussing these at all, immediately turned to suggesting other possibilities. In some couples, the unique integration was then a good answer (e.g., *Time*); in others, the final choice was less appropriate (e.g., *Playboy*). But in all cases of integration, even though the integrative strategy was not verbally formulated by the dyad, it was rapidly adopted, cutting short the discussion of individual preferences.

As a final note on this research, it should be pointed out that the findings signal only a first step in the investigation of transactive processes. Clearly, the results pertain primarily to ad hoc couples who have been made to feel close, not partners in ongoing close relationships. Moreover, the findings arose in a context quite unlike experiments on integrative processes in memory. Because the emphasis of this research was on transactive processes, and not on the accuracy of group retrieval of presented information, it was not necessary to develop these findings in the context of a standard memory paradigm. Until further inquiry is made into the production of unique, integrative knowledge in close relationships, the generality of the observed phenomenon—and its impact on the accuracy of transactive memory—can be anticipated only in broad outline.

Transactive Memory and Intimate Life

We have hinted at an important idea in various ways throughout the chapter, and it is time now to make the proposition explicit: A transactive memory is a fundamental component of all close relationships. We believe that the potential for transactive memory makes intimacy among humans possible, allowing them to develop a form of interdependence with each other that is both lasting and continually in flux. The immediate implications of this idea are twofold: First, a dysfunctional or incompletely operative transactive memory in a relationship should portend the breakdown of closeness; second, many of the personal difficulties that accompany the dissolution of an intimate dyad should be traceable to the absence of transactive memory. Here, we explore each of these implications in turn.

Pathologies of Transactive Memory

Perhaps the most obvious failure of transactive memory would occur if it never got started. Intimacy could not develop in a relationship if the couple never talked, if their initial personal knowledge stores were so disjunct that they had no common ground to discuss, or if they could find no way to put together their ideas into new, group-generated thoughts. In terms of our theoretical analysis, then, intimacy could fail because of a lack of transactive processes, a lack of higher-order linkages that would allow differentiation, or a lack of common lower-order knowledge stores that would allow integration.

Once a relationship has formed, the processes of communication, differentiation, and integration must continue. We suspect that communication will halt in an ongoing partnership, bringing that partnership to an end, when a gross imbalance occurs between the processes of differentiation and integration. As we have already pointed out, extreme differentiation can bring an end to a relationship because it fails to promote the sharing of lower-order information and the consequent development of unique, group-generated knowledge. But just as intimates with too much differentiation can be troubled by too little interdependence, intimates with too much integration can become the victims of too much interdependence.

The danger of integration in transactive memory is its capacity to produce *duplication*. At the outset of the integration process, partners discuss differentially known details about a common topic. In sharing these details, they develop a similar understanding based on modified details from both persons. This similar understanding will lead each partner to remember only some of the details that originated in his or her own memory, and will also convert the higher-order knowledge of the topic held by each partner into a single, shared form. A couple that only conducts integrative discussions will, over time, make many of the higher-order and lower-order integrations that are available across their fields of differentiated knowledge. Such wholesale integration could lead to the very same state of boredom with the relationship that is reached through extreme differentiation; there is nothing new to talk about. Furthermore, if each partner has the same knowledge that the other has, they each *independently* have access to the group memory. Neither partner requires access to the other for any information, and they thus can become functionally isolated from each other despite their apparent closeness. Contrary to its intended effect, then, integration can render transactive memory redundant and unnecessary to the individual.

Duplication can precipitate relationship problems in yet another way. Once considerable duplication has occurred—say, in a couple living together for several years—it can be assumed by partners that their own knowledge is sufficient for group-relevant judgments. In essence, each assumes that the duplication with the other is complete. A partner might know, for example, that the group typically goes out to dinner on Saturday nights, and even knows what the other will prefer to order. Thus, the partner will have no qualms about making dinner reservations for Saturday, unbeknownst to the other, and might even go on to order the entire meal for two while the other is still looking at the menu. This strategy will succeed if the duplication is indeed total—down to the partner's knowledge of which of the six available soups the other will prefer. The strategy will fail, however, whenever duplication is incomplete for any reason. The other may have been exposed to information suggesting that a new soup would be best, or perhaps has just decided that the usual is becoming tiresome. The partner who assumes duplication will often fail to pick up on such subtleties, and in the end, will be rightfully accused of "taking for granted" the other.

In essence, duplication and the assumption of duplication threaten a relationship when partners believe that they know each other very well. This potential endpoint of integrative processes reminds us, then, that couples can become too familiar. It is only when couples do not share everything they know—or at least believe that not everything is shared—that their relationship will be open for further discussion and development. To a degree, this ironic twist in relationship development seems to pose quite a problem. How can couples who remain together for many years keep from becoming duplicates? Perhaps the only way to maintain such "freshness" in the relationship is for each partner continually to seek out domains of knowledge unknown to the other. A renewal of the differentiation of their transactive memory could occur every day—if the partners are willing to be apart, to experience life on their own, and to contribute to the dyad by being at least somewhat independent of it.

Parting With Transactive Memory

A couple may break up because of transactive memory, or their relationship may end in spite of it. What happens to each partner then? Amidst the emotional turmoil that can accompany partnership dissolution (Berscheid, 1983), there may also appear several cognitive effects that can throw the individual into a confused and inefficient state for some time. Certainly, the privilege of discussing events, of coming to a negotiated view of them, and of reacting to them on the basis of this group perspective will be ended. A common feeling accompanying relationship dissolution, then, will be one of indecision. A lone partner who has become used to transactive processes may almost automatically defer judgment on issues as they arise, holding off until an interpretation of events can be transacted. The person will have difficulty forming an independent and personal memory system.

With the loss of the relationship, one also loses access to the differentiated portion of transactive memory held by the other. This loss will be recognized only slowly. As one fails to find phone numbers, recipes, household objects, or the like, it begins to become evident. But more profound losses will be noted as time goes by. One's memory of favorite episodes will fade, almost inexplicably, because the other is not present to supply the differentiated details that one never stored for oneself. One will also lose the benefits of the other's special skills, never again savoring that chocolate mousse or being able to look on a flat tire as a mere inconvenience. Indeed, because transactive retrieval is no longer possible, there will be entire realms of one's experience that merely slip away, unrecognized in their departure, and never to be retrieved again.

Because the other has served often as a context for one's personal encoding of events, there will also be a personal deficit in retrieval. Everything one has learned in the presence of the other, even without depending on the other for transactive encoding or retrieval, will become a bit more difficult to retrieve from one's personal memory. The other has regularly served as a backdrop for one's experience, a part of the setting in which the experience was encoded. And even though the other may have played only a bystander's role in the event, one's encoding of the event is specific to the other's presence and may not allow for retrieval without the other (cf. Tulving & Thomson, 1973). A new partner who shares some qualities with one's former intimate might serve as a substitute context, and so aid one in gaining access to one's own stored information.

Should one become angry at the former partner, yet other changes in personal memory could result. One might renounce certain of the integrations that the group had previously achieved because they continue to be too reminiscent of the relationship. Just as the former dyad's penchant for Sunday afternoon crossword puzzles would be abandoned by the partner, their commonly held views of friends, activities, or experiences would be discarded as well. Similarly, one might attempt to stop speaking of past events in the "group" code—mentioning things that "we" did—and so disguise for oneself and others the degree of one's previous interdependence (cf. Wegner, 1981). The resentful partner could even attempt to develop new domains of expertise (e.g., "No one will ever tell me again that I can't fix a flat!") or let old ones fall into disuse. In this way, it is guaranteed that the original transactive memory developed by the group will no longer fit. Should a reconciliation be attempted, a newly negotiated transactive memory structure would be required—making for extra accommodative work on the part of the less-changed partner and perhaps a "shake-up" of the entire system.

Admittedly, some of these effects could accrue merely by losing contact with a brief acquaintance. The ending of a long-term relationship, however, will surely exact these tolls in every area of one's personal information-processing system. One will have difficulty interpreting events without discussion, and so blindly seek the advice of strangers. One will fail to encode previously differentiated information for oneself, and thus err in coping with all the now-personal information domains. One will abandon the dyad's integrative views of life events, perhaps to adopt less certain or satisfying views that have only the fact that they are one's own to recommend them. And, one will simply lose contact with vast memory domains that one had hoped were personal—but that in reality were transactive, and so ended with the relationship.

Acknowledgments. We are grateful to Norbert L. Kerr, John M. Levine, Richard Machalek, David J. Schneider, William B. Swann, Jr., Robin R. Vallacher, Robert A. Wicklund, and the editor of this volume for their helpful comments.

References

Allport, G. W. (1968). The historical background of modern social psychology. In G. Lindzey & E. Aronson (Eds.), *Handbook of social psychology,* (2nd ed.) (Vol. 1, pp. 1–80). Reading, MA: Addison-Wesley.

Altman, I., & Taylor, D. A. (1973). *Social penetration: The development of interpersonal relationships.* New York: Holt, Rinehart & Winston.

Anderson, J., & Reder, L. (1979). Elaborative processing explanation of depth of processing. In L. S. Cermak & F. I. M. Craik (Eds.), *Levels of processing in human memory.* Hillsdale, NJ: Erlbaum.

Archer, R. L. (1980). Self-disclosure. In D. M. Wegner & R. R. Vallacher (Eds.), *The self in social psychology* (pp. 183–205). New York: Oxford University Press.

Bartlett, F. C. (1932). *Remembering.* Cambridge: Cambridge University Press.

Berscheid, E. (1983). Emotion. In H. H. Kelley et al. (Eds.), *Close relationships* (pp. 110–168). New York: Freeman.

Bertalanffy, L. von (1968). *General system theory.* New York: Braziller.

Cicourel, A. V. (1974). *Cognitive sociology.* New York: Free Press.

Clark, H. H., & Haviland, S. E. (1977). Comprehension and the given-new contract. In R. O. Freedle (Ed.), *Discourse processes: Advances in research and theory* (Vol. 1). Norwood, NJ: Ablex.

Davis, J. H. (1980). Group decision and procedural justice. In M. Fishbein (Ed.), *Progress in social psychology.* Hillsdale, NJ: Erlbaum.

Davis, M. S. (1973). *Intimate relations.* New York: Free Press.

Durkheim, E. (1915). *Elementary forms of the religious life.* New York: Macmillan.

Freyd, J. J. (1983). Shareability: The social psychology of epistemology. *Cognitive Science, 7,* 191–210.

Giuliano, T., & Wegner, D. M. (1983). *Group formation and the integration of transactive memory.* Unpublished manuscript, University of Texas at Austin.

Grice, H. P. (1975). Logic in conversation. In P. Cole & J. L. Morgan (Eds.), *Syntax and semantics* (Vol. 3). New York: Academic Press.

Hart, J. T. (1967). Memory and the memory monitoring process. *Journal of Verbal Learning and Verbal Behavior, 6,* 685–691.

Hayes-Roth, B., & Thorndyke, P. W. (1979). Integration of knowledge from text. *Journal of Verbal Learning and Verbal Behavior, 18,* 91–108.

Hegel, G. W. F. (1910). *The phenomenology of mind* (Trans.). London: Allen and Unwin. (Original work published 1807)

Hertel, P. T. (1982). Remembering reactions and facts: The influence of subsequent information. *Journal of Experimental Psychology: Learning, Memory, and Cognition, 8,* 513–529.

Johnson, M. K., & Raye, C. L. (1981). Reality monitoring. *Psychological Review, 88,* 67–85.

Jung, C. G. (1922). *Collected papers on analytical psychology* (2nd ed.). London: Bailliere, Tindall, and Cox.

Kelley, H. H., Berscheid, E., Christensen, A., Harvey, J. H., Huston, T. L., Levinger, G., McClintock, E., Peplau, L. A., & Peterson, D. R. (1983). *Close relationships.* New York: Freeman.

Kelley, H. H., & Thibaut, J. W. (1978). *Interpersonal relationships: A theory of interdependence.* New York: Wiley-Interscience.

Kerr, N. L. (1981). Social transition schemes: Charting the group's road to agreement. *Journal of Personality and Social Psychology, 41,* 684–702.

Knowles, E. S. (1982). From individuals to group members: A dialectic for the social sciences. In W. J. Ickes & E. S. Knowles (Eds.), *Personality, roles, and social behavior* (pp. 1–32). New York: Springer-Verlag.

Laughlin, P. R. (1980). Social combination processes of cooperative problem-solving groups on verbal intellective tasks. In M. Fishbein (Ed.), *Progress in social psychology.* Hillsdale, NJ: Erlbaum.

LeBon, G. (1903). *The crowd.* London: Allen and Unwin.

Lewis, D. K. (1969). *Convention.* Cambridge, MA: Harvard University Press.

Loftus, E. F., Miller, D. G., & Burns, H. J. (1978). Semantic integration of verbal information into a visual memory. *Journal of Experimental Psychology: Human Learning and Memory, 4,* 19–31.

MacIver, R. M. (1921). *Community.* New York: Macmillan.

McDougall, W. (1920). *The group mind.* New York: Putnam.

Pareto, V. (1935). *The mind and society.* New York: Harcourt-Brace.

Pratt, M. W., Luszcz, M. A., MacKenzie-Keating, S., & Manning, A. (1982). Thinking about stories: The story schema in meta cognition. *Journal of Verbal Learning and Verbal Behavior, 21,* 493–505.

Ross, E. A. (1908). *Social psychology*. New York: Macmillan.

Ross, M., & Sicoly, F. (1979). Egocentric biases in availability and attribution. *Journal of Personality and Social Psychology, 37*, 322–336.

Rousseau, J. J. (1767). *A treatise on the social contract*. London: Becket and DeHondt.

Slamecka, N. J., & Graf, P. (1978). The generation effect: Delineation of a phenomenon. *Journal of Experimental Psychology: Human Learning and Memory, 4*, 592–604.

Spencer, H. (1876). *The principles of sociology*. New York: Appleton.

Tulving, E., & Thomson, D. M. (1973). Encoding specificity and retrieval processes in episodic memory. *Psychological Review, 80*, 352–373.

Tyler, S. W., Hertel, P. T., McCallum, M. C., & Ellis, H. C. (1979). Cognitive effort and memory. *Journal of Experimental Psychology: Human Learning and Memory, 5*, 607–617.

Walker, N., Jones, J. P., & Mar, H. H. (1983). Encoding processes and recall of text. *Memory & Cognition, 11*, 275–282.

Wegner, D. M. (1981, August). *When does the intimate group come to mind?* Paper presented at the meeting of the American Psychological Association, Los Angeles.

Wegner, D. M., & Giuliano, T. (1982). The forms of social awareness. In W. J. Ickes & E. S. Knowles (Eds.), *Personality, roles, and social behavior* (pp. 165–198). New York: Springer-Verlag.

Wundt, W. (1916). *Elements of folk psychology* (Trans.). New York: Macmillan. (Original work published 1910)

Zajonc, R. B. (1960). The process of cognitive tuning in communication. *Journal of Abnormal and Social Psychology, 61*, 159–167.

Chapter 12

Interpersonal Perception in Relationships

Alan L. Sillars

As the eclectic nature of this volume testifies, compatibility in relationships has been approached from a variety of perspectives. However, integrative efforts are rare and it is difficult to keep track of authors who run in different academic circles. Consequently, there are many pockets of research that have developed independently, although they speak to similar issues.

An example of parallel lines of research converging on a similar conclusion is provided by the literature on interpersonal perception. In this literature, different research traditions all point to the conclusion that a general dimension of distorted, inaccurate, or incongruent perception differentiates incompatible relationships from happy, well-adjusted ones. This conclusion is upheld in a number of areas: incongruent personality attributions (e.g., Ferguson & Allen, 1979; Kotlar, 1975; Luckey, 1960); confused, inaccurate, or constricted communication (Gottman, Notarius, Markman, Bank, Yoppi, & Rubin, 1976; Kahn, 1970; Watzlawick, Beavin, & Jackson, 1967); a pattern of blaming and accusing (Bernal, 1978; Madden & Janoff-Bulman, 1981; Wright & Fichten, 1976); "mindreading" (Gottman, Markman & Notarius, 1977; Thomas, 1977); a lack of empathy (Dymond, 1954; Ferreira, 1964; Losee, 1976; Newmark, Woody, & Ziff, 1977; Stuckert, 1963; Taylor, 1967); and incongruent "meta-perceptions" (Bochner, Krueger, & Chmielewski, 1982; Laing, Phillipson, & Lee, 1966). Most (but not all) of these sources attribute incongruent perception to "bias" or "imperceptivity" (i.e., inaccurate or idiosyncratic perception) and assume that such bias is causally related to in-compatibility.

The theory of interpersonal perception is as diffuse as the research literature. McCleod and Chaffee (1973) identify interpersonal perception (though they prefer the term "coorientation") as the common theme in several interpersonal perspectives on human behavior, including consensus theory (Scheff, 1968; Wirth, 1948), symbolic interactionism (Cooley, 1902; Mead, 1934), interpersonal psychiatry (Sullivan, 1953), coorientation theory (Newcomb, 1953), and person perception (Schneider, Hastorf, & Ellsworth, 1979). Transcending these perspectives is a common view of interpersonal perception and social coordination. According to this view, the coordination of different individuals toward one another and toward a common issue is based on (1) the development of shared meaning and (2) the ability of each person to anticipate the perspective of other individuals (Cushman & Whiting, 1972).

Although several theories provide a broad mandate for research on interpersonal perception, this shared interest has not resulted in a cohesive literature. Studies of interpersonal perception within personal relationships are so scattered that a common research agenda addressing basic issues has yet to evolve. In effect, the literature itself illustrates a lack of social coordination. Consequently, relatively little insight has been shed on interpersonal perception within personal relationships beyond the general outlines provided by Berger & Kellner (1964), Hess and Handel (1959), Laing et al. (1966), McCleod and Chaffee (1973), and a few others.

In contrast to the literature cited above, the literature concerning social cognition, attribution, and person perception (e.g., Higgins, Herman, & Zanna, 1981, Kelley & Michela, 1980; Nisbett & Ross, 1980) has considerable theoretical depth and detail. However, the heuristic value of this literature is weakened by the fact that personal relationships have not yet been a central focus of study. In the typical study of person perception, the actor (or perceptual target) and the observer do not know each other, they do not interact, and their perceptions are of relatively minor consequence to the persons involved. These "first impression" relationships established purely for research purposes may differ markedly from personal relationships that have not been arranged by a social science researcher. In naturally occurring personal relationships the actor and observer may have an extensive background of interpersonal meaning, they may be highly interdependent, and their perceptions may have enormous emotional significance. For these reasons, among others, there is a need to clarify how theories of person perception and social cognition apply to personal relationships (see Fincham, 1983, Higgins, Kuiper, & Olson, 1981; Newman, 1981). This effort should acknowledge the special complexity of personal relationships that stems from interpersonal or "interactional" considerations.

Personal relationships are full of contradictions, and this feature contributes to the often puzzling status of research in this area. One of the things we may prize most about long term, close relationships is that they seem to foster a high level of understanding and predictability. It is precisely for this reason that personal relationships can become so thoroughly disorienting when conflict and separation occur (Harvey, Weber, Yarkin, & Stewart, 1982; Weiss, 1975). Although people generally assume that their perceptions of others are accurate, research has shown that interpretations of behavior are actually quite ambiguous, even in the context of close, personal relationships. There are many illustrations of the ambiguity present in personal relationships. For example, married couples may agree only about half the time when asked who usually wins during marital disagreements (Turk & Bell, 1972). Even on such simple and concrete issues as "who takes out the garbage," there may be a wide disparity of perceptions (Frank, Anderson, & Rubinstein, 1980). Other studies suggest that spouses are not very accurate at judging when the other person is lying (Bauchner, 1980) or at estimating the other's feelings and attitudes about marital conflicts (Sillars, Pike, Jones, & Murphy, 1984).

Many factors introduce ambiguity into personal relationships, including behavioral interdependence and causal complexity, the self-confirming nature of attributions about the partner, emotionality, and the absence of consensual coding rules for some behaviors. This chapter explores the influences these factors may have on interpersonal perception and compatibility. From the perspective of this chapter, the study of interpersonal perception should call attention to the interpersonal and interdependent nature of perceptions within relationships. This means that biases in person perception follow from the interpersonal situation as well as from individual-level processes in perception and cognition. Similarly, the implications of interpersonal perception for compatibility depend importantly on the nature of the interpersonal situation (for example, the need for coordination with respect to a particular issue).

The first section of this chapter reviews the distinctive aspects of interpersonal perception within personal relationships. The purpose of this discussion is to provide a general framework for viewing personal relationships—a framework that cuts across different areas and applications of research on interpersonal perception.

The remaining two sections of the chapter consider different levels of interpersonal perception. The second section considers the attribution process within personal relationships. Attributions are constructs used by naive social actors to describe, explain, and predict social interaction (see Heider, 1958). Although the boundaries of this topic are loosely drawn (Ross, 1977), most of the attributional literature directly applicable to personal relationships has to do with the attribution of traits and motives or with the attribution of responsibility and blame for conflict. Biased or incongruent attributions are typically found in conflictual relationships. Attributions often represent deeply felt cognitions about the partner or the relationship, and these cognitions are intrinsically gratifying or punishing. Further, negative and pessimistic attributions may contribute to self-perpetuating, self-confirming interpersonal conflicts.

In the third section of this chapter, the topic of understanding or "empathy" is addressed. Understanding involves the ability to describe another person's perspective (i.e., the accuracy of "meta-perception"). Some might regard this as the most important aspect of interpersonal perception, because empathic ability is widely assumed to mediate a person's flexibility and skill at interpersonal communication (e.g., Argyle, 1969; Mead, 1934; O'Keefe & Sypher, 1981; Piaget, 1926; Wiemann, 1977). However, such apparently straightforward implications can be misleading. Some personal relationships thrive despite little understanding of certain issues. At the very least, the effects of understanding are probably conditioned by the inherent ambiguity of certain perceptions and by the need for coordination with respect to a given issue.

Distinctive Aspects of Personal Relationships

Interpersonal perception in ongoing relationships is especially complex because each individual may simultaneously be the other's most knowledgeable *and* least objective observer. Consequently, although two people may know each other intimately, they can still represent an extreme case of incongruent perception.

In certain fairly obvious respects, people generally do become more predictable and comprehensible to each other during the development of relationships. For example, the increasing depth and breadth of self-disclosure that occurs during relationship development (Altman & Taylor, 1973) may reduce erroneous perceptions caused by cultural and social stereotypes (Berger & Bradac, 1982; Miller & Steinberg, 1975). Communication also may become more efficient as tacit understandings and specialized codes are acquired (Cushman & Whiting, 1972; Knapp, 1978; Morton, Alexander, & Altman, 1976). Further, because ignorance about the psychological and historical context of an act is seen by some attribution theorists as a primary cause of attributional bias (Jones & Nisbett, 1972; Kelley, 1972; Monson & Snyder, 1977), attributions about another person should presumably become more accurate during acquaintance, as information about the context of the other person's behavior is filled in.

Although there are some obvious ways that familiarity may foster understanding, there are also some respects in which familiarity may be misleading. Familiarity increases one's confidence in understanding the other, and this confidence may extend to areas where understanding is not present. Shapiro and Swensen (1969) demonstrated this point when they found that people overestimated how much they knew about their spouses and, conversely, how much their spouses knew about them. This tendency to overestimate understanding may actually reduce understanding because people seek less information when they believe that they already have an accurate knowledge of someone (see Berger & Calabrese, 1975; Pavitt & Cappella, 1979).

Familiarity may also lead to the entrenchment of existing impressions. Weick (1971) suggests that the ability of families to adapt to the new and changing problems of individuals is hampered because family members typically fail to see shifts occurring in individual opinions and behaviors. Instead, they simply assimilate new behavior to old and interpret it in the same way. Of course, similar effects occur outside the context of personal relationships as well (see Nisbett & Ross, 1980; Ross, 1977), but it stands to reason that changes in impressions will be increasingly conservative if impressions have been maintained and supported over a long period of time. Consequently, a period of misperception and confusion is bound to occur in personal relationships when individuals experience personal changes in their attitudes, goals, interests, and so forth.

Two related characteristics of personal relationships with further consequences for interpersonal perception are interdependence and uniqueness. Interdependence refers to the high level of mutual influence and causal complexity that exists in personal relationships. Interdependence is manifested in the development of unique interaction rules, specialized codes, and a joint identity (Cushman & Whiting, 1972; Davis, 1973; Hopper, Knapp & Scott, 1981; Knapp, 1978; Rausch, Barry, Hertel, & Swain, 1974). As interdependence increases, the correspondence between a person's behavior and his or her underlying traits, attitudes, intentions, and perceptions becomes increasingly ambiguous, since behavior may correspond to any or all of several factors, including individual attitudes and traits, past behavior, and negotiated patterns or expectations. This natural confounding of causation has two further consequences for interpersonal perception. First, it becomes more plausible to blame another person for problems when responsibility is ambiguous (see Weary-Bradley, 1978). Second, when people are involved in interdependent situations, they often overlook the effects of their own behavior on others (see Sillars, 1981).

Berger and Kellner (1964) have considered the implications of uniqueness for interpersonal perception in close, personal relationships. These authors suggest that the shared social reality of married couples is fragile to the extent that the relationship is unique and private. As Berger and Kellner point out, the shared, institutionalized perceptions of social groups are far more stable than the unique perceptions of a few individuals. Thus, consensus about important attributions (e.g., the spouse is caring, communicative, and so forth) is more problematic if the rules used to code behavior lack validation and support from other people. A corollary of Berger and Kellner's analysis is that interpersonal perception should be more problematic in nontraditional intimate relationships than in traditional ones. Traditional couples accept the consensual standards that are present in the larger society, thereby making the negotiation of identities less ambiguous. Further, traditional couples stress stability and predictability in their relationships (Fitzpatrick, 1983) and they typically have an extensive social network that is relied on for advice and support (Bott, 1957; Komarovsky, 1964).

A final distinctive quality of personal relationships, especially intimate, long-term relationships, is emotionality. A strong undercurrent of emotionality may exist for a variety of reasons: Personal relationships are highly involving, social constraints on the expression of emotion are relaxed, and people may establish personal relationships partly to dramatize their lives. The results are partially evident in the disheartening statistics on family violence (see Goode, 1971; Straus, 1974). A more mundane result is the relative impoliteness and negativity that spouses display when conversing with each other as opposed to acquaintances (Birchler, Weiss, & Vincent, 1975; Ryder, 1969; Winter, Ferreira, & Bowers, 1973). A third example is the finding that intimates report using more emotional and abrasive conflict strategies with each other than with nonintimates (Fitzpatrick & Winke, 1979).

Emotionality has a variety of implications, most of which can be documented in the social cognition literature. First, self-serving attributional biases are more prevalent when attributions are emotionally involving or threatening (Snyder, Stephan, & Rosenfield, 1978; Weary-Bradley, 1978). A self-serving bias is illustrated by Thompson and Kelley's (1981) research, which found that the members of married and dating couples accepted more personal responsibility for positive events in their relationship than for negative events.

Second, emotional, conflictual behavior is highly salient because of both the greater salience of negative as opposed to positive behavior (see Kanouse & Hanson, 1972) and the inherently vivid qualities of interpersonal conflict. Because salient information is typically given greater emphasis in the attribution process than nonsalient information (see Nisbett & Ross, 1980; Taylor & Fiske, 1978), this tendency to accentuate the negative may help to explain the increasing disillusionment that develops in some relationships. For example, Luckey (1966) found that the interpersonal perceptions of spouses were more negative in older marriages. The longer couples were married, the less likely they were to see their spouse as well thought of, respected by others, self-respecting, independent, firm-but-just, graceful, cooperative, friendly, affectionate, considerate, and helpful. The couples had all been married at least two years, so the results were probably not due to the erosion of prenuptial misconceptions and romantic stereotypes that disappear relatively soon after marriage (the divorce rate peaks at the third year of marriage: see Hicks and Platt, 1970). Instead, it appears that spouses may place increasing emphasis on negative information about their partners following the initial years of their marriage (see also Newman, 1981).

Third, in highly stressful situations, people experience a reduction in their ability to engage in complex, integrated thought, leading to reduced information search, failure to discriminate items of information or points of view, and the perception of only one side of issues (Schroder, Driver, & Streufert, 1967; Suedfeld & Tetlock, 1977). Thus, the stressful nature of emotional conflicts may contribute to a lack of perspective-taking and to increasingly one-sided attributions (see Sillars & Parry, 1982).

Fourth, because overtly expressed attributions are a part of the conversational structure of conflict, they may tend to become more extreme in intense and emotional conflicts. Overtly stated attributions have linguistically pragmatic functions: to insult, justify, criticize, and so forth. Attributions may also express feelings or provide an argument for one's own definition of the relationship (Harvey et al., 1982; Orvis, Kelley, & Butler, 1976). For example, a husband may label his drinking a "release" while his wife calls it an "addiction" (the example is from Orvis et al., 1976). In such instances, attributions are apt to become exaggerated and polarized simply as a reflection of argumentative strategy. Although this point applies mainly to overt statements about attributions, public commitments may, in turn, reinforce private beliefs (see Bem, 1972; Zanna & Cooper, 1976).

Each of the potential effects of emotionality is deserving of more extended treatment, since the role of emotion in social cognition is both poorly understood and highly controversial (see Rogers, 1980; Weary, Swanson, Harvey, & Yarkin, 1980). Still, the examples given are sufficient to show that emotionality may be a pervasive factor in interpersonal perception. Further, the implications of each example are essentially the same—that is, that strong negative emotions are seen as leading to a less accurate, more one-sided, and more negative perception of the partner. Therefore, the potentially volatile nature of intimate conflict may produce extreme examples of imperceptivity.

To summarize: Certain features of the relationship itself can account for ambiguity in interpersonal perception. Ambiguity and imperceptivity may be introduced by familiarity, relationship change, interdependence and causal complexity, uniqueness of coding rules, and emotionality.

Looking beyond features of the relationship that may cloud interpersonal perceptions, we can also distinguish between perceptions that are essentially "self-correcting" in long-term relationships and those that are not. The former consist of perceptions that are easily compared with objective experience and which therefore may be clearly tested. For example, a belief such as "My wife likes her eggs poached" is clearly related to concrete, easily coded behavior, whereas a belief such as "She wants to dominate me" is not. To the extent that the referent of a perception is concrete, easily coded, consensually defined, and stable, congruence of perception is likely to increase with time. On the other hand, if there is an indeterminant relationship between a perception and its referent (that is, the referent is abstract, subtle, interactional, and affectively loaded), then familiarity may have little to do with perceptual congruence. The attribution literature emphasizes the more abstract and interactional forms of perception and this emphasis partly accounts for the frequent observation that attributions are idiosyncratic to an individual's perspective. On the other hand, perceptions of varying abstractness and affective content have been the object of study in the literature on understanding, and these variations may account for some meaningful differences between the results of different studies.

Having considered a number of general factors that affect interpersonal perception, we now turn to the subareas of research on this topic.

Attribution and Compatibility

Attribution theory suggests that humans code behavior according to psychological concepts such as traits, motives, intentions, and so forth. The psychological translation of behavior allows people to anticipate future actions and makes it possible to describe behavior parsimoniously (see Heider, 1958). Although attribution researchers frequently are concerned with the "accuracy" of attributions, it is more relevant in the present context to ask whether attributions are congruent. Presumably, two people are more compatible to the extent that they make complementary attributions that fit into a coherent image of the relationship (see Hess & Handel, 1959) and that confirm each other's perception of self (Goffman, 1959; Morton et al., 1976).

A number of authors have already called attention to the implications of attribution theory for compatibility in relationships (e.g., Doherty, 1981; Fincham, 1983; Harvey et al., 1982; Kelley, 1979; Newman, 1981; Orvis et al., 1976 Sillars, 1981; Wright & Fichten). Indeed, certain implications are so straightforward that they are hard to overlook. Some attributions touch upon the core issues in a relationship (e.g., the partner is loving or unloving, the relationship reflects equity or inequity, the partner is selfish or giving). These attributions are intrinsically satisfying or punishing because they define whether the relationship is meeting its primary goals, such as companionship and security (see Kelley, 1979). Further, the attributions indicate what long-term patterns of behavior can be expected and what the future of the relationship is likely to be. Consequently, attributions are intricately involved with satisfaction and commitment in personal relationships. Attributions also become important to the extent that they affect how dissatisfactions are expressed. At the risk of oversimplifying, human conflicts may become self-perpetuating as a function of rigid, mutually antagonistic attributions developing between two people. As conflict theorists have frequently emphasized (e.g., Deutsch, 1973; Thomas & Pondy, 1977), intense conflicts are characterized by the mutual perception of the other party as hostile and untrustworthy and by the self-confirming behaviors that follow from these perceptions.

The appeal of attribution theory is also based on the straightforward implications of such "attributional biases" as the "fundamental attribution error" (Ross, 1977) or actor-observer difference (Jones & Nisbett, 1972) and several other apparent distortions in human inference (see Berger & Roloff, 1982). There is an undeniable "real life" quality to be found in this part of the attribution literature. The fundamental attribution error, for example, refers to the tendency of observers to overestimate the dispositional causes of an actor's behavior while underestimating the strength of situational causes. One manifestation of this tendency is that general, stable trait labels are preferred over specific behavioral descriptions of people (Kelley, 1979). This "error" helps account for the informal observation by family therapists that spouses often refer to each other in terms that are so vague and overgeneralized that they aggravate marital conflicts (e.g., Thomas, 1977; Weiss, Hops, & Patterson, 1973). It also extends the argument that differentiated perception is a central dimension of interpersonal and spousal competence (Argyle, 1969; Kieren & Tallman, 1972; Wiemann, 1977). Indeed, a study by Fincham and O'Leary

(1983) indicated that undifferentiated attributions were associated with marital distress. Couples seeking counseling attributed their spouse's negative behaviors to more global causes than did couples who were not in couseling.

The actor-observer hypothesis goes a bit beyond the fundamental attribution error in suggesting that people prefer situational explanations for their own behavior and stable, dispositional explanations for the behavior of other people. Again, this idea has considerable commonplace application. Interpersonal conflict is often fueled by each individual's indignation at being the other person's "victim" (i.e., the other person is seen as the causal force). As Watzlawick et al. (1967) have pointed out, people "punctuate" communication sequences differently. Each participant in a conflict may offer simple but conflicting, linear causal interpretations when the causes of action are actually complex, subtle, and interactional. Conflict research provides several examples of this type of bias (Sillars, 1981).

Actor-Partner Attributions

A straightforward implication of the actor-observer hypothesis is that people should place more blame for interpersonal conflicts on their partner in the relationship than on themselves (since their own actions are construed in less dispositional, more situational terms). The same implications follow from the so-called "self-serving bias" in attributions (see Weary-Bradley, 1978). A study by Orvis et al. (1976) supported the expected pattern of actor-partner differences in attributions. The authors found that the members of young couples usually attributed their own behavior during disagreements to unstable, situational causes and their partner's behavior to stable, negative traits. Similarly, in studies of marital dissolution, most divorced and separated individuals blamed the breakup of their marriage on their spouse (Hunt & Hunt, 1977; Newman & Langer, 1981). Several other studies have revealed parallel results for the way that communication and control is perceived within families. In these studies, the actor typically reported a more favorable impression of his or her own behavior than was reported by other family members. For example, parents saw themselves as more self-disclosing (Dalusio, 1972), more affectionate, and less punishing (Zucker & Barron, 1971) than their children perceived them to be. Husbands also thought of themselves as more contractual and less controlling than they were perceived by wives (Hawkins, Weisberg, & Ray, 1980).

Most studies have had people record their attributions on a numerical scale item, thus representing attributions as points along a single continuum. However, attributions may also represent qualitatively different reconstructions of an event. This is illustrated by Weiss' (1975) research on marital separation. Weiss observed that separated spouses tend to provide verbal accounts of their marital breakup with simple, story-like plots. These accounts are highly selective and generally much more coherent than the actual events because, according to Weiss, separated spouses have a pressing need to restore order and predictability to their lives. In one case when a separated husband and wife from the same marriage were both interviewed, their accounts did not overlap. The husband reported that the wife's flirtatiousness precipitated their breakup. The wife reported that the husband would not allow her to return to school. Neither referenced any of the concrete events present in the other person's account. This example illustrates that actor-partner differences in attribution are often considerably more complex than revealed by the typical quantitative attribution study. Actor-partner differences in attributions are established, in part, by qualitative differences in the thematic construction of events by different members of a relationship.

Thus far, the literature we have reviewed suggests that attributional discrepancies are common in personal relationships. Most studies indicate that the partner is more likely to be attributed responsibility for precipitating relationship conflicts, initiating negative communication, and so forth. However, the preceding studies did not directly examine the relationship between attributions and compatibility. Several other studies indicate that actor-partner differences in attributions are greater in conflictual than in non-conflictual relationships. For example, studies by Bernal (1978) and Madden and Janoff-Bulman (1981) indicate that dissatisfied spouses are more blaming of each other than are satisfied spouses. Fincham and O'Leary (1983) did not find any differences in how blaming of their mates satisfied and dissatisfied spouses were, but the authors had couples make attributions about hypothetical rather than real events, so this study may not be comparable to the others.

An additional literature suggests that dissatisfied couples are more discrepant than satisfied couples in their attributions about each other's communicative intent. Specifically, dissatisfied spouses were apt to see hostility in their partner's messages when the partner reported being positive or friendly (Gottman et al., 1976; Kahn, 1970; Noller, 1980). One failure to replicate these results has been reported (Schaap, 1982).

My own research is in agreement with most other studies of attribution in dissatisfying relationships. In two studies of college roommates (Sillars, 1981) and three unpublished studies of married couples (Sillars, 1984), other-directed blame for relationship conflicts was significantly correlated with relationship dissatisfaction, intensity of conflict, and other negative perceptions. In both roomate studies, other-directed blame was greater to the extent that conflicts were more important, overall satisfaction with the relationship was low, and the conflicts were seen as stable or enduring. Other-directed blame was positively correlated with the importance of conflicts in two of the studies involving married couples, and was negatively correlated with marital satisfaction in all three.

These findings are represented in the last column of correlations in Table 12-1, which refers to the discrepancy between wife and husband attributions (i.e., the extent to which other-directed blame exceeded the partner's self-

Table 12-1. Correlations Between Blame, Perceived Importance of Conflicts, and Marital Satisfaction

		Wife's Blame of the Husband	Husband's Blame of the Wife	Discrepancy Between Wife and Husband Blame
Importance of Conflicts to the Wife	Study I	.32*	.03	.33*
	Study II	.61**	.12	.47**
	Study III	.00	−.07	−.05
Importance of Conflicts to the Husband	Study I	.10	.05	.09
	Study II	.39**	−.01	.31*
	Study III	.00	−.10	−.08
Wife's Marital Satisfaction	Study I	−.47**	−.02	−.46**
	Study II	−.61**	−.23	−.54**
	Study III	−.22	−.11	−.28*
Husband's Marital Satisfaction	Study I	−.44**	−.02	−.42**
	Study II	−.53**	−.10	−.37**
	Study III	−.17	.13	−.06

$* = p < .05.$
$** = p < .01$, one-tailed test.

blame).[1] Interestingly, it was primarily the wives' attributions that were responsible for the overall association between blame, satisfaction, and conflict—a finding that is consistent with those of many other studies reviewed by Barry (1970). Barry concluded that the wife's perceptions of a marriage are usually more closely related to marital adjustment or satisfaction than are the husband's perceptions. Barry reasoned that wives may be more sensitive to marital problems because they generally experience a more drastic and stressful role transition during marriage than husbands do.

Although there is convincing evidence that attributions are more discrepant in conflictual, disharmonious relationships than in nonconflictual, harmonious ones, there are nagging doubts about the actual impact of the attribution process. A dominant interpretation is that people are incompatible *because* of

---

[1]Blame was measured by Likert scales that asked who was to blame for different conflicts in the marriage. The anchors were "you much more," "you somewhat more," "both equally or neither," "your spouse somewhat more," "your spouse much more." Each spouse was asked to rate several conflict areas, and the overall attribution score was based on the sum of these ratings. The satisfaction measure is from Spanier (1976). The conflict topics used in the questionnaire and other procedures are described more completely in Sillars, Pike, Jones, and Murphy (1984). There were approximately 40 couples in each of the 3 studies.

attributional problems. In fact, counseling programs have been developed on the basis of this interpretation (see Doherty, 1981; Wright & Fichten, 1976). Another plausible interpretation is that dissatisfaction creates attributional discrepancies (Noller, 1981). For example, other-directed blame may be enhanced by self-serving bias (Weary-Bradley, 1978) or by the effects of stress (Sillars & Parry, 1982) in dissatisfying relationships. It is also possible to interpret the attribution/compatibility relation in noncausal terms. Self-report items pertaining to satisfaction, the importance of conflict, blame, and so forth may intercorrelate simply because they share common semantic dimensions in the perception of subjects or because subjects attempt to maintain a consistent self-presentation (Weary & Arkin, 1981). For example, blaming the partner for conflicts may be part of the subject's justification to the researcher for a low-satisfaction rating.

There is, of course, no reason to assume that there is a single, simple explanation for the attribution/compatibility relation. Harvey et al. (1982) suggest that attributions and compatibility are related through intricate causal loops. This is probably the most reasonable conclusion. Implicit in this interpretation is the idea that attributions affect patterns of social interaction which, in turn, reinforce attributions. There are only a few studies that focus directly on the relation between attributions and interaction patterns; these are discussed in the forthcoming section.

Attributions and Social Interaction

In the classic research by Kelley and Stahelski (1970), people who expressed a competitive orientation toward the Prisoner's Dilemma Game were paired with people who expressed a cooperative orientation. Competitors, who generally assume that others are also competitive, typically elicited a competitive response from partners who were initially cooperative. Thus, a self-fulfilling prophecy was generated by the distrust and misattribution of competitive subjects. Schlenker and Goldman (1978) provided further support for this picture of cooperative and competitive individuals.

These two studies provide simple but clear demonstrations of the process that presumably underlies interpersonal conflict in general. People's actions are based on implicit assumptions about the character of other people, and these assumptions tend to be self-confirming (see Snyder & Gangestad, 1981). As Watzlawick, Weakland, and Fisch (1974) have pointed out, one person's efforts to change another person often result in "more of the same"—anger and hostility, for example, may increase the other person's anger and hostility, and efforts to force togetherness may increase the partner's withdrawal. According to Watzlawick et al. (1974), fundamental change in a relationship occurs only when people come to see the situation in a totally different light (i.e., following "reframing" or attributional change).

Although it is difficult to devise analogues to Kelley and Stahelski's (1970) research within the context of personal relationships, a few studies indicate that behavioral and self-reported manifestations of interpersonal conflict are consistent with individuals' attributions about their partners. Doherty (1982), for example, identified the "attributional styles" of spouses based on their spontaneous comments about other married couples' problems. Wives who attributed problems to the negative personality characteristics of others expressed more disapproval of their husbands during a discussion and had a more "angry" verbal response style on a self-report measure than did wives who had a different attributional style. However, a similar effect was not found for husbands.

In one of the roommate studies reported by Sillars (1981), college dorm residents wrote open-ended accounts describing the most significant conflict they had experienced with their roomate and how it had been handled. People were more likely to say that they avoided discussing issues with their roommates or that they communicated indirectly (for example, by hinting or joking) when (1) conflicts were attributed to stable causes (e.g., the roommate is gay, highly religious, or has a "gossipy personality"), (2) the roommate was seen as uncooperative, and (3) the roommate was blamed for the conflict. If the subjects reported making requests or demands or having arguments, then they were more likely to say that the roommate caused the conflict. If the subjects reported being coercive and emotional, they were more likely to say that the roommate was uncooperative. Self disclosing and mutually supportive conversation about a problem was reported primarily when (1) the conflict was attributed to unstable causes, (2) the roommate was seen as cooperative, (3) subjects blamed themselves more than their roommates for the conflict, and (4) the issue was seen as unimportant.

In a second study, roommates were videotaped while actually discussing conflicts with each other. As in the earlier study, people were far more verbally revealing and supportive when they internalized blame for the conflict, whereas conflict avoidance and verbally competitive statements were more common when the partner was blamed. Attributions were also related to the sequential characteristics of the roommates' conversations. All types of statements were reciprocated at greater than chance probabilities (i.e., a statement was usually followed by a similar statement). However, reciprocity of verbally competitive statements was especially high when the partner was blamed for the conflict and the conflict was seen as stable. Thus, explicit argument was most likely to occur when both people attributed conflicts to the other person's stable, negative traits.

The results of two unpublished couples studies (Sillars, 1984) were largely consistent with those of the roommate studies. (Attribution was not the central focus of this research. See the forthcoming section on "understanding.") When couples blamed each other for their conflicts, there was a higher incidence of "distributive" statements (e.g., faulting, rejection, hostile jokes, and questions) in both studies and a lower incidence of "integrative" statements (e.g., supportive statements, informational questions, self-disclosure, descriptive statements, and statements accepting personal responsibility) in one of the studies. Couples were also more negative and less neutral in their vocal tone when they blamed each other for conflicts.[2] In contrast to the roommate studies, individuals in the couples studies expressed more avoidance statements (e.g., topic shifts, denial of conflict, abstract or ambivalent statements, nonhostile joking) when they blamed themselves rather than their partner for conflicts. Apparently, conflict avoidance had a more positive meaning for many couples than it did for the roommates, possibly because the sample was high in traditionalism and traditional couples appear to respect tactfulness and restraint in their communication (Fitzpatrick, 1977; Sillars, Pike, Jones, & Redmon, 1983).

In sum, when intimate couples and members of other dyads attribute relationship problems to the negative traits of each other, they are then likely to communicate in a negative, verbally competitive or ambiguous manner that often provides the other person with additional confirmation for his or her attributions about the source of these communications. Further, communicative patterns of conflict tend to be self-perpetuating. There is an exceedingly strong tendency for people to reciprocate both the paralinguistic affect and verbal content of the preceding speaker's statement during intimate conflicts (Sillars & Pike, 1984). Therefore, over time, communication patterns generate increasingly greater (self-confirming) evidence for the validity of attributions about the partner. In long-standing conflicts it may be extremely difficult to break this cycle (see Watzlawick et al., 1967; Watzlawick et al., 1974).

It is probably inevitable that attributions typically resemble only the bare outlines of the actual complexity inherent in social interaction. As Heider (1958) emphasized, people fulfill a need for parsimony and predictability by imposing stable, disposition-based structures on complex events. In some instances these disposition-based structures address the core issues in a relationship. For example, can the partner be counted on? Does the relationship reflect fairness and equity? Does the partner value the relationship? People need straightforward answers to these questions, and hence, they provide highly simplified accounts of complex, interactional, and ambiguous events. In compatible relationships the accounts of the different individuals tend to flow together. In incompatible relationships, accounts tend to be antagonistic, bitter,

---

[2]A difference score was computed by subtracting the wife's attribution score from the husband's (after reflecting the wife's score). The resulting score revealed the extent to which spouses blamed each other for marital conflicts (i.e., a high positive score would indicate a classic actor-partner difference, a negative score would indicate that blame was more self-directed than other-directed). Couples were divided into two groups based on the median discrepancy score and a log linear analysis of coded conversations was carried out. There was a significant interaction between the communication codes and attributions in both studies. This effect held for both verbal and paralinguistic communication codes. The specific effects cited cited here were significant according to z-tests on the lambda parameters in the log-linear models.

and blaming of the partner. Although we cannot offer prima facie evidence that the attribution process directly and causally affects compatibility, there are numerous sources of circumstantial evidence linking attributional congruence, patterns of interaction, satisfaction, and other important cognitions about relationships. Moreover, it is intuitively apparent that the truly important attributions about a relationship are so intrinsically a part of general satisfaction that one cannot be changed without influencing the other.

Understanding and Compatibility

Understanding refers to the congruence between one persons's "meta-perspective" (i.e., his or her estimate of the partner's perspective) and the other person's direct perspective (i.e., what the other person actually thinks; see Laing et al., 1966). Some attribution theorists treat understanding as a special case of general attribution processes (e.g., Harvey, Wells, & Alvarez, 1978; Jones & Harris, 1967), but it is more useful for us to treat understanding as a separate phenomenon with a different function. Unlike attribution, understanding involves one person's ability to take the perspective of another person. Attribution and understanding are interdependent in the sense that understanding may potentially allow one to overcome incongruence at the level of direct perspectives (i.e., attributional incongruence) by increasing sensitivity to areas of disagreement and conflict. On the other hand, misunderstanding may lead to a "spiral of reciprocal perspectives," such that one misattribution builds upon another (Laing et al., 1966).

Repeatedly, studies have found a positive association between marital satisfaction or adjustment and measures of understanding (Christensen & Wallace, 1976; Corsini, 1956; Dymond, 1954; Ferguson & Allen, 1978; Laing et al., 1966; Losee, 1976; Murstein & Beck, 1972; Newmark et al., 1977; Stuckert, 1963; Taylor, 1967). Further, there is long-standing acceptance in the social sciences of the belief that understanding facilitates satisfying relationships. At times, this acceptance borders on the ideological (Parks, 1981). However, interpretation of the understanding/compatibility relation is problematic, because little attention has been given to the various measures of understanding or to the different factors that may contribute to the scores derived from these measures. Instead there has been a tendency to treat understanding and its effects in an undifferentiated manner, and this tendency has distracted attention away from several issues.

One issue is methodological. All but a few studies (Corsini, 1956; Dymond, 1954; Newmark et al., 1977) have allowed response similarity to be confounded with understanding. Couples who have a high level of agreement may guess each other's response via projection or the imputation of a similar response to the partner (i.e., the so-called "false concensus" bias in attribution; see Ross, 1977). This process has little to do with "differential accuracy" or understanding of the spouse's unique attitudes and perceptions (see Gage & Cronbach, 1955).

A second issue, related to the first, concerns the extent to which understanding results from active role-taking, as opposed to projection and stereotypic perception. People operate at a concrete level of inference much of the time and may fail to go past the level of direct perspectives, even when encouraged to do so. For example, one of the better documented findings in the area of interpersonal perception is that assumed agreement usually exceeds actual agreement within family and intimate relationships (Byrne & Blaylock, 1963; Good, Good, & Nelson, 1973; Harvey et al., 1978; Knudson, Sommers, & Golding, 1980; Levinger & Breedlove, 1966; Williamson, 1975). This suggests that people use their own direct perspective as a reference for judging other people, even in close relationships where there is a wealth of prior experience that might differentiate the other person. In addition, stereotypic knowledge often provides a sufficient basis for understanding. Most routine interactions do not require perspective-taking and can be carried out simply on the basis of stereotyped cultural and social expectations (see Parks, 1981; Pavitt, 1982). An untested hypothesis that follows from this line of reasoning is that active perspective-taking progressively subsides as relationships become more stable and routine, for example, relationships such as those represented by Fitzpatrick's (1983) traditional couples. In other words, relationships of this type may become highly scripted or "mindless" (Langer, 1978).

A third issue concerns the effect of interpersonal communication on understanding. Most discussions of interpersonal communication and relationship development emphasize the importance of self-disclosure in establishing a common base of private experience in more intimate relationships (e.g., Berger & Bradac, 1982; Miller & Steinberg, 1975; Morton et al., 1976). Altman and Taylor (1973) established the tone for this literature by describing relationship development as a mutual psychological interpenetration of the self, created by reciprocal self-disclosure. Although Altman and Taylor did not intend to address the issues raised in the present chapter, their emphasis calls attention to characteristics of messages (i.e., self-disclosure) as the main determinants of understanding. Similarly, prescriptive manuals on effective communication emphasize the importance of communicating directly, openly, consistently, factually, and so forth (e.g., Miller, Nunnally, & Wackman, 1975; Thomas, 1977). However, there is no previous research I know of that evaluates how people actually use verbal communication to construct or revise inferences about spouses, friends, parents, or other familiar individuals.

Following the reasoning developed earlier in this chapter, there is significant ambiguity in the information provided by direct verbal disclosure, even when such messages are supposedly "well-constructed" (i.e., they are forthright, consistent, documented, etc.). This ambiguity arises from several factors, including the distinctive characteristics of personal relationships that were discussed previously. For example, old impressions are difficult to change, people we presumably know well are not closely monitored for "new" information, coding rules are especially idiosyncratic within intimate relationships, and emotionality may focus attention and bias the interpretation of messages. To this list let us add two further considerations. First, people remember only a small fragment of what they hear in conversations, and what they do remember is a function of prior schemata (Stafford & Daly, 1984). Second, people selectively remember information that is either consistent with or grossly discrepant with existing schemata over schema-irrelevant information (Hastie, 1981). Consequently, recall of conversation is likely to either confirm prior inferences about another person or occasionally lead to the elaboration and differentiation of prior schemata. Rarely will conversation with a very familiar person lead to completely novel insights that are independent of prior expectations.

Verbal communication is subject to a further consideration. Direct, verbal disclosure is restricted in the range of meanings that it is presumed to express. Communication about relationship issues is largely a function of nonverbal expression and indirect, implied meaning rather than direct verbal disclosure. We are reminded by many authors that the process of relationship development is mostly implicit in the way that people communicate (Cushman & Whiting, 1972; Danziger, 1976; Millar & Rogers, 1976; Scheff, 1968; Watzlawick et al., 1967). In other words, a relationship definition may be established without people explicitly talking about it. Further, emotions are inferred primarily from nonverbal behavior (see Harper, Weins, & Matarazzo, 1978; Mehrabian, 1972). In sum, we have several reasons to suspect that verbal communication is not associated with understanding in a straightforward manner.

A fourth and final issue in the literature on understanding is whether understanding is always conducive to compatibility. In some situations greater understanding may increase conflict and dissatisfaction in a relationship—for example, when there are irreconcilable differences (Aldous, 1977; Kursh, 1971) or when benevolent misconceptions previously existed (Levinger & Breedlove, 1966). Some authors even suggest that unclear, tangential, or circumscribed communication is sometimes desirable to prevent understanding and preserve harmony in relationships (Aldous, 1977; Watzlawick et al., 1974).

My collegues and I have carried out three studies of understanding and communication in marriage that illustrate the contingent nature of understanding scores and their meaning. Many of our results contrasted sharply with prevailing assumptions in the literature on understanding. In general, the research suggested that (1) spouses are not highly accurate in judging certain perceptions held by their partner (2) previous studies have probably overgeneralized the relation between understanding and compatibility in marriage, (3) the same inferential "biases" that are generally present in person perception are apparently present in perceptions of communication, and (4) the referent of perception influences the relationships between understanding, communication, and marital satisfaction. The research is very preliminary, however, and these conclusions should be viewed accordingly. Since there are few comparable studies, the results of this research are considered below in some detail.

Couples Studies I and II

In the first two studies (Sillars, et al., 1984), we had spouses record their perceptions of each other and then engage in a conversation about typical marital problems. The understanding scores that were computed from their questionnaire responses differed in two significant respects from the understanding measures used in most previous studies. First, we had spouses guess the importance attributed by their partner to various conflict issues in the marriage. The referent of this task was more global and affective, or feeling-centered, than in other research. Some previous studies have had individuals predict specific attitudes or role perceptions of their spouse (e.g., Laing et al., 1966; Stuckert, 1963), whereas others have evaluated understanding of the spouse's self-perceptions, such as his or her response to a personality inventory (Dymond, 1954; Newmark et al., 1977). Second, understanding scores were computed based on a partial-correlation procedure that eliminated the confound of understanding and agreement (i.e., understanding was the partial correlation between the spouse's rating and a subject's estimate of the spouse's rating, controlling for the subject's own rating; see Wackman, 1973). Simple difference scores (i.e., the imputed response minus the actual response), which are commonly relied on in other research, confound understanding and agreement (see Gage & Cronbach, 1955).

Our procedures apparently had a profound effect on the results. In contrast to previous research, understanding was not positively related to marital satisfaction. In fact, this relation was slightly to moderately negative in both studies.

Though it may seem counterintuitive at first, the negative relation between understanding and satisfaction makes sense when we consider how subjects arrived at their estimate of the spouse's rating. We examined the possible influence of several factors, including projection, stereotypic perceptions, and verbal and nonverbal communication. It was immediately obvious that perceptions of the spouse were based mostly on projection. Perceived agreement was extremely high in both studies and was much higher than actual agreement. Further, the average "raw" understanding (based on a simple correlation between the imputed and actual response of the spouse) was moderate (between .30 and .42 across the two studies), but with agreement partialed out, understanding was very low (between .05 and .19). Thus, people inferred their partner's feelings largely by reference to their own feelings. With this factor statistically controlled, the average level of understanding was little better than chance guessing.

A measure of stereotypic perception was also included in the second study, but this did not prove to be a strong basis for the subjects' inference regarding their spouse's response. People were asked to indicate how husbands or wives in general would respond to the questionnaire items. The assumption was that some individuals, such as traditional couples, might differentiate self from spouse on the basis of gender-linked stereotypes. This was not the case; neither the more traditional couples nor the sample as a whole saw their spouses as highly stereotypic.

Finally, we explored verbal and nonverbal communication patterns associated with understanding. Subjects were divided into more understanding and less understanding groups and a log linear analysis of coded audio-taped conversations was carried out. In the conversations, spouses discussed the same issues that were used in the questionnaires as the stimulus items for perceptions of the spouse (and subsequently used in the computation of understanding scores). There was only one association between a subject's understanding of the spouse and the spouse's communication style that was consistent across the two studies. Specifically, individuals who were better understood by their partners were more negative in vocal tone. Of the verbal communication codes, only verbally competitive acts (faulting, rejection, hostile questions, and so forth) were associated with greater understanding in either study. Affectively neutral informational acts (description, self-disclosure, questions eliciting disclosure, etc.) were not associated with understanding.

The results can be explained by a simple principle that is well-documented in the social cognition literature. In general, the information that was more "immediate" appeared to have had the greatest impact on partners' estimates of their spouses' perceptions. In other words, information that was more "available" (Kahneman & Tversky, 1973), vivid (Nisbett & Ross, 1980), or easily and directly observed (Duck, 1976) had the greatest weight. The most immediate data were the subjects' own feelings and perceptions, since these are easily accessed, emotionally salient, and directly experienced. Consequently, subjects' own feelings were the main point of reference for estimating the partner's feelings.

The next most immediate source of information was the partner's nonverbal (paralinguistic) emotional expression. Nonverbal expression is more image-provoking than verbal communication because of its concreteness and inherently salient qualities. Further, nonverbal behavior is usually assumed by individuals to be a more direct, less censored reflection of an individual's subjective experience (Harper et al., 1978). And, because negative affect is more salient (Kanouse & Hanson, 1972) and more easily recognized than positive or neutral information, it follows that negative affect was the best communicative predictor of understanding. Our coding experience suggested that positive intonation is more subtle and difficult to identify than negative information.

This reasoning may help to explain the negative relationship between understanding and marital satisfaction that Sillars et al. (1984) obtained. Because negative feelings and dissatisfactions are easier to judge accurately than positive or neutral feelings, it follows that people in less satisfying and more conflictual relationships should be better at understanding each other's feelings.

Compared with the nonverbal display of affect, verbal communication is a less salient, less direct reflection of subjective experience. Therefore, verbal explanations may not greatly increase understanding of feelings because verbal disclosure is preempted by more immediate, nonverbal information. However, this principle is obviously tied to the nature of the task. Because specific beliefs and abstract cognitions cannot be expressed through nonverbal communication, verbal disclosure may play a greater role and nonverbal communication a lesser role in more cognitive, less feeling-centered judgment tasks.

Stereotypic knowledge, as we operationalized it, is also a less immediate source of data. However, stereotypic knowledge in the form of concrete personae or prototypes (see Cantor & Mischel, 1977) is more immediate than abstract generalizations and may have a greater effect on estimates of the spouse. Our research did not give this possibility a fair chance because we gave subjects the abstract task of estimating typical gender-related perceptions, rather than eliciting the individual's own stereotypes.

Couples Study III

At this point we only have partial results from the third couples study, but it still provides a useful contrast to the first two studies. In the third study, spouses guessed their partners' attitudes about a variety of companionate and instrumental aspects of marriage (e.g., "In a good marriage people are always honest with each other"; "A neat house is very important"). The judgment items were less feeling centered and more specific than in the first two studies. Correspondingly, there was less of a projection bias. Perceived agreement was nearly the same as actual agreement. Understanding scores were also somewhat higher than in the first two studies, although understanding of companionate topics (affection, communication, irritability, and criticism) was considerably lower, on the average, than understanding of instrumental topics (money, cleaning and caring for the house, leisure activities, and career and work pressures). Similarly, there was mild support for a positive relation between understanding and marital satisfaction, but this applied only to understanding on instrumental topics. These results probably reflect the more complex, less tangible nature of the companionate items. On such ambiguous items, less valid prediction criteria are likely to be employed in judging the spouse's perception, thereby producing low understanding scores and a negligible or even negative relationship between understanding and marital satisfaction.

The research on understanding suggests that underacknowledged aspects of the research context affect the nature of understanding scores and their relation to marital satisfaction. There was not much support in our research for the importance of empathic understanding in marriage. These findings stand in contrast to a formidable coalition of prior research, theory, and popular wisdom about marriage, which suggest that empathic ability is one of the single most important factors in individual and dyadic social competence. The apparent contradiction may be accounted for by three considerations. First, understanding is affected by factors that have little to do with empathy or perspective-taking, such as agreement. Agreement occasionally may be the more important factor in compatibility. Second, the nature of the task may affect the use of less valid prediction criteria. On more abstract and feeling-centered tasks, subjects appear to rely on simple rules of thumb to make predictions about their spouses. In these instances, understanding scores have little, if any, implication for compatibility.

Third, the need for understanding varies a great deal depending on the nature of the topic. This consideration was not addressed in detail by our research, as it was, for example, by Levinger and Breedlove (1966). Levinger and Breedlove suggested that there are often benevolent misconceptions in relationships, such that perceived agreement is more strongly related to marital satisfaction than is actual agreement. This hypothesis was supported in the Levinger and Breedlove study and it fit the data from our first two studies (Sillars et al., 1984). On the other hand, Levinger and Breedlove also reasoned that understanding is more strongly related to compatibility on issues that affect the day-to-day coordination of a couple. Although intuitively reasonable, the latter hypothesis was not clearly supported by Levinger and Breedlove, and little has been done subsequently to identify contexts in which understanding is an essential aspect of compatibility.

Conclusion

Interpersonal perception has been studied from several ostensibly unrelated perspectives and this diversity has contributed to the broad scope of the present discussion. However, there are benefits to be gained from a broad, synthetic approach to interpersonal perception. The conclusions drawn by different researchers, asking somewhat different questions, frequently overlap in their implications. For example, self and other perceptions of communication (e.g., Hawkins et al., 1980) reflect the same differences commonly associated with actor-observer differences in causal attribution. Further, when estimating another person's perspective, individuals appear to assign greater weight or priority to information that is vivid and direct (Sillars et al., 1984), as is the case in other areas of social cognition (Nisbett & Ross, 1980).

As the preceding examples suggest, the person perception/social cognition literature may contribute to our understanding of interpersonal perception in personal relationships. However, this literature does not provide a perspective uniquely tailored to the study of personal relationships. Therefore, sociologists (e.g., Berger & Kellner, 1964; Hess & Handel, 1959), communication theorists (e.g., Cushman & Whiting, 1972; Watzlawick et al., 1967), and others who have devoted their attention primarily to ongoing relationships, command our attention as well.

Authors who focus exclusively on personal relationships emphasize their distinctiveness. Familiarity, interdependence, uniqueness, and emotionality all tend to characterize personal relationships, and each of these factors suggests possible causes of ambiguity in interpersonal perception. Thus, certain features of the relationship itself may explain "biased" or incongruent perception. Intimate partners are capable of both insight and imperceptivity with regard to each other, although the reasons for the former are more self-evident than those for the latter. The "naive" hypothesis generally held by people is that familiarity steadily increases perceptual accuracy, leading to extremely high understanding in most intimate relationships. On the other hand, the less intuitive assumption of this chapter is that interpersonal perception has inherent ambiguity, even in close, personal relationships. Familiarity modifies the basic causes and effects of interpersonal perception, but it does not render interpersonal perception an unproblematic and trivial concern.

Two levels of interpersonal perception were considered in this chapter: the level of direct perspectives (attribution) and the level of meta-perspectives (understanding). Athough these topics reflect distinct research traditions, there are several generalizations that transcend them. First, interpersonal perceptions reflect a need for parsimony in the description, prediction, and explanation of other people's actions. In the attribution literature this principle is reflected in the fact that linear, causal explanations for behavior are often provided when complex, interactional attributions are seemingly more appropriate. In the literature on understanding, parsimony is reflected in the fact that people typically use their own direct perspective as the primary basis for making predictions about the partner, although an "endless spiral" of reciprocal role-taking is depicted by theory (Laing et al., 1966). Perhaps a searching analysis of the partner's perspective is not initiated unless some anomaly in behavior is detected. However, as the earlier discussion suggested, relatively subtle changes in the partner's behavior are likely to be assimilated to previous structures and therefore go unnoticed.

A second common principle is that the level of ambiguity inherent in the referent influences the level of perceptual congruence. Studies of attribution have typically been concerned with social perceptions that are intrinsically ambiguous and problematic—that is, perceptions of abstract, causally complex, and affectively loaded dispositions and events (e.g., good and bad qualities of the partner, communicative intentions, the reasons for interpersonal conflicts). This focus of study probably accounts for the frequent finding that the actor and partner tend to provide opposite and conflicting attributions. Further, in more ambiguous situations (i.e., intense conflict and separation) attribution differences are more extreme. In the understanding literature, it seems that the intrinsic ambiguity of a referent may influence the level of understanding typically achieved, as well as the use of different criteria for predicting the partner's perspective.

Third, general social cognitive biases apparently apply to both attribution and understanding. There has been, of course, a much more systematic exploration of social cognitive biases within the attribution literature. However, the literature on understanding is at least suggestive in indicating that so-called "biases" such as the "false consensus" effect (i.e., overestimation of similarity between self and others) and the "vividness criterion" (i.e., reliance on more vivid or salient information) have an analogue in the way that people use interpersonal communication and other information to estimate the partner's perspective.

Finally, the suggestion that perceptions must fit into a coherent pattern within relationships (Hess & Handel, 1959) probably applies to both attribution and understanding. However, at this point it is not easy to say what type of incongruence represents a bad fit. This conclusion especially applies to the literature on understanding, in which a positive correlation between understanding and relationship satisfaction has been demonstrated many times, but the exceptions to this finding are too important to ignore. Some degree of perceptual incongruence is certainly inevitable in personal relationships and is perhaps even "healthy" (e.g., Kursh, 1971; Levinger & Breedlove, 1966; Parks, 1981). However, the literature does not presently offer a clear picture of the contexts in which interpersonal perception actually does have important consequences for a relationship.

Acknowledgments. Portions of this chapter were facilitated by a grant from the Ohio State University Graduate School. The author gratefully acknowledges the criticisms and suggestions of Bill Ickes and Gifford Weary.

References

Aldous, J. (1977). Family interaction patterns. *Annual Review of Sociology, 3,* 105–135.

Altman, I., & Taylor, D. H. (1973). *Social penetration: The development of interpersonal relationships.* New York: Holt, Rinehart & Winston.

Argyle, M. (1969). *Social interaction.* Chicago: Aldine.

Barry, W. A. (1970). Marriage research and conflict: An integrative review. *Psychological Bulletin, 73,* 41–54.

Bauchner, J. E. (1980). Accuracy in detecting deception as a function of level of relationship and communication history. Unpublished dissertation, Michigan State University.

Bem, D. J. (1972). Self-perception theory. In L. Berkowitz (Ed.), *Advances in experimental social psychology* (Vol. 6). New York: Academic Press.

Berger, C. R., & Bradac, J. J. (1982). *Language and social knowledge: Uncertainty in interpersonal relations.* London: Edward Arnold.

Berger, C. R., & Calabrese, R. J. (1975). Some explorations in initial interaction and beyond: Toward a developmental theory of interpersonal communication. *Human Communication Research, 1,* 99–112,

Berger, C. R., & Roloff, M. E. (1982). Thinking about friends and lovers: Social cognition and relational trajectories. In M. E. Roloff & C. R. Berger (Eds.), *Social cognition and communication.* Beverly Hills, CA: Sage.

Berger, P., & Kellner, H. (1964). Marriage and the construction of reality. *Diogenes, 46,* 1–24.

Bernal, G. (1978). Couple interactions: A study of the punctuation process. Unpublished dissertation, University of Massachusetts.

Birchler, G. R., Weiss, R. L., & Vincent, J. P. (1975). Multimethod analysis of social reinforcement exchange between maritally distressed and nondistressed spouse and stranger dyads. *Journal of Personality and Social Psychology, 31,* 349–360.

Bochner, A. P., Krueger, D. L., & Chmielewski, T. L. (1982). Interpersonal perceptions and marital adjustment. *Journal of Communication, 32,* 135–147.

Bott, E. *Family and social network.* (1957). New York: The Free Press.

Byrne, D., & Blaylock, B. (1963). Similarity and assumed similarity between husbands and wives. *Journal of Abnormal and Social Psychology, 67,* 636–640.

Cantor, N., & Mischel, W. (1977). Traits as prototypes: Effects on recognition memory. *Journal of Personality and Social psychology, 35,* 38–49.

Christensen, L., & Wallace, L. (1976). Perceptual accuracy as a variable in marital adjustment. *Journal of Sex and Marital Therapy, 2,* 130–136.

Cooley, C. H. (1902). *Human nature and the social order.* New York: Charles Scribner.

Corsini, R. J. (1956). Understanding and similarity in marriage. *Journal of Abnormal and Social Psychology, 52,* 327–332.

Cushman, D., & Whiting, G. C. (1972). An approach to communication theory: Toward consensus on rules. *The Journal of Communication, 22,* 217–236.

Dalusio, V. E. (1972). Self-disclosure and perceptions of that self-disclosure between parents and their teenage children. Unpublished dissertation, American International University.

Danziger, K. (1976). *Interpersonal communication.* New York: Pergamon.

Davis, M. S. (1973). *Intimate relations.* New York: Free Press.

Deutsch, M. (1973). *The resolution of conflict: Constructive and destructive processes.* New Haven: Yale University Press.

Doherty, W. J. (1981). Cognitive processes in intimate conflict: I. Extending attribution theory. *American Journal of Family Therapy, 9,* 3–13.

Doherty, W. J. (1982). Attributional style and negative problem solving in marriage. *Family Relations, 31,* 201–205.

Duck, S. (1976). Interpersonal communication in developing acquaintance. In G. R. Miller (Ed.), *Explorations in interpersonal communication.* Beverly Hills, CA: Sage.

Dymond, R. (1954). Interpersonal perception and marital happiness. *Canadian Journal of Psychology, 8,* 164–171.

Ferguson, L. R., & Allen, D. R. (1978). Congruence of parental perception, marital satisfaction, and child adjustment. *Journal of Consulting and Clinical Psychology, 46,* 345–346.

Ferreira, A. J. (1964). Interpersonal perceptivity among family members. *American Journal of Orthopsychiatry, 34,* 64–70.

Fincham, F. D. (1983). Clinical applications of attribution theory: Problems and prospects. In M. Hewstone (Ed.), *Attribution theory: Social and functional extensions.* Oxford, England: Blackwells.

Fincham, F., & O'Leary, K. D. (1983). Causal inferences for spouse behavior in maritally distressed and nondistressed couples. *Journal of Social and Clinical Psychology, 1,* 42–57.

Fitzpatrick, M. A. (1977). A typological approach to communication in relationships. In B. D. Rubin (Ed.), *Communication yearbook* (Vol. 1). New Brunswick, NJ: Transaction Books.

Fitzpatrick, M. A. (1983). Predicting couples' communication from couples' self-reports. In R. Bostrom (Ed.), *Communication yearbook* (Vol. 7). Beverly Hills, CA: Sage.

Fitzpatrick, M. A., & Winke, J. J. (1979). You always hurt the one you love: Strategies and tactics in interpersonal conflict. *Communication Quarterly, 27,* 3–11.

Frank, C., Anderson, O. N., & Rubinstein, D. (1980). Marital role ideas and perceptions of marital role behavior in distressed and nondistressed couples. *Journal of Marital and Family Therapy, 6*, 55–64.

Gage, N., & Cronbach, L. (1955). Conceptual and Methodological problems in interpersonal perception. *Psychological Review, 62*, 411–422.

Goffman, E. (1959). *The presentation of self in everyday life.* Garden City, NY: Doubleday.

Good, L. R., Good, K. C., & Nelson, D. A. (1973). Assumed similarity and perceived intrafamilial communication and understanding. *Psychological Reports, 32*, 3–11.

Goode, W. J. (1971). Force and violence in the family. *Journal of Marriage and the Family, 33*, 624–636.

Gottman, J., Notarius, C., Markman, H., Bank, S., Yoppi, B., & Rubin, M. E. (1976). Behavior exchange theory and marital decision making. *Journal of personality and Social Psychology, 34*, 14–23.

Gottman, J. M., Markman, H., & Notarius, C. (1977). The topography of marital conflict: A sequential analysis of verbal and nonverbal behavior. *Journal of Marriage and the Family, 39*, 461–478.

Harper, R. G., Weins, A. N., & Matarazzo, J. D. (1978). *Nonverbal communication: The state of the art.* New York: John Wiley & Sons.

Harvey, J. H., Weber, A. L., Yarkin, K. L., & Stewart, B. E. (1982). An attributional approach to relationship breakdown and dissolution. In S. Duck (Ed.), *Personal relationships: Dissolving personal relationships.* New York: Academic Press.

Harvey, J. H., Wells, G. L., & Alvarez, M. D. (1978). Attribution in the context of conflict and separation in close relationships. In J. H. Harvey, W. J. Ickes, & R. F. Kidd (Eds.), *New directions in attribution research* (Vol. 2). Hillsdale, NJ: Lawrence Erlbaum.

Hastie, R. (1981). Schematic principles in human memory. In E. T. Higgins, C. P. Herman, & M. P. Zanna (Eds), *Social cognition: The Ontario Symposium* (Vol. 1). Hillsdale, NJ: Lawrence Erlbaum.

Hawkins, J. L., Weisberg, C., & Ray, D. W. (1980). Spouse differences in communication style: Preference, perception, and behavior. *Journal of Marriage and the Family, 42*, 585–593.

Heider, F. (1958). *The psychology of interpersonal relations.* New York: John Wiley & Sons.

Hess, R. D., & Handel, G. (1959). *Family worlds: A psychosocial approach to family life.* Chicago: University of Chicago Press.

Hicks, M. W., & Platt, M. (1970). Marital happiness and stability: A review of research in the sixties. *Journal of Marriage and the Family, 32*, 553–574.

Higgins, E. T., Herman, C. P., & Zanna, M. P. (Eds.). (1981). *Social cognition: The Ontario Symposium* (Vol. 1). Hillsdale, NJ: Lawrence Erlbaum.

Higgins, E. T., Kuiper, N. A., & Olson, J. M. (1981). Social cognition: A need to get personal. In E. T. Higgins, C. P. Herman, & M. P. Zanna (Eds.), *Social cognition: The Ontario Symposium* (Vol. 1). Hillsdale, NJ: Lawrence Erlbaum.

Hopper, R., Knapp, M. L., & Scott, L. (1981). Couples' personal idioms: Exploring intimate talk. *Journal of Communication, 37*, 23–33.

Hunt, M., & Hunt, B. (1977). *The divorce experience.* New York: McGraw-Hill.

Jones, E. E., & Harris, V. A. (1967). The attribution of attitudes. *Journal of Experimental Social Psychology, 3*, 1–24.

Jones, E. E., & Nisbett, R. E. (1972). The actor and the observer: Divergent perceptions of the causes of behavior. In E. E. Jones & others (Eds.), *Attribution: Perceiving the causes of behavior.* Morristown, NJ: General Learning Press.

Kahn, M. (1970). Nonverbal communication and marital satisfaction. *Family Process, 9*, 449–456.

Kahneman, D., & Tversky, A. (1973). On the psychology of prediction. *Psychological Review*, *80*, 237–251.

Kanouse, D. E., & Hanson, L. R. (1972). Negativity in evaluations. In E. E. Jones & others (Eds.), *Attribution: Perceiving the causes of behavior*. Morristown, NJ: General Learning Press.

Kelley, H. H. (1972). Attribution in social interaction. In E. E. Jones & others (Eds.), *Attribution: Perceiving the causes of behavior*. Morristown, NJ: General Learning Press.

Kelley, H. H. (1979). *Personal relationships: Their structure and processes*. Hillsdale, NJ: Lawrence Erlbaum.

Kelley, H. H., & Michela, J. L. (1980). Attribution theory and research. *Annual Review of Psychology*, 31, 457–501.

Kelley, H. H., & Stahelski, A. J. (1970). Errors in perceptions of intentions in a mixed-motive game. *Journal of Experimental Social Psychology*, *6*, 379–400.

Kieren, D., & Tallman, I. (1972). Spousal adaptability: An assessment of marital competence. *Journal of Marriage and the Family*, *34*, 247–255.

Knapp, M. L. (1978). *Social intercourse: From greeting to goodbye*. Boston: Allyn & Bacon.

Knudson, R. A., Sommers, A. A., & Golding, S. L. (1980). Interpersonal perception and mode of resolution in marital conflict. *Journal of Personality and Social Psychology*, *38*, 251–263.

Komarovsky, M. (1964). *Blue collar marriage*. New York: Random House.

Kotlar, S. L. (1965). Middle-class marital role perceptions and marital adjustment. *Sociology and Social Research*, *49*, 284–291.

Kursh, C. O. (1971). The benefits of poor communication. *Psychoanalytic Review*, *58*, 189–208.

Laing, R. D., Phillipson, H., & Lee, A. R. (1966). *Interpersonal perception: A theory and a method of research*. New York: Springer-Verlag.

Langer, E. J. (1978). Rethinking the role of thought in social interaction. In J. H. Harvey, W. J. Ickes, & R. F. Kidd (Eds.), *New directions in attribution research* (Vol. 2). Hillsdale, NJ: Lawrence Erlbaum.

Levinger, G., & Breedlove, J. (1966). Interpersonal attraction and agreement. *Journal of Personality and Social Psychology*, *3*, 367–372.

Losee, G. D. (1976). An investigation of selected interpersonal and communication variables in marital relationships. Unpublished dissertation, University of Illinois.

Luckey, E. B. (1960). Marital satisfaction and its association with congruence of perception. *Marriage and Family Living*, *22*, 49–54.

Luckey, E. B. (1966). Number of years married as related to personality perception and marital satisfaction. *Journal of Marriage and the Family*, *28*, 44–48.

Madden, M. E., & Janoff-Bulman, R. (1981). Blame, control, and marital satisfaction: Wives' attributions for conflict in marriage. *Journal of Marriage and the Family*, *43*, 663–674.

McCleod, J. M., & Chaffee, S. H. (1973). Interpersonal approaches to communication research. *American Behavioral Scientist*, *16*, 469–499.

Mead, G. H. (1934). *Mind, self and society*. Chicago: University of Chicago Press.

Mehrabian, A. (1972). *Nonverbal communication*. Chicago: Aldine Atherton.

Millar, F. E., & Rogers, L. E. (1976). A relational approach to interpersonal communication. In G. R. Miller (Ed.), *Explorations in interpersonal communication*. Beverly Hills, CA: Sage.

Miller, G. R., & Steinberg, M. (1975). *Between people*. Chicago: Science Research Associates.

Miller, S., Nunnally, E. W., & Wackman, D. B. (1975). *Alive and aware: How to improve your relationships through better communication*. Minneapolis: Inter-personal Communication Programs, Inc.

Monson, T. C., & Snyder, M. (1977). Actors, observers, and the attribution process. *Journal of Experimental Social Psychology*, *13*, 89–111.

Morton, T. L., Alexander, J. F., & Altman, I. (1976). Communication and relationship definition. In G. R. Miller (Ed.), *Explorations in interpersonal communication*. Beverly Hills, CA: Sage.

Murstein, B. I., & Beck, G. D. (1972). Person perception, marriage adjustment, and social desirability. *Journal of Consulting and Clinical Psychology*, *39*, 396–403.

Newcomb, T. M. (1953). An approach to the study of communicative acts. *Psychological Review*, *60*, 393–404.

Newman, H. (1981). Communication within ongoing intimate relationships: An attributional perspective. *Personality and Social Psychology Bulletin*, *7*, 59–70.

Newman, H., & Langer, E. J. (1981). Post divorce adaptation and the attribution and the attribution of responsibility. *Sex Roles*, *7*, 223–232.

Newmark, C. S., Woody, G., & Ziff, D. (1977). Understanding and similarity in relation to marital satisfaction. *Journal of Clinical Psychology*, *33*, 83–86.

Nisbett, R., & Ross, L. (1980). *Human inference: Strategies and shortcomings of social judgment*. Englewood Cliffs, NJ: Prentice Hall.

Noller, P. (1980). Misunderstandings in marital communication: A study of couples' nonverbal communication. *Journal of Personality and Social Psychology*, *39*, 1135–1148.

Noller, P. (1981). Gender and marital adjustment level differences in decoding messages from spouses and strangers. *Journal of Personality and Social Psychology*, *41*, 272–278.

O'Keefe, D. J., & Sypher, H. E. (1981). Cognitive complexity measures and the relationship of cognitive complexity to communication: A critical review. *Human Communication Research*, *8*, 72–92.

Orvis, B. R., Kelley, H. H., & Butler, D. (1976). Attributional conflict in young couples. In J. H. Harvey, W. J. Ickes, & R. F. Kidd (Eds.), *New directions in attribution research* (Vol. 1). Hillsdale, NJ: Lawrence Erlbaum.

Parks, M. R. (1981). Ideology in interpersonal communication: Off the couch and into the world. In M. Burgoon (Ed.), *Communication yearbook* (Vol. 5). New Brunswick, NJ: Transaction Books.

Pavitt, C. (1982). Conceptual issues in the communication/coorientation accuracy relationship. Paper presented at the Speech Communication Association convention, Louisville, Kentucky.

Pavitt, C., & Cappella, J. N. (1979). Coorientational accuracy in interpersonal and small group discussions: A literature review, model, and simulation. In D. Nimmo (Ed.), *Communication yearbook* (Vol. 3). New Brunswick, NJ: Transaction Press.

Piaget J. (1926). *The language and thought of the child*. New York: Harcourt Brace.

Rausch, H. L., Barry, W. A., Hertel, R. K., & Swain, M. A. (1974). *Communication, conflict and marriage*. San Francisco: Jossey-Bass.

Rogers, T. B. (1980). Models of man: The beauty and/or the beast? *Personality and Social Psychology Bulletin*, *6*, 582–590.

Ross, L. (1977). The intuitive psychologist and his shortcomings: Distortions in the attribution process. In L. Berkowitz (Ed.), *Advances in experimental social psychology* (Vol. 10). New York: Academic Press.

Ryder, R. (1969). Husband-wife dyads versus married strangers. *Family Process*, *7*, 233–238.

Schaap, C. (1982). Communication and adjustment. Lisse, Netherlands: Swets & Zeitlinger, B. V.

Scheff, T. (1968). Negotiating reality: Notes on power in the assessment of responsibility. *Social Problems*, *16*, 3–17.

Schlenker, B. R., & Goldman, H. J. (1978). Cooperators and competitors in conflict: A test of the "triangle model." *Journal of Conflict Resolution*, *22*, 393–410.

Schneider, D. J., Hastorf, A. H., & Ellsworth, P. C. (1979). *Person perception.* Reading, MA: Addison-Wesley.

Schroder, H. M., Driver, M. J., & Streufert, S. (1967). *Human information processing.* New York: Holt, Rinehart & Winston.

Shapiro, A., & Swensen, C. (1969). Patterns of self-disclosure among married couples. *Journal of Counseling Psychology, 16*, 179–180.

Sillars, A. L. (1981). Attributions and interpersonal conflict resolution. In J. H. Harvey, W. J. Ickes, & R. F. Kidd (Eds.), *New directions in attribution research* (Vol. 3). Hillsdale, NJ: Lawrence Erlbaum.

Sillars, A. L. (1984). *Attributions and marital communication.* Unpublished research. Ohio State University.

Sillars, A. L., & Parry, D. (1982). Stress, cognition and communication in interpersonal conflict. *Communication Research, 9*, 201–226.

Sillars, A. L., & Pike, G. R. (1984). Reciprocity in marital communication. Unpublished manuscript, Department of Communication, Ohio State University.

Sillars, A. L., Pike, G. R., Jones, T. S., & Murphy, M. A. (1984). Communication and understanding in marriage. *Human Communication Research, 10*, 317–350.

Sillars, A. L., Pike, G. R., Jones, T. J., & Redmon, K. (1983). Communication and conflict in marriage. In K. Bostrom (Ed.), *Communication yearbook* (Vol. 7). Beverly Hills, CA: Sage.

Snyder, M., & Gangestad, S. (1981). Hypothesis-testing processes. In J. H. Harvey, W. J. Ickes, & R. F. Kidd (Eds.), *New directions in attribution research* (Vol. 3). Hillsdale, NJ: Lawrence Erlbaum.

Snyder, M., Stephan, W. G., & Rosenfield, D. (1978). Attributional egotism. In J. H. Harvey, W. J. Ickes, & R. F. Kidd (Eds.), *New directions in attribution research* (Vol. 2). Hillsdale, NJ: Lawrence Erlbaum.

Stafford, L., & Daly, J. A. (1984). Conversational memory: The effects of recall mode and memory expectancies on remembrances of natural conversations. *Human Communication Research, 10*, 379–402.

Straus, M. (1974). Leveling, civility and violence in the family. *Journal of Marriage and the Family, 36*, 13–29.

Stuckert, R. (1963). Role perception and marital satisfaction: A configuration approach. *Marriage and Family Living, 25*, 415–419.

Suedfeld, P., & Tetlock, P. (1977). Integrative complexity of communications in international crises. *Journal of Conflict Resolution, 21*, 169–184.

Sullivan, H. S. (1953). *The interpersonal theory of psychiatry.* New York: W. W. Norton.

Taylor, A. B. (1967). Role perception, empathy, and marriage adjustment. *Sociology and Social Research, 52*, 22–34.

Taylor, S. E., & Fiske, S. T. (1978). Salience, attention, and attribution: Top of the head phenomena. In L. Berkowitz (Ed.), *Advances in experimental social psychology* (Vol. 11). New York: Academic.

Thomas, E. J. (1977). *Marital communication and decision making: Analysis, assessment and change.* New York: The Free Press.

Thomas, K. W., & Pondy, L. R. (1977). Toward an "intent" model of conflict management among principal parties. *Human Relations, 30*, 1089–1102.

Thompson, S. C., & Kelley, H. H. (1981). Judgments of responsibility for activities in close relationships. *Journal of Personality and Social Psychology, 41*, 469–477.

Turk, J. L., & Bell, N. W. (1972). Measuring power in families. *Journal of Marriage and the Family, 34*, 215–222.

Wackman, D. B. (1973). Interpersonal communication and coorientation. *American Behavioral Scientist, 16*, 537–550.

Watzlawick, P., Beavin, J., & Jackson, D. D. (1967). *Pragmatics of human communication: A study of interactional patterns, pathologies, and paradoxes.* New York: W. W. Norton.

Watzlawick, P., Weakland, J., & Fisch, R. (1974). *Principles of problem formation and problem resolution.* New York: W. W. Norton.

Weary, G., & Arkin, R. M. (1981). Attributional self-presentation. In J. H. Harvey, W. Ickes, & R. F. Kidd (Eds.), *New directions in attribution research* (Vol. 3). Hillsdale, NJ: Lawrence Erlbaum.

Weary, G., Swanson, H., Harvey, J. H., & Yarkin, K. L. (1980). A molar approach to social knowing. *Personality and Social Psychology Bulletin, 6,* 56–62.

Weary-Bradley, G. (1978). Self-serving biases in the attribution process: A re-examination of the fact or fiction question. *Journal of Personality and Social Psychology, 36,* 56–71.

Weick, K. E. (1971). Group processes, family processes, and problem solving. In J. Aldous et al., (Eds.), *Family problem solving: A symposium on theoretical, methodological and substantive concerns.* Hinsdale, IL: Dryden Press.

Weiss, R. L., Hops, H., & Patterson, G. R. (1973). A framework for conceptualizing marital conflict: A technology for altering it, some data for evaluating it. In L. A. Hamerlynck, L. C. Hundy, & E. J. Mash (Eds.). *Behavior change: Methodology, concepts, and practice.* Champaign, IL: Research Press.

Weiss, R. S. (1975). *Marital separation.* New York: Basic Books.

Wiemann, J. J. (1977). Explication and test of a model of communicative competence. *Human Communication Research, 3,* 195–213.

Williamson, L. K. (1975). Self and other: An empirical study of interpersonal perception in dyadic marital communication systems. Unpublished doctoral dissertation, Temple University.

Winter, W. D., Ferreira, A. J., & Bowers, N. (1973). Decision making in married and unrelated couples. *Family Process, 12,* 83–94.

Wirth, L. (1948). Consensus and mass communication. *American Sociological Review, 13,* 1–15.

Wright, J., & Fichten, C. (1976). Denial of responsibility, videotape feedback and attribution theory: Relevance for behavioral marital therapy. *Canadian Psychological Review, 17,* 219–230.

Zanna, M. P., & Cooper, J. (1976). Dissonance and the attribution process. In J. H. Harvey, W. J. Ickes, & R. F. Kidd (Eds.), *New directions in attribution research.* Hillsdale, NJ: Lawrence Erlbaum.

Zucker, R. A., & Barron, F. H. (1971). Toward a systematic family mythology: The relationship of parents' and adolescents' reports of parental behavior during childhood. Paper presented at the Eastern Psychological Association convention, New York.

Part V

Perspectives on Marital Interaction

Chapter 13

Compatibility in Marriage and Other Close Relationships

George Levinger and Marylyn Rands

Will Owen, an ambitious graduate student from New York City, be successful in courting Paula, a summer farm worker from rural Pennsylvania? And, if they should marry each other, how well will they get along together? Questions such as these are the stuff of soap operas. They are also likely to concern each of us in our everyday lives.

The questions here lead to other questions: How shall we conceive of compatibility in close relationships such as friendship or marriage? And what theory and findings inform our knowledge of this topic? In this chapter, we first define what we mean by a close relationship, marriage in particular, and then analyze compatibility in that context. Subsequently, we examine selected research on mate selection and the maintenance of marriage.

Theoretical Analysis

Defining the Close Relationship

Almost everyone has an implicit definition of a close relationship. It would probably include terms such as "intimate," "enduring," or "committed." Yet precise definitions have been surprisingly hard to formulate, partly because of the multiplicity of types and functions of relationships. One approach is to focus on the kind and degree of interdependence between two persons. Interdependence can refer to causal interconnections in partners' affect, thoughts, and actions; each of these can then be classified according to their frequency, diversity, strength, and duration (Kelley, Berscheid, Christensen, Harvey, Huston, Levinger, McClintock, Peplau, & Peterson, 1983). Thus, a *close* relationship, such as marriage, is one that has relatively frequent, diverse, strong, and enduring interconnections of affect, thoughts, and actions.

A high level of closeness, then, implies that each partner is able to affect the other deeply. The closer a pair, the more the partners' behaviors, plans, and outcomes are causally interconnected, and the less able is either partner to act independently of the other. If one truly cares for another, then one usually considers his or her outcomes in relation to one's own, and this consideration is reflected in one's own plans and behavior.

Interactive events and their connections. The basic elements of a pair relationship, then, are interconnected events and patterns of events (Kelley et al., 1983). Events consist of discrete changes in one or both members' actions, thoughts, or feelings; *interactive* events are traceable to actions or occurrences in the other partner. For example, one partner's smile may be traced to the other's earlier tone of voice, and in turn will enhance the other's feeling of pleasure and anticipation of future interaction. Figure 13-1, adapted from Kelley et al. (1983), illustrates how each pair member's chain of events is causally connected to the other's chain. The two vertical chains (under P, for person, and O, for other, respectively) refer to *intra*chain connections—i.e., temporal changes in thoughts, feelings, or actions of either P or O, as affected by their own previous events. The arrows that point *between* these two chains (from P's to O's chain and vice versa) refer to *inter*chain connections, wherein partners influence each other's plans, emotions, or behaviors. Later we discuss how each partner's influence on the other's intrachain sequences is central to the concept of pair compatibility. For the moment, note that this perspective on pair interaction emphasizes the immediate or short-term dynamics of interdependence.

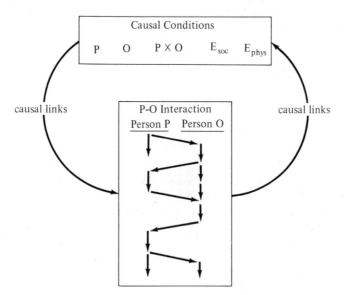

Figure 13-1. A causal model of pair interaction. Person-Other interaction is affected by, and in turn affects, relatively stable causal conditions, which include P's and O's personal characteristics (P and O), their relationship's attributes (P × O), and their environmental characteristics (E_{soc} and E_{phys}). Adapted from Kelley et al. (1983, p. 57).

Causal conditions and long-term linkages. Closeness is also affected by stable and enduring "causal conditions," which consist of continuing personal, relational, and environmental attributes. Causal conditions endure over considerable time and do not fluctuate in the manner of interactional events. Examples of enduring *personal* conditions include personality traits, skills, habits, attitudes, and long-range goals. *Relational* conditions are P $\times$ O factors such as the two partners' shared history, mutual knowledge, or attitude similarity. *Environmental* conditions consist of both social and physical components (E_{soc} and E_{phys}). Examples of E_{soc} conditions are the size or supportiveness of an acquaintance network or the nature of cultural norms; examples of E_{phys} conditions are the noisiness or crowdedness of one's neighborhood. The stability of such causal conditions affects the stability of the entire relationship; instability in important conditions (e.g., in either partner's personal goals or employment) can lead to significant relational changes.

Relationships can be examined at two levels: the level of events and the level of causal conditions. At the event level, one can observe the temporal patterning of P's and O's respective actions, thoughts, and feelings. Each single event may be connected to past and future events within each actor's own chain of events; it may also be connected to the other's events. This level of interpersonal patterning—as exemplified in Figure 13-1—will here be called the *micro*level. The microlevel refers to immediate interaction processes and detailed analyses thereof.

Causal linkages can also be noted with regard to enduring attributes or causal conditions. For example, similar age or similar recreational preferences are associated with the choice of friends. It is tempting to attribute a causal character to such interpersonal similarity, to assume that such personal attributes "cause" the interpersonal actions. This level of analysis will here be called the *macro*level, which refers to broad structural variables and patterns of variables. Patterned interconnections at both the microlevel and macrolevel are central to our conception of pair compatibility.

Compatibility and Incompatibility

Close relationships are characterized by interdependence, by the members' strongly and diversely interconnected chains of events. In other words, each partner is subject to the other's influence in a wide variety of situations and times. Given such diversity, it is likely that intimate partners will at least occasionally encounter conflicts in goals, beliefs, emotions, or actual behavior. Achieving and maintaining pair harmony is a major challenge of interpersonal relationships.

Defining compatibility. We here define pair compatibility as the ratio of facilitating to interfering events between P and O. This definition derives from Kelley et al.'s (1983, p. 34) discussion of "interchain facilitation versus interference." If one assumes that P's behavior is directed toward a goal, then the causal connections from O's to P's chain may either *facilitate* or *interfere* with progression toward that goal, or it may have no effect at all. In facilitation, interchain causal connections promote the partner's desired action sequences and outcomes; in interference, interchain connections disrupt them. Examples of O's interfering behavior would include confusing, unsettling, or distracting P, attacking P's self-image, or interrupting P's plans or activities.

In this chapter, pairs perceived to have high overall facilitation/interference (F/I) ratios are considered highly compatible, or as promoting each other's goals or action sequences. Those with low F/I ratios are defined as low in compatibility, or as not furthering these aims. This definition links the topic of compatibility to Deutsch's (1973) conceptualization of conflict, defined as the occurrence of "incompatible actions." Conflict, according to Deutsch, derives from a mismatching either between goals or between ways of reaching goals. It can occur either within one partner's (intrapersonal) or between two partners' (interpersonal) goal orientations. Our present emphasis is on *inter*personal issues, but if either member of a relationship is seriously conflicted *intra*-personally, this conflict is likely to have *inter*personal repercussions. Pair compatibility is difficult to achieve and to maintain under conditions where one or both partners have serious unresolved personal problems, or where either has important conflicting demands from his or her kin, friends, work environment, or from the broader sociocultural context.

Ratios of facilitation to interference are only one way of conceiving interchain causal connections. One can also consider the *amount* of facilitation and interference. Two pairs may have equal F/I ratios (e.g., 10:1) but differ greatly in the number of their respective events—say 10,000/1000 as against 20/2. The first pair has an established history of facilitation, the second does not. High absolute amounts of facilitative interchain connections, over a long time period, suggest stability. Low amounts, over a long period, indicate a casual or a distant relationship; over a short period, they indicate little shared experience.

Facilitation and interference need not affect both partners equally. Effects of an action may be facilitative for one partner while interfering with the other's "sequence." For example, a husband may feel that his protective advice to his wife confirms that he is a concerned husband, but she may feel that he is patronizing her and questioning her competence.

Not all "facilitative" actions lead to pleasurable results. For instance, each partner's words may set off mutual strings of familiar, well-rehearsed argu-ments, and thus "facilitate" the predictable escalation of a marital quarrel, as is often the case in "conflict-habituated" couples (Cuber & Harroff, 1965). Furthermore, not all "interference" has negative consequences. For example, an automobile passenger, seeing an oncoming vehicle at an intersection, might yell "Stop!" This would interfere with the driver's immediate action chain, but help avoid longer-lasting damage to the car, driver, and passenger. In considering facilitation and interference, therefore, we must take into account the relative importance or value of the facilitated versus interfered-with actions and goals.

Macrolevel versus microlevel compatibility. Almost all the sociological literature about mate selection, marital compatibility, and homogamy is couched at the macrolevel—an implicit acknowledgment that partners' immediate thoughts, feelings, and actions are rooted in long-lasting, general conditions. It seems to be assumed that similarity in background leads partners to react to each other in a predictable and facilitative fashion. Nevertheless, that assumption is often rendered untrue over the course of a relationship. The present chapter, therefore, emphasizes the importance of microlevel compatibility and incompatibility—that is, facilitation and interference in regard to immediate events.

To distinguish further between microlevel and macrolevel analysis, it is helpful to consider Ajzen and Fishbein's (1980, p. 79) causal model for predicting individual behavior. Their model suggests that a series of variables affects an individual's action toward another person. The farther a variable is removed from the specific behavior at the end of this series, the less definite are its effects. At the *beginning* of the series are different sorts of "external variables," such as people's demographic characteristics, relations with significant others in their social environment, personality traits, and general attitudes or values. These "external variables" correspond roughly to Kelley et al.'s (1983) enduring causal conditions. Ajzen and Fishbein (1980) note that we cannot be sure how such general variables are linked to a particular behavior. Macrovariables frequently prove to be unreliable predictors of specific actions.

In contrast, Ajzen and Fishbein have shown that variables near the *end* of the chain are much better predictors. These variables pertain directly to specific goals (intentions) or behaviors in a particular context. For example, a wife's feelings about her husband's current complaint are a much better predictor of what she will do next than her education or her religion. In view of the specificity and transitoriness of these variables, they are here labeled microvariables. This heading subsumes each partner's beliefs and expectations (thoughts) about self's or other's actions and outcomes. Consequent to these thoughts are evaluations ($+/-$ feelings) about particular behaviors or the other's attitudes regarding those behaviors. Nearest to the specific behavior are intentions about what one will actually do in the given situation; Ajzen and Fishbein have demonstrated that indices of such intentions lead to the highest predictability of the corresponding action.

If Ajzen and Fishbein's model is applied to interpersonal compatibility, it becomes evident that the sources of interpersonal compatibility or incompatibility are found both outside and inside the dyad. The effects of the external variables, however, are mediated by the partners' thoughts and feelings, as well as by their goals regarding the interaction. Compatibility, according to our definition, is located at the behavioral end of the causal series, where it is associated most directly with microlevel variables. Unfortunately, little research has been done to describe behaviors or to analyze pair dynamics at this end point. Instead, much of the research on compatibility—in regard to both mate selection and marital continuity—has referred to macrolevel variables, such as "homogamous" background or personality complementarity (Kerckhoff, 1974). From our present viewpoint, it is not at all surprising that such macrolevel determinants would be only weakly correlated with subsequent marital outcomes (see Burgess & Wallin, 1953; Huston & Levinger, 1978; Lewis & Spanier, 1979), or that interpersonal similarity and complementarity have shown inconsistent associations with long-term pair stability (Hill, Rubin, & Peplau, 1976; Levinger, 1983).

Recapitulation. Compatibility as defined here refers mainly to the ratio of facilitating to interfering events in two partners' overall interaction. If couples are preselected on important macrovariables, as typically occurs during the mate selection process (Kerckhoff, 1974), then microlevel interaction is especially salient for examining compatibility in established pairs. Nevertheless, mutual congruence at the macrolevel is also valuable: If two partners' outcome preferences correspond in most domains, and if they are skilled in coordinating their mutual plans and behaviors, it is likely that they can facilitate each other's goalward movement with relatively little interference. The process of mate selection, to which we now turn, is concerned with the development of such congruence.

Compatibility in Mate Selection

Western society assumes that marital partners are free to select each other on whatever bases they believe are important. Considering how varied such pairings could be when people are granted maximal freedom, it is noteworthy that mate selection tends to be rather predictable. For instance, much evidence suggests that people who choose each other as permanent partners tend to be similar in a variety of personal and social characteristics. Thus, married couples are likely to be more homogeneous than randomly matched pairs in characteristics such as residential background (Katz & Hill, 1958), age (Kerckhoff, 1974), race (Burma, 1963; Heer, 1974), education (Kerckhoff, 1974), or socioeconomic background (Hollingshead, 1950; Rubin, 1968). Religion, which used to be an extremely important matching factor, today appears much less important (Murstein, 1980). Each of these matching factors is a macrovariable that influences mate selection only indirectly through the effects of mediating variables.

The Causal Influence of Macrovariables

In an important analysis of the "social context" of mate selection, Kerckhoff (1974) has argued that understanding the process of mate selection requires us to "take into account more than the personal characteristics of the two people involved" (p. 75). Not only does the larger social setting delimit contact between "prospective spouse-candidates," but it also defines what is valued in a prospective spouse and what is to be the nature of the relationship itself. Marriage, in most cultures, implies a commitment to live together permanently or at least for the indefinite future. In Western middle-class culture, people also expect marriage to provide strong mutual attachment. Even within Western culture, however, couples differ in their pattern of marriage. Some adopt a pattern based on traditional norms, an "institutional" (Burgess & Wallin, 1953) or "parallel" pattern (Bernard, 1964); each such partner "lives primarily in a male or female world . . . and neither violates the boundaries of the other's world" (Bernard, 1964, p. 687). Other couples adopt a marriage pattern labeled "companionate" (Burgess & Wallin, 1953) or "interactional" (Bernard, 1964); the interactional model "demands a great deal more involvement in the relationship. . . . Companionship, expression of love, recognition of personality (as distinguished from mere role performance) are among the specifications of this pattern" (Bernard, 1964, p. 688).

Although different sets of partner attributes may be valued in interactional versus parallel marriages, all relational development is to some extent affected by the partners' propinquity and their similarity on macrovariables such as age, race, or religion. Since the effects of these variables have been well reviewed elsewhere (e.g., Kerckhoff, 1974; Udry, 1974), we here examine only two such variables—racial and religious similarity—in order to illustrate the present analysis.

Racial and religious similarity. Historically, in America and elsewhere, both racial and religious similarity have been extremely important screens in the selection of marriage partners. In some American states, interracial marriage was legally forbidden until the removal of such laws during the 1950s. Interreligious marriages, though not legally forbidden, were generally disapproved and often associated with family bitterness and divisiveness.

Today, interracial marriage is less unusual than formerly, but absolutely it is still rare. In 1960, 0.4% of all marriages in the United States were interracial, according to the race classification used by the U.S. Census; in the 1970 Census, 0.7% were interracial (Carter & Glick, 1976); and in the 1980 Census, such racial categories were no longer employed. Although population statistics for interreligious marriages are even harder to estimate, all reports indicate that they have risen markedly over the last few decades. What factors account for these contrasting trends?

An explanation may invoke slow-changing norms concerning race and fast-changing norms for religion. Racial discrimination, even though it has lessened greatly in the legal system, strongly resists change. Not only do people remain suspicious of others who look different physically, but racial differences are linked historically to differences in social class, residence, education, and economic opportunities and resources. One's racial features are determined genetically and do not change over time. In contrast, one's religious affiliation is independent of one's genetic features and is susceptible to alteration. Although some persons hold their religious beliefs rigidly throughout their lifetime, others hold them so weakly that they may undergo dramatic change.

Given the fixity of race and the plasticity of religion, intermarrying racially versus religiously has quite different implications: Interracial partners retain their public skin differences, whereas interreligious partners either can privately deemphasize their religious beliefs or change toward a common orientation. Further, whereas the offspring of interracial unions are marked visibly by their parents' genetic makeup, children from interreligious marriages can develop their personal faith in their own unique fashion.

In other words, interracial couples not only may face strong deterrents initially, but are likely to continue encountering outside interferences. Norms to which growing individuals are exposed may suggest that people of other races are different in important, perhaps fearsome ways. Such negative norms have the following sorts of consequences: (1) Initially, they help maintain low spatial propinquity between members of different races; in turn, low equal-status contact interferes with the development of trustful, rewarding interaction. (2) Later, even if frequent and continuing contact should develop, interracial partners are more likely to have disjoint and even antagonistic personal networks; such competing affiliations can either actively or passively interfere with the building of a good relationship, raising its costs for one or both members. (3) If, despite such obstacles, the partners intend to form a lasting union, they will probably meet new normative pressures from families and friends. (4) If those influences are survived, a married couple must later contend with recurring difficulties in regard to differential occupational discrimination between husband and wife, possible residential discrimination, and new problems during successive stages of child rearing.

Such normative pressures do *not necessarily* lead to interactive incompatibility, but they may exacerbate interpersonal difficulties when those difficulties do arise. If these normative obstacles are not faced early in a couple's relationship, they may be sources of future trouble. Indeed, interracial marriages have consistently been found more divorce-prone than same-race marriages (Carter & Glick, 1976). Note, however, that "interracial" mixtures differ widely both in their nature (e.g., Asian-Caucasian vs. Black-Caucasian) and in their implication for harmony or discord.

General implications. Racial and religious similarity are merely two instances of macrolevel factors that affect the building of a permanent relationship. They affect initial perceptions of another's availability, eligibility, and desirability, but they do not inevitably have a huge impact on later interaction. Before considering such interaction in general, we now turn to the case of one particular married couple.

The Case of Paula and Owen

Our illustrative couple is a composite of two actual couples interviewed by Levinger, Faunce, and Rands in a 1976 unpublished study of "successful" married pairs. Overall, Paula and Owen developed an extremely compatible marriage, marked by stability and mutual pleasure. At various points during courtship and marriage, however, they had to cope with various differences, irritations, and conflicts.

Their first meeting. Owen and Paula met on a rainy Saturday at a lakeside community where each had come for the weekend to visit friends. Standing in the lunch line at a barbecue, they started talking and discovered mutual friends in Paula's hometown. This led to an animated conversation and to sitting together at lunch. That afternoon it started to rain, so Owen took Paula for a drive through the nearby wet and misty forests, which he greatly enjoyed. Paula seemed more attentive and interesting than anyone he had met in years, even though she was a lot younger than he. For her part, Paula found Owen fascinating: he had been to places she had only dreamed of visiting and he spoke so well about his experiences. She was impressed that he was a graduate student; she herself had just finished her junior year at college and was working on a farm that summer. After their excursion, they gave each other a warm hug, warmer than anything they might have expected from knowing each other only 4 hours.

That evening the rain stopped. After everyone else had gone to bed, the two of them decided to go out for a walk. As they approached the lake, the moon began to break through the clouds, casting a glitter on the water. It seemed magical. Walking along the shore, they each marveled privately at how comfortable they were with each other, how they walked with the same rhythm, and could either talk easily or be silent without embarrassment. This felt like no ordinary date; they seemed so well tuned to each other. When they parted that night, each continued to think about the other; both looked forward to breakfast together. The next morning their encounter was again a special one, so much so that Owen decided to drive Paula back to her hometown—ostensibly to visit his old friends there, but really because he wanted to extend their time together.

Analysis. We can consider Paula and Owen's encounter both at the macrolevel and at the microlevel. Their backgrounds revealed both similarities and dissimilarities. Both were interested in modern literature; both enjoyed nature; both were healthy and vigorous. They also had mutual friends. Furthermore, they could talk each other's language and found each other appealing. There were, however, some salient personal differences: Paula came from a small town, Owen from a big city. She grew up in a conservative Methodist family in which religion was very important; he came from an agnostic family with few rituals. She had worked on farms since she was 11; he had always lived in the city and his work experiences were in an office, and now at a university. Her parents were happily married and living together; his father and mother were divorced, and his father had had little contact with the family for a number of years. She was 20, he 25.

These macrolevel differences, though, had little effect on their first encounter. If anything, they made the other more interesting. Primary was the synchrony of their thoughts and feelings: they "clicked" in their interaction and thoroughly enjoyed their sense of attunement. In our present language, Paula and Owen's interchain connections promoted desired action sequences and outcomes. Their interaction showed high facilitation and little interference.

Later courtship. Their relationship subsequently advanced more slowly. Although they spent several more summer weekends together, at the end of August Paula went back to college for her senior year and Owen went off in a different direction to graduate school. They did not see each other again until Christmas. After this separation, they were amazed at how good it felt being together, so much so that Owen was led to talk about marriage. Although Paula did not feel ready for it, she was excited by the idea and by Owen's feeling of commitment.

However, as Owen began to talk openly about marriage, Paula began to have serious doubts about the idea of a permanent bond. She became worried about whether they could continue to get along so well, about what her parents thought of Owen, about their religious dissimilarity, and about several other matters. Her feelings communicated themselves to Owen enough for him to back off; he told her that perhaps she needed more time, that maybe they ought to see different people before they made any permanent commitment. Sadly, Paula agreed.

During the next weeks and months, however, both of them continued to be preoccupied with thoughts about the other. They found themselves writing and calling each other far more than they had anticipated, and were unable to enjoy the company of alternate partners. And one day they discovered, quite independently, that each of them had visited a Unitarian church and had enjoyed the service and the atmosphere there; they began to wonder whether the Unitarians could help them to bridge their religious differences.

During spring vacation they saw each other again. They spent hours discussing things that they saw as roadblocks to their relationship. Finding more shared ground now than at Christmas, especially in ethical and religious matters, cheered them greatly. Then, one day they realized that they were ready to make a commitment; and soon after, Paula and Owen announced their plans to get married.

Analysis. Despite the differences in Owen and Paula's backgrounds, they felt so comfortable with each other during their everyday interaction that this aspect of their relationship dominated. Even while they deplored their lack of communality in some important areas, they were developing ways of dealing with their differences and were unconsciously building stronger links of interdependence. Their attempt at separation failed because they soon realized how interlinked they had become over the months of their acquaintance, so much so that it was painful to live without each other.

Other couples may find their differences unresolvable or their attempts to work out problems unsuccessful. Many such pairings dissolve before the partners decide to get married. In other cases, where the partners enter marriage with unresolved differences or with little practice in joint problem solving, couples are likely to face more difficulty in developing a high level of compatibility. Paula and Owen's successful relationship seems based in large part on their earlier willingness to face important issues directly.

Microlevel Interaction

The case presented above can also help to illustrate the occurrence of interactive microevents. For example, in their first meeting in the lunch line, Owen and Paula were not only aware of who and where they were (personal and environmental macroconditions), but also of the extent to which the other's immediate responses were interesting and appropriate. The extent to which the other's actions matched one's own actions, tone, and mood affected each person's subsequent responses. When Paula later felt that Owen and she were well "attuned," it indicated a high degree of facilitative meshing between their internal chains of events. Still later, when they were "working through" their religious differences, they were doing preventive work on macrolevel differences that they feared might later interfere with their enjoyment of each other at the microlevel.

There has been little empirical research on microlevel interaction during courtship. Studies of self-disclosure have addressed the issue of reciprocal openness and communication, and it is generally assumed that disclosure increases over the course of a developing relationship (e.g., Altman & Taylor, 1973; Levinger & Snoek, 1972). Research on communication during courtship, however, has almost always been cast at the macrolevel (e.g., reports of aggregate disclosures or agreements) rather than at the microlevel (e.g., observations of interaction). Many interesting questions about the role of microlevel interaction in courtship remain to be investigated (see Berscheid, Chap. 6 in this volume; Duck, 1977; Levinger, 1983), but the very tentativeness of relationship building at this stage resists observational study. Nevertheless, we can further examine the contrast between macrolevel and microlevel analyses by comparing two different theoretical models of mate selection.

Two Contrasting Models of Mate Selection

Robins (1983) has distinguished between two contrasting models of marital choice, which he calls the "compatibility testing model" (CT model) and the "interpersonal process model" (IP model). The CT model has enjoyed the favor of the mainstream family-sociology researchers, but the IP model draws more on recent social psychological theorizing and comes nearer to our present approach.

Both models accept the importance of endogamous norms that serve to limit a person's pool of available and eligible partners during the initial search process. The CT model, however, views individual partners primarily as information appraisers who subject another person to increasingly selective appraisals as

information filters in. In contrast, the IP model emphasizes the joint contributions of both partners to the buildup of a relationship. It assumes that partners in
courtship each invest increasingly more of themselves in the pairing, and that as
time goes on the self-other boundary becomes progressively less distinct and the
pair's meanings and expectations become jointly defined. Thus, a major
difference between the two models is that the CT model treats the other's
contribution to the relationship as relatively fixed, whereas the IP model
assumes a circularity whereby Person-Other interaction itself becomes an
entity which can in turn affect each partner's personal and environmental
qualities—e.g., moods, attitudes, values, and arrangements with the outside
world. Robins' (1983) analysis further illuminates the differences between these
macrolevel and microlevel approaches.

The compatibility testing model. The CT model suggests that persons employ
increasingly deeper psychological criteria for judging another's compatibility.
The more information they discover that confirms their sense of compatibility,
the more they increase their commitment to the relationship and eventually to
marriage. This model implies a general sequence of "filters" through which
information is processed (see Levinger, 1983, pp. 328–330). Presumably, at
the beginning of a relationship, one's information about the other is limited to
his or her social status and physical appearance; later one learns about the
partner's attitude and value similarity, and still later about "need fit" or role
compatibility. Filtering models of mate selection suggest that all couples follow
a similar causal sequence on their developmental path: From point to point in
this sequence, a partner's attributes either pass or fail the successive screenings,
and accordingly one either increases or decreases one's personal involvement.
    Two sorts of difficulties confront this model of mate selection. First, there is
no direct *empirical* evidence that confirms the operation of this process in actual
pairs. Although there is evidence that most of the factors are indeed correlated
with the probability of marriage—and it is logical that some factors (e.g.,
propinquity) have to operate sooner than others (e.g., role compatibility)—there
is no convincing research evidence for the sequential screening process itself. In
fact, findings from one important longitudinal study suggest that personal and
social characteristics continue to exert significant effects throughout the
courtship (Hill et al., 1976).
    Second, there is no *theoretical* consensus that people test compatibility via a
fixed set of sequential filters. Current theorizing (e.g., Kelley et al., 1983)
suggests that relationships are open systems that are formed and maintained via
circular causal processes. In other words, a relationship is only partly
determined by the partners' initial personalities and environments; their ensuing
interactions also have substantial effects. We turn now to the IP model, which
focuses specifically on those circular causal effects.

The interpersonal process model. The IP model considers early relational
development as affected by the same spatial and normative criteria as the CT
model, but it emphasizes the importance of cumulative interaction later in a

relationship. Later relational progress is considered primarily due to rewarding interpersonal events, to the interchain meshing of intrachain sequences, and to the couple's successive self-definitions and redefinitions.

Other causal conditions include the individuals' personal attitudes and feelings toward the partner and the relationship, the social supportiveness of their environment, and the growth of facilitative interconnections in the dyad. Only recently has significant quantitative research (Braiker & Kelley, 1979; Huston, Surra, Fitzgerald, & Cate, 1981; Robins, 1983) yielded substantive data for illuminating these processes. Nevertheless, qualitative case studies of couples such as Paula and Owen support the plausibility of this interactive model.

Compatibility in Marriage

How does the concept of compatibility apply to actual married couples engaged in their everyday lives? Marital compatibility is the degree to which spouses continue to facilitate, rather than interfere with, each other's individual and relational goals. Because of its emergent nature, marital compatibility depends on the continuation of processes begun before marriage.

During courtship, low F/I ratios encourage relationship termination. After marriage, however, relationships often continue even if spouses appear incompatible; the barriers to termination have increased so that they may make even unhelpful relationships continue indefinitely. Indeed, there are varieties of continuing marriages with widely differing combinations of ratios and amounts of facilitation and interference. Figure 13-2 depicts four types of such marriages, differing in their combination of high or low compatibility and high or low interdependence. The four types include (1) fully satisfying interactional unions, the contemporary ideal; (2) compatible, but less intimate parallel

CLOSENESS

(Amount of Interdependence)

		High	Low
COMPATIBILITY	High	Interactional Marriage	Parallel Marriage
(Ratio of Facilitating to Interfacing Interaction)	Low	Conflict-Habituated Marriage	Empty-Shell Marriage

Figure 13-2. Classification of marital types. Closeness refers to the *amount* of interdependence, indicated by the frequency, diversity, and strength of the spouses' interconnected actions, affects, and thoughts. Compatibility refers to the *ratio* of their facilitating to interfering actions, affects, and thoughts.

marriages; (3) less satisfying conflict-habituated marriages; and (4) unsatisfying but persisting empty-shell marriages (Cuber & Harroff, 1965; Rands,
Levinger, & Mellinger, 1981).

This section first presents some spouses' impressions about compatibility in
their own marriages, gleaned from interviews with a sample of "successfully"
married couples. It then examines examples of specific macrolevel and
microlevel variables as they may affect marital compatibility.

Spouses' Own Descriptions

In an interview study of 16 seemingly successful long-married couples
(Levinger, Faunce, & Rands, 1976), spouses were asked what had contributed most to their high marital satisfaction. Two general conclusions
emerged.

First, most spouses considered their compatibility a process rather than an
end product, an achieved rather than an ascribed state. One wife defined as
"compatible" two people who are "able to get along without too many
differences of opinion and who are also not constantly fighting." Another wife
said: "Marriage is not a constant; it's an ever-changing, growing, moving-ahead
kind of process."

Second, facilitation often requires effort. Some couples' behaviors, thoughts,
and feelings mesh easily; such couples (or all couples during particularly
harmonious periods) may need to devote little attention to getting along
together. In other cases or at other times, adequate meshing requires
considerable effort. If marriage partners take the course of least effort, mutual
facilitation seems likely to decrease over time and interference to increase. As
social relationships tend toward entropy, they will weaken or dissolve unless
active forces are exerted to maintain them (Levinger & Snoek, 1972, p. 15).
Nonetheless, having similar goals and similar preferences probably reduces the
frequency of misunderstanding each other's desires or motives, as well as the
likelihood of hindering the realization of each other's goals.

Relationship "work" and marital satisfaction. Do spouses who must "work"
to get along with each other thereby value their marriage more, or do they value
it less than those whose harmony appears effortless? This question is hard to
answer. For one thing, some effort was reported as necessary for maintaining
even the smoothest relationship. Furthermore, wide differences among couples
make generalization difficult. These interviews with married couples did suggest
that conscious effort does not diminish marital satisfaction. Consider the
responses of one highly successful pair to the question "What do you think is
the most important thing about being married?" The husband answered
". . . the problems we've shared and solved," while his wife said, "It's a
willingness on the part of both husband and wife to do a lot of giving."

Another husband answered this question by saying, "You have to weigh what
you want against what your wife wants; if there is any conflict between those

goals, then you have to be able to cooperate to solve it." Other spouses commented as follows: "We work at it"; "I work as hard as I can to keep up my end of the deal, and I expect the same from her too"; ". . . working with somebody"; and ". . . working together and sharing." This theme of effort and mutual problem solving in maintaining the quality of marriage appeared in more than half of the responses of these long-married spouses.

The Influence of Macrolevel Variables

Macrolevel variables are important during mate selection and their influence remains so during marriage. Personal characteristics such as age, education, or race remain influential. And environmental variables such as family support and neighborhood norms provide the context in which a married pair carries on its daily interaction. We now look briefly at two illustrative macrovariables, role complementarity and network support.

Role complementarity. Traditionally, wives have assumed major housekeeping and child-care responsibilities, while husbands have provided economic sustenance. Although both sets of roles still need to be performed, contemporary couples often depart from such a traditional division of labor. The question then becomes: How *should* these responsibilities be divided?

The traditional division of marital roles is characteristic of the parallel marriage. The more clearly spouse roles are separated, the more easily a household can be maintained without much interaction. And, if both spouses perform their duties to the other's satisfaction, life will proceed smoothly and with little interference. This is a functional advantage of parallel marriages. Difficulties arise only when things go wrong in the performance of tasks or if either spouse begins to desire a greater degree of marital interdependence. That is, if either spouse disappoints the other, their inexperience in discussing mutual problems can aggravate the trouble. For example, a wife who feels that her husband is not properly fulfilling his outside role as family provider may, deliberately or not, begin to withhold sexual affection; in turn, the husband may feel that his wife's coldness is a reason for his withholding spending money. Such a pattern can lead to spiraling conflict. In contrast, interactional couples presumably have a greater capacity for resolving such a conflict before it escalates.

This analysis suggests how a macrolevel condition, the manner in which spouses structure their family responsibilities, can affect microlevel interaction. Role division indirectly affects communication, mutual influence, and the nature and frequency of disagreement. At times, a given role arrangement will facilitate interaction, rendering smooth the partners' progress toward mutual goals. At other times, the same arrangement will impair interaction, especially if the partners are locked into inflexible patterns or if they fail to meet their responsibilities. Depending on the couple and the situation, a given form of role complementarity may be either positively or negatively associated with marital quality (Lewis & Spanier, 1979; Yogev, 1982). An example from Paula and Owen's case helps illustrate this potential for inconsistency.

Before their wedding, Paula and Owen discussed their future family roles. They decided that until their first child was born they would share housekeeping and income-earning responsibilities. Owen would continue work toward his doctorate, financed by a research grant, and Paula would find a job as a librarian. They would share the daily cooking and cleanup, and alternate other jobs such as laundry and house cleaning. They planned to cook together to have extra time for talking over the day's activities. In other words, they were trying to establish an interactive marital style.

This egalitarian format worked well during the early months of their marriage. Subsequently, however, it was disrupted whenever Owen had to work late and could not come home for dinner, or when he felt so pressured that house-cleaning chores seemed unimportant. Even when he did try to do his share of the cleaning, usually on weekends, his standards of neatness and cleanliness failed to meet Paula's. For a considerable time, this led to irritation for Paula and guilt for Owen. Finally, on a vacation weekend, they had time to talk about this problem, and they realized that their initial expectations did not fit their present situation. Their resolution of this problem led them toward a more traditional role division, in which Owen merely *tried* to do his share whenever possible, but it did greatly lessen subsequent marital tension. Years later, after societal norms had changed and Owen's career had stabilized, he and Paula again developed a more egalitarian pattern.

Social network influences. Another macrolevel variable that affects microlevel events is the "social support" experienced by the two spouses. Social networks change following marriage, as spouses accommodate each other's friends and relatives. Initially, there is a loosening of ties with one's own family and single friends and increased socializing with other couples (Boissevain, 1974; Shulman, 1975). In addition, spouses may interact more with their kin than they did before marriage, especially after they have children (Brandwein, Brown, & Fox, 1974; Spicer & Hampe, 1975).

Individual well-being is strongly affected by social membership and participation. Friendships provide a sense of belonging, information about appropriate behavior, and simple sociability; kinship and attachment networks provide emotional support and a sense of reliable alliance (Komarovsky, 1964; Weiss, 1974). Marital well-being is also affected by the spouses' kin and friendship networks. To the extent that others support their life-style and values, their own interaction is made easier. When others differ in important values or actions, however, conflict may occur between the spouses. For example, a wife may feel that her mother-in-law's Sunday visits cut into the couple's personal time and may criticize her husband for allowing this intrusion. Meanwhile, the husband may resent his wife's making it difficult for him to spend time with his mother on Sundays as he did before marriage.

If the partners' relations to their social networks mesh well, there is no conflict and little need for discussion. If, however, their respective relations interfere, communication about these differences becomes necessary. In this way, network compatibility affects microlevel interaction. Furthermore, members of the network sometimes exert direct or indirect pressure on spouses to conform to outside norms. In fact, the closer the attachment, the greater the pressure (Ridley & Avery, 1979). Thus, marital interaction is affected by network interaction. For an illustration, we turn briefly to Paula and Owen.

Paula and Owen found that most of their friends supported their role-sharing and Paula's decision to take a job and delay having children. Owen's mother, however, was unsupportive. She frequently made such comments as, "I'll be so glad when Paula can stop working and take care of things properly."

After several tense interactions, Paula and Owen discussed the issue. Owen was able to confirm his agreement with their decision and to allay Paula's defensiveness. The next time his mother criticized Paula's working, Owen answered her with a joke that defused the issue and showed both Paula and his mother where he stood.

The Influence of Microlevel Variables

Person-Other interaction involves the reciprocal effects of P's and O's thoughts, feelings, and behaviors. Although no single study has attempted to examine all these aspects simultaneously, they are implicit in studies of marital communication and conflict. Three empirical studies support the finding reported earlier that many successful spouses believe that compatibility reflects processes more than end products.

A survey of conflict-resolution styles. In one study (Rands et al., 1981), a large sample of young married pairs answered questions about the kinds of conflict they tended to encounter, their style of dealing with conflict, its usual outcome, and their marital satisfaction. Four main conflict-resolution types were found: (I) Nonintimate–Aggressive, (II) Nonintimate–Nonaggressive, (III) Intimate–Aggressive, and (IV) Intimate–Nonaggressive. Type I spouses, who perceived their interaction as largely aggressive and not intimate, were generally least satisfied with their marriage. Type IV spouses were, on the average, the most satisfied; the two middle types were intermediate in their marital satisfaction. Nevertheless, the study revealed that no single way of dealing with conflict was alone associated with high marital satisfaction.

Most satisfied were spouses who characterized their altercations as high in confrontation, but low in verbal attack, as well as "very likely" to end in intimacy. When openness occurred in an atmosphere of trust, the expression of conflict seemed to draw these spouses closer together. These marriages exemplified Bernard's (1964) interactional pattern.

Next most satisfied were spouses who also avoided verbal attack, but who felt less intimate. Such spouses have sometimes been labeled as "passive-congenial" (Cuber & Harroff, 1965). They were lower on interpersonal expressiveness, but fairly high in marital satisfaction. Their marriages corresponded most nearly to Bernard's (1964) parallel pattern.

Almost equally satisfied, and significantly above average, were spouses who did not eschew attacking each other, but who said that their conflicts tended to end in intimacy. These spouses saw themselves as confrontative, but not destructively so. Their marriages followed a mainly interactional pattern.

Thus, the study found multiple paths toward high as well as toward low marital satisfaction. Several different patterns of conflict resolution were associated with each. One important point is that confronting versus avoiding styles had different implications for spouses differing in intimacy. For spouses who felt highly intimate, confronting an argument appeared to increase satisfaction; for those low in intimacy, it seemed to reduce it. In some relationships, spouses viewed conflict as an opportunity to engage each other; in others, they saw it as a threat to harmony and personal security.

Observed patterns of conflict resolution. The above data were derived from spouses' limited self-reports. Another study, by Raush, Barry, Hertel, and Swain (1974), coded direct observations of couple interaction during the role-play of conflict situations. Especially pertinent is their comparison of seven "harmonious" and six "discordant" couples. The six discordant pairs displayed considerable avoidance and aggression; some pairs showed one of these styles predominantly, whereas others showed both in alternation. The harmonious couples fell into two groups, "one very adept at expressing and dealing with hostility and conflict, the other engaging in the avoidance of conflict" (Raush et al., 1974, p. 174).

Although this study did not examine ratios of facilitative to interfering acts, it did assess the overall frequency of behaviors differing in concern for the other (e.g., compromising vs. attacking). Discordant pairs exhibited either of two patterns: Either the two spouses showed a pattern of attack and counterattack, or they avoided all signs of conflict and overtly behaved like "lambs"; however, the submissive lambs (especially husbands) often later acted like tigers, becoming "far more coercive and attacking" than other spouses (p. 174). Thus, this observational study also found that intimate interaction tends to range between joint problem solving, on the constructive side, and aggression and problem avoidance, on the nonconstructive side.

Sequential analyses of marital interaction. If the ability to resolve differences is a key index of compatibility, how may this ability be measured objectively? A valuable answer to this question has recently been provided by Gottman's (1979) observational research on marital interaction. Employing sensitive observational and statistical techniques, he showed that spouses in "distressed" marriages—as compared to those in "nondistressed" unions—showed more negative and less positive affect, particularly in their nonverbal behavior, and more reciprocity in their negative affect.

Through the microanalytic coding of both verbal and nonverbal acts, and a focus on affective cues, Gottman was able to assess not only overt behavior but also thoughts and feelings. He found, for example, that both distressed and nondistressed spouses occasionally "mindread" the meaning of their partner's actions; but a distressed spouse's mindreading tended to imply criticism, whereas a nondistressed spouse's mindreading functioned mainly as a feeling probe.

Because Gottman's sequential analyses focused directly on the *inter*active aspects of P–O behavior chains, he could locate points in pair interaction where conflicts seemed either to begin or to end. Whereas nondistressed couples often used "validation" or acceptance in response to one member's complaint or expressed difficulty, distressed couples were more likely to exhibit chains of "cross-complaining"—chains that failed to lead to satisfying conclusions. In other words, when satisfied pairs engaged in "metacommunication" (i.e., communicated about their conflicts), they were frequently able to rapidly terminate an unpleasant interactive sequence; in contrast, dissatisfied spouses' attempts to communicate "about" a conflict often served to perpetuate the dispute.

An actual relationship. Let us now look at an example from early in Paula and Owen's marriage, which helps to illustrate processes involved in resolving differences. Their own words are informative:

Owen: I had been having some hard days, getting a lot of pressure from my dissertation adviser, and things were not going well. I'd been up all night at the lab working on a particularly difficult problem, and I hadn't been able to solve it. So I was feeling distracted and anxious when I came home for a short break the next morning. I told Paula that my work had to be finished and turned in by five o'clock that afternoon.

Paula: I'd also been feeling anxious and unhappy about some things going on at work. I needed to talk with Owen, but he hadn't been available. So, after he said that, I especially looked forward to relaxing together that evening and having a chance to talk.

Owen: I came home around six that evening, still feeling very tense. We had a simple supper together and talked for a while about what had been going on at the lab. Then I started to feel restless and said I needed to go. I wanted to visit my mother, as I hadn't seen her in a while, and I was feeling neglectful about it.

Paula: I couldn't believe what Owen was saying. Here I was expecting to talk or go out somewhere, and he was starting to say goodbye. I told him it wasn't fair.

Owen: As soon as I said it, I saw the hurt look on Paula's face and remembered that I'd implied I'd have time with her that evening. She got very quiet and I could feel myself worry about her thoughts. So I asked her what she was thinking, and she said, "When you do things like that, it makes me feel you don't care about me the way you used to."

Paula: Yes, since an evening together was important to me, I couldn't understand why it wasn't important to Owen. But he apologized, and I saw that he felt bad about my hurt feelings. I asked him if he really wanted to go, and he said, "No," he wanted to spend the time with me.

I was glad he did, because I would have felt bad if he'd gone, even though I would have understood. But then, all evening I couldn't stop feeling that he was only spending the time with me because he was feeling guilty about forgetting. Also, knowing he was tired and under lots of pressure, I felt selfish about keeping him.

Owen: We still get into things, even now, where she interprets my mood and I interpret hers. Most of the time, that works pretty well, because we're both pretty considerate. But this was one time when it didn't work so well, because we both kept thinking the other was unhappy. Even when we went out for a drink and tried to have a good time, we both felt preoccupied.

Paula: A week or two later, when Owen's pressure had let up, we talked about this situation. We realized that we'd made ourselves miserable by worrying about the other. We agreed to try to be clearer about our feelings in the future, so we wouldn't have such misunderstandings.

Analysis. This excerpt from our interviews illustrates the operation of both macrolevel and microlevel variables. The context of each partner's personal anxieties and preoccupations, Owen's long-standing concern with his mother, and his current exhaustion all set the stage for a misunderstanding. The pair's initial interaction was more interfering than helpful: Neither member was meeting the other's goals and both experienced unpleasant emotions as a result. Their subsequent discussion, however, showed that each was fundamentally attuned to the other's concerns and that each was able to modify his or her behavior to adapt to the other.

The sequence also shows an instance of spouses' "mindreading" behavior, wherein partners attribute feelings to each other (Gottman, 1979). Mindreading can often indicate empathy and understanding, as it did here, but as in this case, it can also contribute to additional distress if attributions of negative feelings temporarily destroy the partners' spontaneous enjoyment of their interaction.

Finally, this piece of interaction is a small instance of constructive conflict resolution. As one of our acquaintances recently said, "What counts in making a happy marriage is not so much how compatible you *are*, but how you *deal with incompatibility*." Dealing with seemingly small problems before they can grow into big problems seems to be a valuable characteristic of happy couples. And since such problems are inevitable in any close, ongoing relationship, it is a skill that is likely to be exercised repeatedly in the lifetime of a marriage.

Conclusion

"Closeness," in marriage and in other pair relationships, has here been defined as the extent of the partners' interdependence. "Compatibility" has referred to a pair's overall ratio of facilitation to interference occurring between the partners' chains of thoughts, feelings, and behaviors. According to our circular-process model, both long-term macroconditions and short-term microevents pertain to a pair's compatibility, but macrolevel variables affect it only indirectly.

There are several advantages to this definitional approach. First, it places an emphasis on proximal variables, which have elsewhere been shown to have a greater correlation with actual behavioral outcomes than have distal variables.

Second, it accords with subjective experience. People often experience their relationships as a continuous flow of responses between their own and their partner's thoughts, feelings, and actions. This definition helps to clarify amorphous statements such as "We get along well together."

Third, this approach not only draws on Kelley et al.'s (1983) circular-loop model of close relationships, but it also places the analysis of compatibility within the conceptual domain of family process analysis (e.g., Raush et al., 1974; Watzlawick, Beavin, & Jackson, 1967). Pair members' interconnected chains of action and reaction become the focal points for such an examination. Conceivably, the approach thereby furthers the operational testing of existing interactional theories.

Having reviewed those advantages, we can also reconsider the limitations in previous theory and research on compatibility. For example, marital compatibility has sometimes been equated with either a couple's stability or its closeness. Our conception suggests that although both stability and closeness may be correlated with high compatibility, neither will alone assure it. Thus, a stable relationship may be devoid of much helpfulness (e.g., the empty-shell marriage), and a close relationship may be highly conflictual (e.g., the conflict-habituated marriage). In other words, studies of marital stability or intimacy do not necessarily reveal very much about compatibility.

Furthermore, research on compatibility has usually been couched at the macrolevel rather than the microlevel of analysis. There are several reasons for this tendency. For one thing, similarity in background characteristics does correlate positively with the durability of marriages. Furthermore, it is far easier to collect data on personal backgrounds or environmental contexts than to observe ongoing pair interaction; in the absence of a compelling theoretical reason for doing so, one would rather avoid such a laborious task.

This chapter has indicated, however, that it is necessary both theoretically and practically to build a bridge between macrolevel and microlevel analyses. Regarding the marriage of Paula and Owen, for example, it would be impossible either to forecast its development or to describe its subsequent adaptation without carefully looking at its ongoing interaction. Moreover, as is shown in our theoretical model, the macroconditions are themselves amenable to changes mediated by occurrences at the microlevel. We hope, therefore, that this approach to marital compatibility stimulates further conceptual work so that appropriate empirical studies can be designed.

Acknowledgments. We thank Ann Levinger, Ted Huston, and Michael Johnson for their helpful comments on a previous version of this chapter.

References

Ajzen, I., & Fishbein, M. (1980). *Understanding attitudes and predicting behavior.* Englewood-Cliffs, NJ: Prentice-Hall.

Altman, I., & Taylor, D. A. (1973). *Social penetration: The development of interpersonal relationships.* New York: Holt, Rinehart, & Winston.

Bernard, J. (1964). The adjustment of married mates. In H. T. Christensen (Ed.), *Handbook of marriage and the family.* Chicago: Rand McNally.

Boissevain, J. (1974). *Friends of friends: Networks, manipulators, and coalitions.* Oxford, England: Basil Blackwell.

Braiker, H. B., & Kelley, H. H. (1979). Conflict in the development of close relationships. In R. L. Burgess & T. L. Huston (Eds.), *Social exchange in developing relationships.* New York: Academic Press.

Brandwein, R. A., Brown, C. & Fox, E. M. (1974). Women and children last: The social situation of divorced mothers and their families. *Journal of Marriage and the Family, 36,* 498–514.

Burgess, E. W., & Wallin, P. (1953). *Engagement and marriage.* Philadelphia: Lippincott.

Burma, J. C. (1963). Interethnic marriage in Los Angeles, 1948–1959. *Social Forces, 42,* 156–165.

Carter, H., & Glick, P. C. (1976). *Marriage and divorce: A social and economic study* (rev. ed.). Cambridge, MA: Harvard University Press.

Cuber, J. F., & Harroff, P. B. (1965). *The significant Americans: A study of sexual behavior among the affluent.* New York: Appleton-Century.

Deutsch, M. (1973). *The resolution of conflict: Constructive and destructive processes.* New Haven, CT: Yale University Press.

Duck, S. W. (1977). *The study of acquaintance.* Gower: Farnborough.

Gottman, J. M. (1979). *Marital interaction: Experimental investigations.* New York: Academic Press.

Heer, D. M. (1974). The prevalence of black-white marriage in the United States, 1960 and 1970. *Journal of Marriage and the Family, 36,* 246–258.

Hill, C. T., Rubin, Z., & Peplau, L. A. (1976). Breakups before marriage: The end of 103 affairs. *Journal of Social Issues, 32,* (1), 147–168.

Hollingshead, A. B. (1950). Cultural factors in the selection of marriage mates. *American Sociological Review, 15,* 619–627.

Huston, T. L., & Levinger, G. (1978). Interpersonal attraction and relationships. *Annual Review of Psychology, 29,* 115–156.

Huston, T. L., Surra, C. A., Fitzgerald, N. M., & Cate, R. M. (1981). In S. Duck & R. Gilmour (Eds.), *Personal relationships: Vol. 2. Developing personal relationships.* London: Academic Press.

Katz, A. M., & Hill, R. (1958). Residential propinquity and marital selection: A review of theory, method, and fact. *Marriage and Family Living, 20,* 27–34.

Kelley, H. H., Berscheid, E., Christensen, A., Harvey, J. H., Huston, T. L., Levinger, G., McClintock, E., Peplau, L. A., & Peterson, D. R. (1983). *Close relationships.* San Francisco: Freeman.

Kerckhoff, A. C. (1974). The social context of interpersonal attraction. In T. L. Huston (Ed.), *Foundations of interpersonal attraction.* New York: Academic Press.

Komarovsky, M. (1964). *Blue-collar marriage.* New York: Random House.

Levinger, G. (1983). Development and change. In H. H. Kelley et al., *Close relationships.* San Francisco: Freeman.

Levinger, G., Faunce, E. E., & Rands, M. (1976). [Interviews with spouses from "successful" marriages]. Unpublished raw data.

Levinger, G., & Snoek, J. D. (1972). *Attraction in relationship: A new look at interpersonal attraction.* Morristown, NJ: General Learning Press.

Lewis, R. A., & Spanier, G. B. (1979). Theorizing about the quality and stability of marriage. In W. R. Burr, R. Hill, F. I. Nye, & I. L. Reiss (Eds.), *Contemporary theories about the family* (Vol. 1). New York: Free Press.

Murstein, B. I. (1980). Mate selection in the 1970s. *Journal of Marriage and the Family, 42,* 777–792.

Rands, M., Levinger, G., & Mellinger, G. (1981). Patterns of conflict resolution and marital satisfaction. *Journal of Family Issues, 2,* 297–321.

Raush, H. L., Barry, W. A., Hertel, R. K., & Swain, M. A. (1974). *Communication, conflict, and marriage.* San Francisco: Jossey-Bass.

Ridley, C. A., & Avery, A. W. (1979). Social network influences on the dyadic relationship. In R. L. Burgess & T. L. Huston (Eds.), *Social exchange in developing relationships.* New York: Academic Press.

Robins, E. J. (1983). *An empirical test of the compatibility testing model of marital choice.* Unpublished doctoral dissertation proposal, The Pennsylvania State University.

Rubin, Z. (1968). Do American women marry up? *American Sociological Review, 33,* 750–760.

Shulman, N. (1975). Life cycle variation in patterns of close relationships. *Journal of Marriage and the Family, 37,* 813–821.

Spicer, J. W., & Hampe, G. D. (1975). Kinship interaction after divorce. *Journal of Marriage and the Family, 37,* 113–119.

Udry, J. R. (1974). *The social context of marriage* (3rd ed.). Philadelphia: Lippincott.

Watzlawick, P., Beavin, J. H., & Jackson, D. D., (1967). *Pragmatics of human communication.* New York: Norton.

Weiss, R. S. (1974). The provisions of social relationships. In Z. Rubin (Ed.), *Doing unto others.* Englewood Cliffs, NJ: Prentice-Hall.

Yogev, S. (1982). Happiness in dual-career couples: Changing research, changing values. *Sex Roles, 8,* 593–605.

Chapter 14

Assessment and Treatment of Incompatible Marital Relationships

William C. Follette and Neil S. Jacobson

For much of its history, marital therapy has been an orphan child. Though marital distress has long been one of the more common reasons for seeking counseling, services have been provided by several sources including the cleric counselor, the lawyer seeing his or her clients in the midst of divorce, the family practitioner, the psychoanalyst, and the psychologist. Marital counseling developed out of necessity rather than research or theory. In 1929 Abraham and Hannah Stone founded the Marriage Consultation Center in New York, and Paul Popenoe began the American Institute of Family Relations in Los Angeles shortly thereafter. By 1938 a paper on the psychoanalysis of married couples had been published (Oberndorf, 1938). Still, it was not until 1948, with the increase in divorce following World War II, that a text solely on marriage counseling was written (Cuber, 1948). Even by 1960 fewer than 100 articles had been written on marriage counseling, and by 1972 fewer than 30 outcome studies had been reported (Gurman, 1973a, 1973b). The history of marital therapy has been summarized by Prochaska and Prochaska (1978) and Jacobson and Bussod (1983). Marital therapy has undergone a slow evolution indeed.

But all this has changed dramatically since the early 1970s. There are currently at least 10 journals devoted primarily to marital and family therapy and research. A number of professional associations have been formed. There is considerable debate between paradigms on the pros and cons of different treatment approaches (cf. Gurman & Knudson, 1978; Gurman, Knudson, & Kniskern, 1978; Jacobson & Weiss, 1978), and the research proliferates with more and more controlled outcome studies appearing all the time. In short, there are plenty of candidates applying for the rights to adopt and nurture this once orphan clinical area.

In the earliest days of clinical treatment, therapists did not have a particularly useful model of how to counsel couples. The psychoanalytic approach conceptualized marital distress in terms of the neurotic needs of two individuals coming in conflict (Mittleman, 1944). This view of individual psychopathology led to a treatment program wherein both members of a dyad were seen *separately* so that each individual's problems could be treated in the traditional analytic manner. Therapy was done separately (concurrent marital therapy) so that the presence of the spouse would not interfere with the development of powerful transference between the individual and the therapist (Mittleman, 1948).

During the 1960s, psychoanalytic theorists began to argue that the presence of both members of a dyad in a particular therapy session would not necessarily undermine the therapeutic transference required for the effective resolution of individual pathology. Thereafter, conjoint marital therapy became a more and more common method of treatment (cf. Jackson, 1959; Sager, 1966). More recently, it has been suggested that the analytic approach could be useful in treating marital distress without necessarily focusing solely on each individual's pathology. Instead, the *relationship* was considered a legitimate focus of the therapy. Gurman (1978) has stated, for example, that "marital conflict can occur in the absence of significant individual pathology in either or both marital partners" (p. 454). It is the emphasis on the relationship and conjoint therapy that most distinguishes marital therapists as a group from other mental health professionals (Prochaska & Prochaska, 1978). In fact, the potential risks in treating marital discord when only one spouse is willing to participate have been described with some consensus (Gurman & Kniskern, 1978a; Hurvitz, 1967).

Systems theory has been applied to the theory and treatment of marital distress since the mid-1960s. Systems theory subsumes a number of models that adapt concepts from cybernetics to the analysis and treatment of families. One of the central postulates of most systems theories is that families are entities that have a life of their own, and cannot be adequately understood simply through knowledge of individual family members; in other words, the whole is more than the sum of its parts. Family systems have rules that define the structural relationships as well as the function of each family member, and these structures and functions determine the behavior of each member. According to systems theory models, people cannot be changed in isolation from the family system.

A major influence in the contemporary systems movement has been the Mental Research Institute in Palo Alto, California, where the focus has been on conceptualizing family interactions using communication theory. Contributors to this perspective have included Don Jackson and Gregory Bateson, who developed the double bind theory of schizophrenia (Bateson, Jackson, Haley, & Weakland, 1956). Their contributions have led to a number of family theory approaches, the most common of which is strategic therapy (e.g., Haley, 1963). One can review the theoretical models and work of other contributors elsewhere (Sluzki & Ransom, 1976; Watzlawick, Beavin, & Jackson, 1967).

Minuchin's (1974) structural family therapy is another major force among the systems theorists and practitioners. This approach assumes that behavior is determined by the external social environment. Social systems consist of subsystems, one of which is the marital subsystem. Subsystems have structures, some of which are functional and others of which are dysfunctional. Therapy focuses on modifying the dysfunctional structures.

Family Systems Theory was developed by Murray Bowen (1966). It was later to be referred to as the Bowen Theory, in part because Bowen saw substantial differences between his theory and the general systems theory (Bowen, 1976). This theoretical formulation also posits that one's behavior represents an interaction among systems. In this case the systems exist within the person. One system is a lower-order emotional system. This system interacts with a second, higher-order intellectual system. These systems exist within a person, and their interactions with other persons and structures (e.g., a family or a dyad) can trigger conflicts for both the person and the system. It is suggested that behavior has strong roots in the past since the pattern of relationships that a person engages in is influenced by the behavior patterns of family members including parents, grandparents, and even great-grandparents (Steinglass, 1978). Delineation of the historical development of a pattern is important in helping one determine the meaning of current events.

The influence of the systems theorists has been significant in marital therapy. Whereas the psychodynamic paradigm found a way ultimately to treat marital distress, it was the systems pioneers who developed a conceptual model for understanding the relationship between two persons as an entity in itself. They also noted that factors external to the individuals and their relationship could exert powerful influences upon a couple. On the other hand, systems theorists were primarily what their name implied—theorists. Actual controlled clinical tests based on the theory were rare. Family therapists have been able to conceptualize marital distress using the theory, but predictions and empirical research have been slow to follow.

During the late 1960s and early 1970s, behavior therapy was in its heyday. There was much enthusiasm for understanding complex behaviors by applying learning principles. Intervention took the form of specifying behaviors related to the problem and modifying those behaviors until it was agreed that change had been effected. Behavior therapy was generally atheoretical. All that was assumed was that behavior was learned. What was dysfunctional could be changed through relearning.

Two major occurrences opened the way for behavior therapists to focus on marital distress. The first was the elaboration of social exchange theory by Thibaut and Kelley (1959). This theory suggested that interpersonal relationships are formed and maintained partly on the basis of the rewards derived from the relationship balanced against the costs of maintaining the relationship. This conceptualization prompted behaviorists to think of interactions in terms of the delivery of reinforcers and punishers. Hence, in the context of marriage, distress could be thought of as a high ratio of punishing to reinforcing contingencies delivered by each spouse.

The second major influence was the work of Patterson and his colleagues (e.g., Patterson, 1971, 1974). Their work specifically applied learning and behavior modification principles to the understanding and treatment of family interactions in which child behavior disorders were present. This work clearly demonstrated that family interaction patterns were not too complex to yield to behavioral technologies. Children could learn dysfunctional behavior patterns partly because parents inadvertently reinforced them or failed to properly punish them, while they also failed to adequately reinforce more appropriate behaviors. Treatment followed a functional analysis of the problematic behavior, and focused on reducing the deviant behavior while strengthening alternative, desirable behaviors (Jacobson & Bussod, 1983). Since the late 1970s, formal treatment programs making use of functional analyses and conditioning procedures to conceptualize and treat marital distress have been specified and are readily available to the practitioner (e.g., Jacobson & Margolin, 1979; Stuart, 1980).

In spite of a fairly long history with rapidly accelerating research and theory, there is no single agreed-upon way of conceptualizing the origins of marital distress, no single best method of treating marital distress, and indeed no clear-cut agreement on whom or what the focus of therapy ought to be. There is no mainstream marital therapy, but rather a multitude of marital therapies. But in spite of the diversity of opinion and practice, the fact is that—regardless of theoretical orientation—much of what is done in therapy is quite similar across approaches. In part, this is because practical considerations limit what the therapist is able to do. The following discussion of therapy for marital distress will focus on elements that are used by more than one paradigm, although our explanations of them will make use primarily of a social-learning approach.

Marital Therapy

There are certain constraints that affect the way that therapy is delivered to a distressed couple. It is in part these constraints that force some degree of similarity among treatment approaches. Perhaps the primary fact that has to be reckoned with is that most marital therapy is short-term. About two-thirds of marital therapy interventions last fewer than 20 sessions (Gurman, 1973b, 1978; Gurman & Kniskern, 1978b). This means that one's therapeutic goals have to be set realistically, with targets that are often more circumscribed than one might wish. Therapy may be considered a high-cost behavior for a spouse who perceives that the current relationship provides little satisfaction and that other alternate relationships are possible. Therefore, such a spouse with a high comparison level for alternatives (Kelley & Thibaut, 1978) may not be willing to stay in long-term therapy. The goals of short-term therapy are to reduce the immediate distress that the couple is experiencing and to reintroduce some of the positive experiences that the couple once shared. Such a strategy is consistent with the goals specified for short-term psychotherapy interventions (Butcher & Koss, 1978). The initial stages of the treatment help form the expectations needed for additional change to occur.

Couples are often in the midst of an acute crisis when they enter therapy. They are decidedly discontent with their current situation and want things to be different. Unlike some other life problems for which people seek help, couples have at their disposal a remedy for their distress which they can play as a trump card: divorce. Though divorce may have significant costs to both clients and offspring in the more distant future, it is frequently the course of action taken (Stuart, 1980). Therefore, the therapist does not have the luxury of being a passive facilitator of insight, but instead must reduce the immediate sense of turmoil and set a clear target for therapy that is relevant for the couple (Butcher & Maudal, 1976).

Mutual hostility often accompanies distressed couples into therapy. Gaining cooperation in treatment despite this hostility and mistrust requires an active, directive approach at times. Behaviors or attitudes that retard therapy progress must be modified early so that the couple does not drop out of treatment. This may be a particularly difficult task for a therapist accustomed to a nondirective, passive style. Doing therapy with two clients instead of one can present other problems as well. In the beginning of therapy, arguments can erupt quickly as each person tries to ensure that his or her point is made. Again, a more assertive role is demanded of the therapist.

Another consideration affecting therapy is the perspective the clients may have on the nature of the problem. For the client, the problem exists at the present moment in time. By focusing on the past as an explanation of the present, the therapist may appear to clients as failing to fully appreciate their current distress and their perception of the spouse's contribution to it. Gurman (1978) argues that this phenomenon requires the marital therapist to be present-centered rather than past-centered. Problems that arose in the distant past have led to contingencies operating in the present that maintain them. Attending to the couple's current situation helps the therapy seem most relevant.

Because of the above considerations, therapy often emphasizes short-term treatment goals, acute problem reduction, and skills training. If the couple finds therapy immediately rewarding and decides to stay in treatment, then the goals of the therapy can be expanded. If the couple leaves therapy having experienced clear benefits, they can be encouraged to consolidate their gains outside therapy and later return for more work. It is important to have therapy be a "success experience" so that couples are not reluctant to seek additional help if needed. This does not mean that therapists may not choose to engage in long-term therapy if they believe it is necessary, feasible, and useful. It does mean that when long-term interventions are planned, one still runs the risk of high attrition unless early experiences are clearly beneficial and relevant to the couple's perceived needs. It is simply realistic, not defeatist, to be aware of what would happen to a couple if they dropped out of therapy after the typical 16 to 20 sessions. Would they then be likely to seek help again or not?

Behavioral Marital Therapy as an Example

Having described some of the factors that influence how therapy with couples is conducted, we will now focus specifically on the major components of one type of marital therapy—behavioral marital therapy (BMT). This choice is made for two reasons. First, it is the paradigm preferred by the present authors and the one with which they are most experienced. Second, it is the therapy modality that has been subjected to the most empirical testing. Several empirical studies demonstrating the efficacy of BMT or related therapies have been performed.

Efficacy. There have been few controlled studies that directly compare the efficacy of BMT with nonbehavioral approaches to marital problems. Primarily because of this fact, Gurman and Kniskern (1978b) argue that the superiority of therapy based on social-learning approaches has yet to be established. Although their point is certainly well-taken, there are also relatively few controlled studies in the literature that test the effectiveness of nonbehavioral techniques. If data on the effectiveness of other modalities were available, then at least a meta-analysis could be performed to compare the effect sizes of various treatment approaches (Smith & Glass, 1977).

Another problem is the lack of *specified* nonbehavioral marital therapies. If therapists and/or researchers are unable to formulate some sort of treatment manual, controlled-outcome studies are difficult to evaluate even if they should be performed. Techniques do not have to be rigid or invariant in order to be testable, yet so far, at least, well-designed comparative studies of nonbehavioral techniques are rare.

Although there are different versions of behavioral marital therapy, relatively structured treatment manuals do exist to be tested (e.g., Jacobson & Margolin, 1979; Liberman, Wheeler, deVisser, Kuehnel, & Kuehnel, 1980, Stuart, 1980). Moreover, there is an expanding body of literature that demonstrates the effectiveness of BMT in comparison to various waiting-list or nonspecific control groups (e.g., Baucom, 1982; Crowe, 1978; Emmelkamp, van der Helm, MacGillavry, & van Zanten, 1984; Hahlweg, Revenstorf, & Schindler, 1982; Jacobson, 1977, 1984; Margolin & Weiss, 1978; Turkewitz & O'Leary, 1981).

Although BMT appears to be effective, the available evidence does not clearly identify exactly what the active components are. Many of the above studies compare individual components of behavior therapy with a combination of these components and some type of control group. The studies to date appear to show that both the individual components and the combinations of those components are more effective than the control group conditions. However, these studies generally have not shown the combined treatment groups to be significantly more powerful than the component treatments. It is too early to fully interpret these findings since there are several methodological factors that may account for the failure to detect differential outcomes. Such factors probably include technique overlap among the component groups and the lack of statistical power to detect differences should they exist. A more complete discussion of the state of outcome research in BMT can be found in Jacobson, Follette, and Elwood (1984).

Assessment of marital functioning. One of the factors that has made possible the proliferation of BMT outcome studies has been the emphasis placed on the ongoing assessment of the treatment interventions. Goals are set and the couple's progress toward these goals is repeatedly assessed. This means that data for outcome research are often readily available.

Assessment occurs even when the therapy is not part of a larger study. Both the therapist and the couple have established criteria on which to evaluate progress. If all the goals of therapy are met but the couple still remains unsatisfied with the relationship, a new functional analysis of the problem can occur and the targets for therapeutic intervention can be modified.

Stuart (1980) has proposed five guidelines for therapists to use in the assessment of "troubled" marriages. First, Stuart suggests that assessment should be parsimonious so as to expedite therapy. Recalling our earlier discussion of the brief nature of most marital therapies, this is a particularly relevant point. Parsimonious does not necessarily mean simplistic, however. A complicated assessment may be in order if it provides significantly more useful information. An assessment that slows therapy or produces attrition generally cannot be considered satisfactory.

Second, assessment should be multidimensional. Marital distress is often adequately understood only when the relationship has been examined from several perspectives; certainly the behaviors and complaints of both spouses should be assessed. Moreover, it is rare that long-standing difficulties in one area of the relationship do not affect other areas. For example, chronically poor communication may interfere with the development or maintenance of a satisfying sexual relationship. In the ideal case, successful treatment should result in improvement in all areas of functioning. However, problems that derive from one source (such as poor communication in this example) may become self-perpetuating (functionally autonomous) and need to be addressed specifically in therapy.

Stuart's third criterion is that assessment should be linked to a theory of intervention. One ought not to assess what one does not intend to use in therapy. In research settings, however, adherence to this principle is not always possible.

Fourth, the assessment of marital distress should be situation-specific. Mischel (1968) has argued that behavior is a function of past history, current contingencies, and the current stimulus conditions. If assessment is done only in the therapy room, then all one can be certain of is that change has taken place *in the therapy room*. The issue of generalization to other environments must be assessed and not assumed. The therapist may well act as a major moderating variable for the couples' behavior. Though a couple can solve problems and negotiate change under the watchful eye of therapist, it may be beyond the couple to do so at the end of a hard day at work, with the infant crying in the background.

Finally, participation in the assessment process must be of value to the couple in and of itself. The relevance of the assessment process should be made clear to the couple. Presenting assessment data to them in a positive fashion is helpful.

An assessment process that adheres to these suggestions is likely to promote the establishment of rapport between therapist and clients early in the therapeutic process. Some assessment devices may be useful to the therapist even though the clients may not understand why. In such cases it is incumbent on the therapist to explain how the information may be useful in facilitating improvement in the relationship.

Assessment devices. There is such a vast array of assessment tools available to the clinician and researcher in this area that we can only describe a subset of them. The subset we have chosen are those that meet the above criteria and/or have been extensively used in the outcome literature.

There are many measures of marital adjustment in the literature. The most commonly used global measure of this construct is the Locke-Wallace Marital Adjustment Scale (MAS) (Locke & Wallace, 1959). The MAS is a 15-item scale that measures overall satisfaction, amount of disagreement, mutual activity and responsibility, and attitudes about the decision to marry. Scores range from 2 to 161, with scores below 100 indicative of marital distress. The MAS has discriminant, content, and concurrent validity, and acceptable internal consistency. Its major drawback is that it is significantly correlated with measures of social desirability.

Spanier (1976) reviewed measures of marital adjustment and listed 17 different instruments. In an attempt to improve the measurement of the construct, Spanier took all the items ever used in any scale to measure adjustment, discarded redundant items and items without content validity, added some items that he thought had been ignored until then, and then analyzed the remaining pool of approximately 200 items. Based on responses from working-class and middle-class Pennsylvania residents, 40 items that discriminated married and divorced couples were then factor analyzed. Thirty-two items with factor loadings greater than .30 were retained in the final instrument. What resulted was the Dyadic Adjustment Scale (DAS), a measure which contained four factors: dyadic consensus, dyadic satisfaction, dyadic cohesion, and affectional expression. Cronbach's alpha for the DAS is .96. To date, the DAS is probably the psychometrically soundest measure of marital adjustment available. However, the correlation between the 32-item DAS and the 15-item MAS is about .86 for married couples and .88 for divorced respondents, suggesting that these two instruments are virtually interchangeable.

The above measures are not always the most useful instruments for clinical use. Also available is Marital Precounseling Inventory (MPCI), a multidimensional tool developed by Stuart and Stuart (1973) for use in an operantly based treatment program. This largely unresearched device is used at pretest and can also be administered at intervals during therapy. The MPCI is intended to familiarize clients with the type of information the therapist will be seeking while focusing on positive aspects of both spouses' behaviors (Stuart, 1976). It surveys 12 areas of functioning, including (1) desire for positive change in the spouse's behavior, (2) positive behaviors emitted by the individual's spouse, (3) perceived desires of the spouse for self-change, (4) goals for self and marriage, (5) recreational interests, both self and shared, (6) interactions involving child-rearing practices, (7) distribution of power in the relationship concerning decision-making issues, (8) effectiveness of communication, (9) quality of sexual interaction, (10) commitment to the relationship, (11) assessment of resources, and (12) general areas of satisfaction in the marriage. The couple's responses to the MPCI allow the therapist to plan treatment and evaluate change. Jacobson and Margolin (1979) comment on the self-change-promoting aspects of the instrument as well as the fact that it helps the couple focus on their own relationship's strengths.

Also recognizing the need for multidimensional assessment and using a format familiar to clinicians, Snyder (1979) developed a 280-item true/false-format instrument called the Marital Satisfaction Inventory (MSI). Taking an approach much different from that of Stuart, Snyder used classical (as opposed to latent-trait) test-construction techniques to develop an 11-scale profile of marital satisfaction for both the husband and wife. The psychometric approach to the problem and the resulting instrument can be likened to the Minnesota Multiphasic Personality Inventory (MMPI). The inventory contains a validity scale based partly on the Marlowe-Crowne Social Desirability Scale (Crowne & Marlowe, 1960), called conventionality (CNV), that appears to measure naive image manipulation or a tendency to see the relationship in unrealistically glowing terms. There is also a measure of global distress (GDS). The remaining nine dimensions assess marital interaction and are as follows: general affective communication (AFC), problem-solving communication (PSC), quality and quantity of leisure time together (TTO), disagreement about finances (FIN), sexual dissatisfaction (SEX), sex-role orientation (ROR), history of family and marital disruption (FAM), dissatisfaction with children (DSC), and conflict over child-rearing (CCR). The scores on these scales are plotted on a profile in *T*-score form with both spouses' data appearing on the same plot. Elevations and problem areas are easily highlighted.

The MSI's component scales have acceptable internal consistency (.80 to .97) and the entire inventory has a test-retest reliability of about .89. The MSI also has discriminant validity based on comparisons of samples of couples in marital therapy with matched controls. It remains to be seen whether the MSI is confounded with social desirability as defined by Edwards (1957) and measured with his SD scale. Whether the MSI will be used in developing actuarial predictions for profile types or whether configurations will be studied in a different manner than individual scale scores also remains to be seen. In any event, Snyder's psychometric approach offers one alternative to more strictly behavioral assessments of marital dysfunction.

The Spouse Observation Checklist (SOC) was developed at the University of Oregon by Weiss and Patterson and their colleagues, and has undergone several modifications (Christensen & Nies, 1980; Jacobson, Follette, & McDonald, 1982; Jacobson & Moore, 1981; Patterson, 1976; Weiss, Hops, & Patterson,

1973). In the version we use, there are 408 behaviors divided into 12 categories. The items are a rather comprehensive list of possible behaviors that the spouses can perform individually or as a couple. The SOC is filled out at the end of each day by each spouse separately. Each records whether the behavior occurred and the valence of the behavior as perceived by the spouse recording the events (i.e., was the impact of the behavior positive, neutral, or negative?). At the same time the SOC is completed, a rating of daily satisfaction with the marriage is obtained using a 9-point scale. Used in this way, the SOC allows the couple and the therapist to examine what occurs and how it impacts each partner and the relationship. These data are typically used to demonstrate the relationship between marital satisfaction and the frequency of positive or negative events. The length of the checklist is its primary liability.

The Areas of Change Questionnaire (AOC) is another tool devised by Weiss, Patterson, and their associates (Weiss et al., 1973; Weiss & Margolin, 1977). It assesses marital satisfaction by inquiring how much change would be welcomed by each partner in 34 areas. Each spouse responds to the prompt "I want my partner to: [for example] spend time keeping the house clean." The responses can range from −3 (much less) to +3 (much more). In addition to rating the degree of change desired, each spouse can mark items of particular significance and thus provide additional information to the therapist.

It is argued that the AOC provides an exceptionally precise sample of satisfaction in behaviorally specific terms (Weiss & Birchler, 1975). Whether the AOC provides additional information to ratings of global satisfaction is unclear, however. Weiss et al. (1973) have shown the AOC and the MAS to have a significant negative correlation ($r = -.69$). Margolin, Talovic, and Weinstein (1983) have demonstrated the discriminant validity of the instrument, but also question its behavioral specificity. In addition, they point out that while the AOC may pinpoint problem areas, a more thorough assessment yielding more detailed information is still necessary. This criticism calls into question the actual utility of the AOC.

The Marital Status Inventory (Weiss & Cerreto, 1975) is a 14-item measure of a couple's readiness for divorce. The true/false items on the MSI, which represent the apparent readiness of the couple to consider and carry out the separation process, include behavioral statements such as "I have set up an independent bank account in my name . . . " to "I have filed for divorce. . . . " There are also items relating to the cognitive processes involved, such as "I have occasionally thought of divorce or wished that we were separated . . . " and "I have considered who would get the kids. . . . " The MSI provides clinically useful information about the degree of commitment each spouse maintains to the relationship. Certainly a high score on the MSI would be an indication for the therapist to assess with the couple whether their purpose for seeking therapy was to improve the relationship or to facilitate the divorce. To date, the predictive validity of the MSI has not been established.

Whereas many of the above assessment devices tend to be behaviorally specific regarding what is presently occurring in a relationship, there are another set of assessment procedures that are designed to assess some of the instrumental processes that a couple might use to resolve problems. These procedures focus on communication and problem-solving skills—another domain in which distressed and nondistressed couples clearly perform differently (see Gottman, 1979).

The prototype assessment procedure for examining communication processes in couples is the Marital Interaction Coding System (MICS), developed by Patterson, Weiss, and their associates (Hops, Wills, Patterson, & Weiss, 1972). The MICS is an observational coding system used by trained raters. Thirty-second blocks of a couple's videotaped conversation are rated on 29 categories of behavior that have been grouped into 6 larger categories. The categories are problem-solving behaviors, problem-descriptive behaviors, negative verbal behaviors, negative nonverbal behaviors, positive verbal behaviors, and positive nonverbal behaviors. The MICS is used to examine the interactional patterns of a couple. The interaction is coded so that conditional probabilities can be computed for each class of responses. Analyses of these conditional probabilities have shown, for example, that once a spouse engages in negative behaviors, the probability of more negative behaviors ensuing increases for distressed, but not for nondistressed, couples.

There have been many studies demonstrating the discriminant validity of the MICS (e.g., Billings, 1979; Vincent, Weiss, & Birchler, 1975). However, while Jacobson (1977) was able to demonstrate changes in interactions using the MICS in problem-solving based treatments, the reliability and validity of the instrument remain open to question (see Jacobson, Elwood, & Dallas, 1981).

Another interaction-coding system, The Couples Interaction Scoring System (CISS), was developed to examine not just the content of an interaction, but also the context of the message and the affect used in the exchange (Gottman, 1979; Gottman, Markman, & Notarius, 1977). The CISS breaks down videotaped interactions into thought units instead of simple time-determined units as is done with the MICS. A thought unit may be a phrase or a sentence, and such units can be reliably identified and coded. There are eight content codes in the CISS. They are: agreement (AG), disagreement (DG), communication talk (CT), mind-reading (MR), proposing solutions (PS), summarizing other (SO), summarizing self (SS), and feelings about a problem (PF). Affect and context codes are rated as positive, neutral, or negative.

Gottman's contributions to the understanding of marital interactions include innovative methods of data analysis. Using lag-sequential and time-series analyses, Gottman has examined in detail the patterns of responding in distressed and nondistressed relationships (see Gottman, 1979) and has used his findings to design a therapy based upon his and others' empirical findings.

Clearly, the MICS and the CISS are of little practical use to the clinician in the ongoing assessment of therapy. Both devices were created for researchers to study the process of dyadic interactions. Their primary use is to gather descriptive information and identify change in larger outcome studies. At this time there is no practical, validated tool to use during the course of therapy to objectively assess communication patterns or problem solving skills.

Validity. In most cases the aforementioned assessment tools possess discriminant validity. That is, the tools have been developed to discriminate between nondistressed couples and distressed couples who present for therapy or respond to some type of recruitment campaign. Items are generated and those that differentiate the two groups are retained, while the others are discarded. Several of the instruments possess face validity, a feature that helps meet Stuart's criteria for making evaluation and assessment a sensible experience for the couple. However, none of the self-report instruments have been shown to be devoid of the tendency to elicit the social-desirability response set described by Edwards (1957).

Virtually none of the assessment devices described above have established predictive validity. That is, we do not yet know if changing one's score on, for example, the AOC filled out in the clinic is related in the long run to marital longevity and happiness. Further, studies using categories derived from the MICS to assess marital interactions occurring in the home have not demonstrated the ecological validity of these measures (e.g., Robinson & Price, 1980).

Many of the above instruments are intercorrelated in spite of the fact that they appear to sample several domains of behavior. The instructions, therapy situation, cognitive set of the clients, and/or the researcher may all act to elicit a common response set from the client. The resulting intercorrelations and restriction of range on the different measures may hamper our ability to make fine discriminations between couples and between treatments.

Clinical Application of Behavioral Marital Therapy

In this section we will describe the behavioral marital therapy approach that is used at the University of Washington in the Center for the Study of Relationships. Its major components are commonly used by many marital therapists.

Behavior exchange. Because couples are generally in considerable distress when they seek therapy, quick change to make the relationship more pleasant is often necessary to buy time for the therapy to progress. Behavior exchange (BE) strategies are designed to increase the frequency of positive behaviors emitted by each spouse. Such strategies follow a reinforcement model of relationships. During the pretreatment assessment, a list of pleasing behaviors that already occur in the relationship is developed. Such behaviors may be identified from the Spouse Observation Checklist or by direct interview with each spouse. Often these positive behaviors occur at a very low rate. BE attempts to increase the frequency of these pleasing behaviors as well as identify and develop new domains of potentially reinforcing exchange.

It has been shown that couples' marital satisfaction is linked to the occurrence of recent positive and negative behaviors (Jacobson, Follette, & McDonald, 1982; Margolin, 1981; Wills, Weiss, & Patterson, 1974). Negative behaviors tends to have particular impact on couples and be reciprocated quickly (Gottman, Markman, & Notarius, 1977; Raush, 1965; Weiss, Hops, & Patterson, 1973). Unless there is physical abuse occurring in the relationship, it is generally not desirable to attempt to directly engineer a reduction in the rate of negative behaviors. The reduction of such behaviors often requires the use of aversive-control contingencies, including negative reinforcement and punishment. Couples are all too familiar with such techniques in their existing relationship, and do not need to see them as an integral part of accomplishing desired goals. Instead, it is important to increase the rate of positive behavior exchange.

The use of positive behavior control is a good precedent to set early in therapy. Both spouses are charged with increasing the rate of their own positive behaviors and/or increasing the daily satisfaction experienced by the partner. Depending on the degree of collaboration between partners, each spouse has the option of deciding for himself or herself how to better please the partner. Or each partner may ask the other for specific suggestions as to how to increase the frequency of positive behaviors or increase the other's daily satisfaction rating. The therapist often directs the client to increase pleasant but low-cost behaviors.

There are several ways of accomplishing behavior exchange. Jacobson and Margolin (1979) have used the Spouse Observation Checklist plus a Likert Daily Satisfaction Rating to help facilitate an increase in positive reciprocity. Stuart (1980) uses a technique called "caring days." Couples are asked to act "as if" they cared for each other. Each person builds for the other spouse a list of pleasing behaviors from which to choose. Stuart recommends an initial list of 18 items and suggests that each person continually add to it. Then each spouse is asked to emit at least five of the behaviors from the list each day. All of the items included on the list must be positive, specific, and small behaviors that are not the subject of major conflict.

There are several benefits that accrue from using these techniques. First, even subjects who already maintain a high rate of positive behavior exchange can experience increased satisfaction early in therapy. Those with lower rates of spontaneous exchange can have specific behaviors made available to them from lists or suggestions from the partner. Most techniques allow the person emitting the behavior to select what exactly he or she wishes to do to increase the partner's satisfaction. This process lets each spouse emit behaviors that they deem to be of reasonable "cost." In addition, the receiver is not in a position to discount what the partner does as having been a case of "doing what he or she was told." One spouse may ask the other for information about what is or is not positive. When this occurs, it is an opportunity for the receiver of the behavior to learn to be specific in describing what is pleasing. This may involve the receiver's learning to say "Give me a hug when you come home after work" instead of "Quit taking me for granted all the time."

Behavior exchange frequently leads to an increase in short-term satisfaction with the relationship. It also provides evidence that each partner's feelings about the relationship and his or her spouse are, in fact, reactive. Often couples begin therapy thinking that things are always the same—rotten. This task can provide evidence to the contrary.

The behavior exchange method emphasizes two additional features of BMT. First the therapy encourages "positive tracking," a process whereby the couple increases the positive aspects of the relationship without focusing on negative occurrences. Second, the therapy teaches couples to attend to the present and future while trying to leave the past in the past.

Early behavior exchange strategies emphasized contingency contracting such as the "quid pro quo" contract wherein one partner alters his or her own behavior in exchange for a desired alteration in his or her partner's behavior (Stuart, 1969; Weiss, Birchler, & Vincent, 1974). It soon became evident that there were two problems with such contracts. One problem is that distressed couples are already under immediate reciprocal control by reward and punishment (e.g., Gottman, 1979), whereas nondistressed couples appear to be under the control of long-term contingencies. Another problem is that fixed ratio schedules or reinforcement (especially a FR1 schedule, when reinforcement is delivered after each behavior) are the easiest to extinguish should the contingencies not be delivered. Because trust in a relationship is partly dependent on seeing that positive behaviors are reciprocated over the long run even if not in the short term, practitioners (Jacobson, 1983b; O'Leary & Turkewitz, 1978; Stuart, 1980) have begun to emphasize unilateral but parallel changes in each spouse in recognition of the fact that long-term positive exchange is more representative of nondistressed marital behavior than is immediate exchange.

Problem solving and communications training. Whereas the therapeutic importance of behavior exchange strategies is not universally accepted by everyone engaging in marital therapy, the need to enhance and improve communications and problem-solving skills has been discussed by authors of many different theoretical orientations (e.g. Ables & Brandsma, 1977; Guerney, 1977; Satir, 1967). There are studies describing communication problems in unsatisfactory relationships dating back to Terman (1938). Locke (1951) described differences in communication between happily married couples and couples who divorced. The relationship between marital adjustment and communication quality was documented by Hobart & Klausner (1959), and many other studies have supported the correlation between marital distress and poor communication patterns or skills. Whether the poor communication is cause, effect, or both has yet to be definitively answered in a longitudinal study. For the purposes of treatment, that question may be less important than the fact that good skills are a prerequisite for improvement in therapy.

Couples frequently cite poor communication as part of their problem when they seek therapy. Introducing the rationale for such training in general is therefore quite simple because it has face validity for most couples. Guerney (1977, see especially p. 63) offers a positive rationale for the need for good communication skills. It is common for couples to agree with the general need for good communication skills but still fail to see their own specific deficits when communication exercises are performed.

Marital therapy emphasizes the use of communication skills to express feelings, reflect the feelings of one's spouse, negotiate change, and resolve conflicts. The choice of what function to emphasize depends upon the orientation of the therapist and the needs of the clients. In cases where the partners complain of being unable to get what they want from the other person, early exercises may emphasize communication skills as a vehicle to induce change.

After the rationale is given to clients, the appropriate behaviors that constitute good communication skills are presented by using either a written manual, a didactic session, or modeling by the therapist. Regardless of how the information is presented, there is a great deal of role-playing, behavioral rehearsal, in-session practice, homework, and feedback from the partner and the therapist. Often the therapist will observe interactions, and when problems arise, step in and role-play or model the appropriate behavior. This is particularly common in the early stages of communication training since escalation into argument can be extremely rapid. If there is a history of dysfunctional communication, certain phrases or voice tones can serve as conditioned stimuli that elicit a conditioned affective response of anger or anxiety.

During communication training, the clients are taught to make a clear distinction between the intent and the impact of what the partner has said. Again, it is often the case that the listener will focus on how a statement was made instead of what was said. The listener first is taught to attend to the content of the communication by physically facing the partner and using appropriate facial expression and body language. The listener is also taught to paraphrase the content of what was just said. Accurate paraphrasing indicates that the intent was understood. When one paraphrases, one rephrases what was heard without interjecting a value judgment about the content or style of what was said. Couples are taught to use the key words that the initiator of the communication used. This is particularly important when the communicator expresses a feeling.

During this process the listener may ask for clarification and is encouraged to get feedback on the accuracy of the paraphrase. Couples can gather information about how to please each other during the behavior exchange exercises. Information about feelings can also be communicated. Sometimes couples are so poor at expressing feelings that it is necessary to supply them with a written list of the feelings they might possibly have (Gottman, Notarius, Gonso, & Markman, 1976).

The person initiating the conversation is also instructed to use appropriate skills so that the burden of being civil is shared by both partners. But the idea is emphasized that it is reasonable to have different viewpoints on a subject. One way that spouses can be taught to recognize the validity of each other's point of view is to have them preface their statements with self-referencing "I" statements of the form "I feel . . . "or "From my perspective . . . ", and so on. This helps them share feelings even when they are trying to solve problems. It also minimizes the tendency to start sentences with accusatory structures such as "you always . . . " or "you make me. . . . " In addition, the use of personal statements promotes self-disclosure and increases intimate exchanges. For some couples, it has been a long time since either partner has revealed his or her own reactions to the other in a nonaccusatory way. Some clients find it an unusually pleasant experience to express a feeling and have it reflected back to them without getting attacked or ridiculed.

The use of "I" type statements are also useful in conveying other information to the partner. Specifically, such statements can be made to pinpoint specific circumstances that are associated with particular feelings. Couples are encouraged to make use of communication of the form "I feel hurt and ignored when you make a social commitment without asking me first." It is also powerful and constructive when the listener paraphrases this as "When I make commitments without even asking you first, it makes you feel hurt, is that right?" By promoting an atmosphere where it is safe to express feelings, where truth exists in each person's experience, and where intent is understood, the therapist helps to minimize mind-reading, cross-complaining, and mutual accusation. A great deal of homework, homework debriefing, and in-session time is devoted to such exercises.

Communication skills can be applied toward any goal defined by the couple and therapist. A common next step is to introduce problem-solving skills that build on the communication training. In an approach detailed elsewhere (Jacobson & Margolin, 1979), problem solving is taught in two stages. The first stage is problem definition. Making clear, specific statements of the problem is taught. The couple is told to discuss one and only one problem at a time. One spouse is allowed to bring up the problem while the other is instructed not to cross-complain or try to usurp the session. Each speaker is encouraged to try to define the problem in the smallest, most specific terms possible. When it is the listener's turn to respond, he or she should begin the response with some sort of paraphrase of the other's remark, making sure to get verification of the accuracy of the paraphrase.

It is of paramount importance in these sessions that the listener does not make inferences about the motivation of the other. Often spouses act as though they have perfect knowledge of the motivations of their partner, leading them to make premature inferences and judgments. Statements like "You don't like it when I come home late because you're insecure" are actively discouraged. At this point in the task it is important only that the spouse does not like the behavior. Each spouse gets to initiate problem-solving sessions so that each can bring up topics to be resolved.

Of course, verbal abuse is prohibited. Often couples are only vaguely aware of the impact of their verbal "jabs." These abusive communications may also include nonverbal components such as facial expression, body language, and the like. Gottman (1979) has shown that the major portion of negative affect is communicated using nonverbal behaviors, and attention is paid to this fact during the sessions. To help encourage a more positive exchange, we suggest that spouses begin problem-definition phases with statements of positive aspects of the partner's behavior. This is especially useful if there if something positive related to the problem being discussed. An example would be a statement like "I feel very supported by you when you tell the children to behave when I ask them to do something. I also feel that I don't get as much help with the children as I would like."

The solution-generation phase can provide opportunities to develop novel solutions to problems. Often couples are stuck in a rut and fail to generate imaginative or even practical solutions to problems. One way to facilitate new solutions is to use brainstorming techniques. Brainstorming is the part of the solution-generation phase during which each person can generate ideas regardless of how absurd or impractical they might be. The task is to come up with ideas without worrying about their utility. A list is generated without either party injecting editorial commentary.

Once the list of possible solutions is generated, the couple proceeds to a discussion of the merits of the proposed solutions. Since absurd solutions are sometimes generated during brainstorming ("We can send the kids to camp and move without leaving a forwarding address"), they are immediately eliminated from the solution list if *both* people agree they are absurd. If at least one spouse does not think the solution is patently absurd, then the evaluation process begins. The one who proposed the solution explains why it was offered and what its potential benefits are. The couple evaluates each idea based on the solution's apparent likelihood of helping to solve the problem. Items from the list are eliminated if it is agreed that the solution would not contribute to resolving the problem, or if the potential costs outweigh the benefits.

At the end of this process, the couple will have a list of one or more remaining solutions. From this list, the couple chooses one or more of the alternatives after discussing their acceptability. Some therapists make use of a written contract constructed by the couple that details the elements of the solution, including specific statements of who does what and when. The couple may be as specific as they wish, but vagueness is discouraged since vague agreements often lead to failure. It can be helpful to have the couples write in specific contingencies to be invoked if specific events occur that might hinder the implementation of their solutions.

Throughout the behavior exchange, communication training, and problem-solving phases of therapy, the tasks begin with low demand for major concessions or changes. As therapy progresses, there is gradual movement from minor problems to more major concerns. Whereas, early on, changes in behavior and style can be primarily self-initiated, in the later stages there is a movement toward changing at the request of the spouse. These major changes occur only after there has been a history of collaboration established during therapy. The goal of behavioral marital therapy is to promote collaboration and generalization of the skills learned in therapy (Jacobson, 1981).

In addition to modeling, behavioral rehearsal, and role-playing, the therapist will often engage in what is called trouble-shooting. Trouble-shooting is indicated when partners are bickering and fighting a lot at home. Couples often complain that there is nothing they can do to alter the course of events during these arguments. Trouble-shooting is, in part, an intensive effort to challenge the notion that nothing can be done once problems have occurred. It teaches the couple that they have a much wider variety of response options than they seem to see at first glance.

Trouble-shooting takes the form of debriefing an aborted interchange between the couple. Spouses are made to go step by step through a disagreement, stating what was occurring for them and their partner and then developing alternative behaviors that could have helped them to avoid a destructive interchange. When one person cannot generate an alternative behavior, the therapist may ask the partner what could have been done. At times it may be necessary for the therapist to model alternatives. This trouble-shooting process occurs often throughout the therapy. As the therapy progresses, the spouses may trouble-shoot naturally when they recognize that escalation is taking place.

Current Issues

Though behaviorally based marital therapies have demonstrated effectiveness, they still do not provide benefit for all distressed relationships (Jacobson, Follette, Revenstorf, Baucom, Hahlweg, & Margolin, 1984). There are cases in which it seems that the positive aspects of the relationship are virtually ignored while the spouses focus on past transgressions or perceptions. Increasing attention has been paid to the importance of cognitive factors in treating dysfunctional couples (for a review, see Berley & Jacobson, 1984).

Behaviorally based therapies are time-limited and the therapist does not have adequate control over all the contingencies in the couple's environment. Dynamically based therapies are often limited in their scope because of similar constraints. Adding a cognitive component to therapy may help couples find alternate, constructive ways of interpreting each other's behaviors.

We have noted that couples in therapy exhibit a tendency to credit outside factors when a spouse emits positive behaviors, while at the same time attributing the spouse's negative behaviors to internal factors. A laboratory analogue study using distressed and nondistressed couples has supported our clinical observation (Jacobson, McDonald, Follette, & Berley; in press): Distressed spouses do indeed find it difficult to give appropriate credit to their partners for behavioral improvements. Alerting couples to the tendency to make faulty attributions may facilitate progress in therapy.

Distressed couples are particularly reactive to the occurrence of negative behaviors, and such behaviors have a great deal of impact on their satisfaction ratings (Jacobson, Follett, & McDonald, 1982). The work of Tversky and Kahneman (1973) may help us understand the reason for spouses' focusing on negative aspects of each other's behavior. They have demonstrated that one's judgment of the likelihood or frequency of a particular event may be influenced by the relative availability of the event in memory—an influence which they call "the availability heuristic." Availability is influenced by factors other than objective reality. Perceptual saliency, or the vividness and completeness of recall, affects estimates of the frequency of behaviors. When a spouse says, "You always say hurtful things in front of my parents," he or she is exaggerating. This exaggeration is based on the tendency to recall and generalize from highly vivid past experiences.

In therapy we have not dealt directly with this problem. We encourage and model positive tracking whereby couples are taught to notice positive aspects of an interchange while minimizing the importance of negative features. We have not yet formally added strategies to teach our clients to recognize and overcome faulty inferences that may be interfering with the therapy. An emphasis on positive tracking may not be sufficient in itself to overcome the tendency to recall more vivid negatively-toned experiences.

Cognitive theorists have also discussed what is termed the representativeness heuristic (see Nisbett and Ross, 1980, for a detailed presentation of these topics). In making judgments about a situation (e.g., a relationship), one assesses the degree to which the most obvious features of the situation are representative of one's presumptions about what the situation should be like. For some couples, their expectation of what constitutes a relationship is itself problematic. Some couples have idealized views of what a marriage should be (perhaps a rose-colored view of their parents' marriage) and are disappointed by their own reality. Others are constantly comparing their current relationship to the days when the relationship was first forming and there was an emphasis on play, sex, and pleasure-giving. By comparison, they are disappointed in the state of their years-old marriage.

To date, marital therapists have had little to say about how to deal with faulty perception of what constitutes a viable relationship. Doing so smacks of the value judgments that most therapists attempt to avoid whenever possible. On the other hand, not addressing this issue fails to recognize the importance of a factor that may fundamentally affect a couple's satisfaction with the outcome of therapy.[1]

---

[1]Recently, debate about what are reasonable goals for marital therapy has begun to appear in the marital literature (cf. Jacobson, 1983b; Margolin, 1983). As this discussion proceeds and empirical data are gathered on the degree of change couples can comfortably make and maintain as a result of therapy, therapists will be better able to help couples establish both realistic and satisfying goals for their relationship.

In behavior exchange therapies, partners are taught to notice the relationship between their own behavior and the reaction evident in their spouses' satisfaction rating. This is usually done empirically. One can chart satisfaction and positive behaviors and show it to the couple. Kelley (1973) has suggested that people recognize and reasonably use the relationship between two events in making causal attributions. But Nisbett and Ross (1980) provide a summary of evidence that people are not particularly skillful at detecting the covariation between events or identifying causal relationships. A modification of the behavior exchange components of therapy that recognizes this weakness and teaches couples to become better observers and investigators of their relationship may be a useful adjunct to therapy.

In our clinical work, we have recognized that couples have their own "idiosyncratic cognitive sets and schemata" (Jacobson, 1984b). A formal component of therapy that examines these schemata and their contributions to both distress and positive change is needed (Arias, 1982; Epstein, 1982; Fincham, in press; Jacobson, 1984; Kopel & Arkowitz, 1975; Schindler & Vollmer, 1984).

Beck, Rush, Shaw, and Emery (1979) have said that depressives manifest systematic errors in their thinking and that such faulty information processing leads to depression. Their therapy provides ways of correcting the depressives' faulty logic about themselves and the world. The degree to which distressed couples make the same kinds of errors is not clear, but it does seem clear that arbitrary inference, selective abstraction, overgeneralization, magnification and minimization, and dichotomous thinking all exist in distressed couples. Whether or not these logical errors are the cause or result of distress has not been studied. Most marital therapy to date seems to have addressed these problems on an ad hoc basis. Because the depression literature indicates that a treatment strategy for altering dysfunctional cognitive processes already exists, an appropriate modification of this strategy may be a useful addition to marital therapy.

Individual and Marital Therapy

Often a couple will come to therapy with a distressed relationship and/or with one of the partners manifesting an apparently individual complaint such as depression or substance abuse (Gurman & Knudson, 1978; Knudson, Gurman, & Kniskern, 1979). While this may be common in clinical practice, most marital therapy outcome studies exclude couples in which one partner manifests significant individual psychopathology. Yet, in many cases, significant relationships between marital conflict and individual pathology have been reported. This is certainly the case with regard to depression, in that many studies have documented the joint occurrence of depression and relationship problems (e.g., Brown & Harris, 1978; Coleman & Miller, 1975; Weiss & Aved, 1978; Weissman & Paykel, 1974). Other studies have suggested that disruption of an intimate relationship can induce depression (Cooke, 1981; Paykel, Myers, Dienelt, Klerman, Lindenthal, & Pepper, 1969; Finlay-Jones, 1981).

Some theorists have even conceptualized and constructed therapies for depression with an emphasis on interpersonal relationships (Klerman & Weissman, 1982). In Klerman and Weissman's approach, however, the depressed person alone is the primary focus of therapy. Coyne (1976a, 1976b) has argued that depression is maintained in part by the way the depressed person interacts with others, but as yet no controlled clinical trials have been completed that systematically compare the efficacy of marital therapy with individual therapy in the treatment of individual disorders. There are few studies actually identifying the effects of marital distress on the individually based treatment, though Rounsaville, Weissman, Prusoff, and Herceg-Baron (1979) reported that marital distress was associated with poor response to their interpersonal therapy for depression.

The idea of treating individual disorders with marital therapy is beginning to attract attention. Often only one spouse actively seeks therapy while the partner reluctantly acquiesces. In such cases the initiating spouse will frequently try to form an alliance with the therapist to treat his or her spouse's "problem." This can complicate the therapy.

How to treat individual problems and marital distress concurrently may depend on the nature of the problem and the theory that the therapist uses to explain the disorder. If one were to take a cognitive-behavioral approach to the treatment of depression and integrate it into marital therapy, the "marriage"of the two therapies might be relatively straightforward. Using behavior exchange principles to increase the frequencies of positive behaviors for the depressed spouse should have salutary effects for both the depression and the marital distress. Communication training might be expected to positively influence the social stimulus value of the depressed client (Coyne, 1976a). And problem-solving strategies might benefit the relationship as well as increase the sense of control that the depressive has over his or her environment (Seligman, 1975).

What remains to be worked out is how to combine individual therapy sessions with conjoint therapy. In some sessions there is no logical reason to include a spouse. For example, if a distressed spouse is also being treated for agoraphobia that is contributing to the marital distress, there may be no reason to include the other spouse when relaxation training is being taught. We are currently experimenting with concurrent individual sessions as an adjunct to conjoint sessions. Clearly, ancillary clinical problems can contribute to marital distress and it may be most expedient to treat both types of problems simultaneously.

It was pointed out earlier that individual therapy for marital distress generally leads to poor outcome (Gurman & Kniskern, 1978a). We see no reason to depart from the conjoint treatment of marital dysfunction as a primary strategy. An individual format to address relationship problems seems to imply that only one spouse has a problem. There are times, however, when the best interests of the individuals and the relationship are in conflict, and clinical innovations are still needed in such cases (Jacobson, 1983b).

Sexual Dysfunction and Marital Therapy

Couples who seek either sex therapy or marital therapy have some degree of both sexual problems and relationship discord in about three-quarters of the cases (Sager, 1976). Couples who seek services at sex therapy clinics or marital therapy clinics seem to have similar degrees of both sexual and marital problems (Frank, Anderson, & Kupfer, 1976), regardless of which type of service they seek. Melman and Jacobson (1983) report that in a sample of 48 couples seeking marital therapy, two-thirds had "a significant sexual concern or dysfunction." This sample excluded couples whose presenting complaint was a circumscribed sexual dysfunction. O'Leary and Arias (1983) report sexual problems in about 40% of a sample 44 consecutive cases presenting for marital therapy. Interpretation of the high coincidence of marital and sexual complaints is complicated by a possibly high base rate of sexual complaints in the normal population (Frank, Anderson, & Rubinstein, 1978).

The treatment for specific sexual dysfunction has been described by Masters and Johnson (1970). Although they state that the real patient in their treatment is the relationship itself, little is said about conflict resolution, cooperative behavior exchange, or communication. In fact, couples with significant marital distress were excluded from their pioneering studies (Zilbergeld & Evans, 1980).

It has been suggested that different typologies of couples with marital and sexual difficulties should be considered (Sager, 1976). Couples who have primary sexual dysfunction and resultant marital distress may be candidates for sex therapy first. Couples who experience increasing marital distress with a resulting decrease in satisfactory sexual experiences may benefit from beginning with marital therapy. Some researchers have observed that marital discord (and especially, hostility) interferes with effective sex therapy (Roffe & Britt, 1981; Stuart & Hammond, 1980).

On the other hand, there may be cases in which sexual dysfunction and marital dysfunction are relatively unrelated (Berg & Snyder, 1981; Hartman, 1980a, 1980b). The results of some clinical studies examining the effects of sex therapy on marital functioning have likewise been equivocal. Some studies find generalized benefits (Chesney, Blakeney, Chan, & Cole, 1981; Crowe, Gillan & Golombok, 1981; Foster, 1978), whereas others do not (Everaerd & Dekker, 1981).

Studies that have examined the effects of marital therapy on sexual problems have yielded disappointing results. O'Leary and Arias (1983) found that couples in BMT improved their sex lives, though their ratings of sexual satisfaction still remained lower than those of a normal control group. In a study reported by Melman and Jacobson (1983), couples who had sexual complaints at the beginning of marital therapy showed little improvement in these sexual problem areas despite improvements in other areas of relationship functioning. The authors point to several factors that may have affected the results, including inattention by the therapist. In the cases of the O'Leary and Arias study and the Melman and Jacobson study, no specific sex therapy was offered.

For couples presenting for marital therapy, improving communication skills and attending to the marital relationship itself will not typically lead to improvement in sexual interactions. In cases of concomitant marital and sexual difficulties, both sets of problems should be addressed by using techniques designed to treat the specific problems of each type.

Conclusion

Both the assessment and treatment of incompatible marital relationships are still in relatively early stages of development. We have attempted to summarize the current status of both and elaborate a bit on the clinical practice of behavioral marital therapy. Other therapeutic approaches continue to evolve also. It remains to be seen as to whether or not they generate empirically based research on treatment outcome. Future directions will focus on a number of issues that research has only begun to address. More and better designed outcome research is needed to identify what types of techniques work best for what types of couples. Prediction studies and process research are needed to aid in the understanding of change mechanisms, and to identify predictors of positive outcome. Finally, much work remains to be done in the area of treatment development. The treatment of marital problems has only recently entered the scientific stage. We have gotten off to a good start, but we still have a long way to go.

References

Ables, B. S., & Brandsma, J. M. (1977). *Therapy for couples*. San Francisco: Jossey-Bass.

Arias, I. (1982, December). Cognitive processes influencing marital functioning. Paper presented at the annual convention of the American Psychological Association, Washington, DC.

Bateson, G., Jackson, D. D., Haley, J., & Weakland, J. (1956). Toward a theory of schizophrenia. *Behavioral Science, 1*, 251–264.

Baucom, D. H. (1982). A comparison of behavioral contracting and problem-solving/communication training in behavioral marital therapy. *Behavior Therapy, 13*, 162–174.

Beck, A. T., Rush, A. J., Shaw, B., & Emery, G. (1979). *Cognitive therapy of depression*. New York: Guilford Press.

Berg, P., & Snyder, D. K. (1981). Differential diagnosis of marital and sexual distress. *Journal of Sex and Marital Therapy, 7*, 290–295.

Berley, R. A., & Jacobson, N. S. (1984). Causal attributions in intimate relationships: Toward a model of cognitive behavioral marital therapy. In P. Kendall (Ed.), *Advances in cognitive-behavioral research and therapy*. (Vol. 3). New York: Academic Press.

Billings, A. (1979). Conflict resolution in distressed and nondistressed married couples. *Journal of Consulting and Clinical Psychology, 47*, 368–376.

Bowen, M. (1966). The use of family theory in clinical practice. *Comprehensive Psychiatry, 7*, 345–374.

Bowen, M. (1976). Theory in the practice of psychotherapy. In P. J. Guerin (Ed.), *Family therapy: Theory and practice*. New York: Gardner Press.

Brown, G. W., & Harris, T. O. (1978). *Social origins of depression: A study of psychiatric disorder in women*. New York: Free Press.

Butcher, J. N., & Koss, M. P. (1978). Research on brief and crisis-oriented therapies. In S. L. Garfield & A. E. Bergin (Eds.), *Handbook of psychotherapy and behavior change* (rev. ed.). New York: Wiley.

Butcher, J. N., & Maudal, G. R. (1976). Crisis intervention. In I. B. Weiner (Ed.), *Clinical methods in psychology*. New York: Wiley.

Chesney, A. P., Blakeney, P. E., Chan, F. A., Cole, C. M. (1981). The impact of sex therapy on sexual behaviors and marital communication. *Journal of Sex and Marital Therapy*, 7, 70–79.

Christensen, A., & Nies, D. C. (1980). The Spouse Observation Checklist: Empirical analysis and critique. *The American Journal of Family Therapy*, 8, 69–79.

Coleman, R. E., & Miller, A. G. (1975). The relationship between depression and marital maladjustment in a clinical population: A multitrait-multimethod study. *Journal of Consulting and Clinical Psychology*, 43, 647–651.

Cooke, D. J. (1981). Life events and syndromes of depression in the general population. *Social Psychiatry*, 16, 181–186.

Coyne, J. C. (1976a). Depression and the response of others. *Journal of Abnormal Psychology*, 85, 28–40.

Coyne, J. C. (1976b). Toward an interaction description of depression. *Psychiatry*, 39, 28–40.

Crowe, M. J. (1978). Conjoint marital therapy: A controlled outcome study. *Psychological Medicine*, 8, 623–636.

Crowe, M. J., Gillan, P., & Golombok, S. (1981). Form and content in the conjoint treatment of sexual dysfunction. *Behavior Research and Therapy*, 19, 47–54.

Crowne, D. P., & Marlowe, D. (1960). A new scale of social desirability independent of psychopathology. *Journal of Consulting and Clinical Psychology*, 24, 349–354.

Cuber, J. (1948). *Marriage counseling practice*. New York: Appleton-Century-Crofts.

Edwards, A. L. (1957). *The social desirability variable in personality assessment and research*. New York: Holt, Rinehart and Winston.

Emmelkamp, P., van der Helm, M., MacGillavry, D., & van Zanten, B. (1984). Marital therapy with clinically distressed couples: A comparative evaluation of systems-theoretic, contingency contracting and communication skills approaches. In K. Hahlweg & N. S. Jacobson (Eds.), *Marital interaction: Analysis and modification*. New York: Guilford Press.

Epstein, N. (1982). Cognitive therapy with couples. *American Journal of Family Therapy*, 10, 5–16.

Everaerd, W., & Dekker, J. (1981). A comparison of sex therapy and communication therapy: Couples complaining of orgasmic dysfunction. *Journal of Sex and Marital Therapy*, 7, 278–289.

Fincham, F. D. (in press). Clinical applications of attribution theory: Problems and prospects. In M. Hawthorne (Ed.), *Attribution theory: Extensions and applications*. Oxford: Blackwells.

Finlay-Jones, R. (1981). Showing that life events are a cause of depression: A review. *Australian and New Zealand Journal of Psychiatry*, 15, 229–238.

Foster, A. L. (1978). Changes in marital-sexual relationships following treatment for sexual dysfunctioning. *Journal of Sex and Marital Therapy*, 4, 186–197.

Frank, E., Anderson, C., & Kupfer, D. J. (1976). Profiles of couples seeking sex therapy and marital therapy. *American Journal of Psychiatry*, 133, 559–562.

Frank, E., Anderson, C., & Rubinstein, D. (1978). Frequency of sexual dysfunction in normal couples. *New England Journal of Medicine*, 299, 111–115.

Gottman, J. M. (1979). *Marital interaction: Experimental investigations*. New York: Academic Press.

Gottman, J. M., Markman, H., & Notarius, C. (1977). The topography of marital conflict: A study of verbal and nonverbal behavior. *Journal of Marriage and the Family, 39*, 461–477.

Gottman, J. M., Notarius, C., Gonso, J., & Markman, H. (1976). *A couple's guide to communication*. Champaign, IL: Research Press.

Guerney, B. G. (1977). *Relationship enhancement*. San Francisco: Jossey-Bass.

Gurman, A. S. (1973a). Marital therapy: Emerging trends in research and practice. *Family Process, 12*, 45–54.

Gurman, A. S. (1973b). The effects and effectiveness of marital therapy: A review of outcome research. *Family Process, 12*, 145–170.

Gurman, A. S. (1978). Contemporary marital therapies: A critique and comparative analysis of psychoanalytic, behavioral and systems theory approaches. In T. J. Paolino & B. S. McCrady (Eds.), *Marriage and marital therapy: Psychoanalytic, behavioral and systems theory perspectives*. New York: Bruner/Mazel.

Gurman, A. S., & Kniskern, D. P. (1978a). Deterioration in marital and family therapy: Empirical, clinical and conceptual issues. *Family Process, 17*, 3–20.

Gurman, A. S., & Kniskern, D. P. (1978b). Research in marital and family therapy: Progress, perspective, and prospect. In S. L. Garfield & A. E. Bergin (Eds.), *Handbook of psychotherapy and behavior change* (rev. ed.). New York: Wiley.

Gurman, A. S., & Knudson, R. M. (1978). Behavioral marriage therapy: I. A. psychodynamic-systems analysis and critique. *Family Process, 17*, 121–138.

Gurman, A. S., Knudson, R. M., & Kniskern, D. P. (1978). Behavioral marriage therapy: IV. Take two aspirin and call us in the morning. *Family Process, 17*, 165–180.

Hahlweg, K., Revenstorf, D., & Schindler, L. (1982). Treatment of marital distress: Comparing formats and modalities. *Advances in Behavior Research and Therapy, 4*, 57–74.

Haley, J. (1963). Marriage therapy. *Archives of General Psychiatry, 8*, 213–234.

Hartman, L. M. (1980a). The interface between sexual dysfunction and marital conflict. *American Journal of Psychiatry, 137*, 576–579.

Hartman, L. M. (1980b). Relationship factors and sexual dysfunction. *Canadian Journal of Psychiatry, 25*, 560–563.

Hobart, C. W., & Klausner, W. J. (1959). Some social interactional correlates of marital role disagreements, and marital adjustment. *Marriage and Family Living, 21*, 256–263.

Hops, H., Wills, T., Patterson, G. R., & Weiss, R. L. (1972). *Marital Interaction Coding System*. Unpublished manuscript, University of Oregon and Oregon Research Institute.

Hurvitz, N. (1967). Marital problems following psychotherapy with one spouse. *Journal of Consulting and Clinical Psychology, 31*, 38–47.

Jackson, D. (1957). Family interaction, family homeostasis and some implications for conjoint family psychotherapy. In J. Masserman (Ed.), *Individual and family dynamics*. New York: Grune and Stratton.

Jacobson, N. S. (1977). Problem solving and contingency contracting in the treatment of marital discord. *Journal of Consulting and Clinical Psychology, 45*, 92–100.

Jacobson, N. S. (1981). Behavioral marital therapy. In A. S. Gurman & D. P. Kniskern (Eds.), *Handbook of family therapy*. New York: Brunner/Mazel.

Jacobson, N. S. (1983a). Beyond empiricism: The politics of marital therapy. *The American Journal of Family Therapy, 11*, 11–24.

Jacobson, N. S. (1983b). Expanding the range and applicability of behavioral marital therapy. *The Behavior Therapist, 6*, 189–191.

Jacobson, N. S. (1984a). A component analysis of behavioral marital therapy: The relative effectiveness of behavior exchange and communication/problem-solving training. *Journal of Consulting and Clinical Psychology, 52,* 295–305.

Jacobson, N. S. (1984b). The modification of cognitive processes in behavioral marital therapy: Integrating cognitive and behavioral intervention strategies. In K. Hahlweg & N. S. Jacobson (Eds.), *Marital interaction: Analysis and modification.* New York: Guilford Press.

Jacobson, N. S., & Bussod, N. (1983). Marital and family therapy. In M. Hersen, A. E. Kazdin, & A. S. Bellack (Eds.), *The clinical psychology handbook.* London: Pergamon Press.

Jacobson, N. S., Elwood, R., & Dallas, M. (1981). The behavioral assessment of marital dysfunction. In D. H. Barlow (Ed.), *Behavioral assessment of adult disorders.* (pp. 439–479). New York: Guilford.

Jacobson, N. S., Follette, W. C., & Elwood, R. W. (1984). Research on the effectiveness of behavioral marital therapy: Methodological and conceptual critique. In K. Hahlweg & N. S. Jacobson (Eds.), *Marital interaction: Analysis and modification.* New York: Guilford Press.

Jacobson, N. S., Follette, W. C., & McDonald, D. W. (1982). Reactivity to positive and negative behavior in distressed and nondistressed married couples. *Journal of Clinical and Consulting Psychology, 50,* 706–714.

Jacobson, N. S., Follette, W. C., Revenstorf, D., Baucom, D. H., Hahlweg, K., & Margolin, G. (1984). Variability in outcome and clinical significance of behavioral marital therapy: A reanalysis of outcome data. *Journal of Consulting and Clinical Psychology, 52,* 497–504.

Jacobson, N. S., & Margolin, G. (1979). *Marital therapy: Strategies based on social learning and behavior exchange principles.* New York: Brunner/Mazel.

Jacobson, N. S., McDonald, D. W., Follette, W. C., & Berley, R. A. (in press). Attributional processes in distressed and nondistressed married couples. *Cognitive Therapy and Research, 9.*

Jacobson, N. S., & Moore, D. (1981). Spouses as observers of the events in their relationship. *Journal of Clinical and Consulting Psychology, 49,* 269–277.

Jacobson, N. S., & Weiss, R. L. (1978). Behavioral marriage therapy: III. "The contents of Gurman et al. may be hazardous to our health." *Family Process, 17,* 149–164.

Kelley, H. H. (1973). The process of causal attribution. *American Psychologist, 28,* 107–128.

Kelley, H. H., & Thibaut, J. W. (1978). *Interpersonal relations: A theory of interdependence.* New York: Wiley.

Klerman, G. L., & Weissman, M. M. (1982). Interpersonal psychotherapy: Theory and research. In A. J. Rush (Ed.), *Short-term psychotherapies for depression.* New York: Guilford Press.

Knudson, R. M., Gurman, A. S., & Kniskern, D. P. (1979). Behavioral marriage therapy: A treatment in transition. In C. M. Franks & G. T. Wilson (Eds.), *Annual review of behavior therapy* (Vol. 7). New York: Brunner/Mazel.

Kopel, S. & Arkowitz, H. (1975). The role of attribution and self-perception in behavior change: Implications for behavior therapy. *General Psychological Monographs, 92,* 175–212.

Liberman, R. P., Wheeler, E. G., deVisser, L., Kuehnel, J., & Kuehnel, T. (1980). *Handbook of marital therapy.* Plenum Press: New York.

Locke, H. J. (1951). *Predicting adjustment in marriage: A comparison of a divorced and happily married group.* New York: Holt.

Locke, H. J., & Wallace, K. M. (1959). Short marital adjustment and prediction tests: Their reliability and validity. *Marriage and Family Living, 21,* 251–255.

Margolin, G. (1981). Behavior exchange in happy and unhappy marriages: A family cycle perspective. *Behavior Therapy, 12,* 329–343.

Margolin, G. (1983). Behavioral marital therapy: Is there a place for passion, play, and other non-negotiable dimensions? *The Behavior Therapist, 6*, 65–68.

Margolin, G., Talovic, S., & Weinstein, C. D. (1983). Areas of change questionnaire: A practical approach to marital assessment. *Journal of Clinical and Consulting Psychology, 51*, 920–931.

Margolin, G., & Weiss, R. L. (1978). A comparative evaluation of therapeutic components associated with behavioral marital treatment. *Journal of Consulting and Clinical Psychology, 46*, 1476–1486.

Masters, W., & Johnson, V. (1970). *Human sexual inadequacy*. Boston: Little-Brown.

Melman, K. N., & Jacobson, N. S. (1983). Integrating behavioral marital therapy and sex therapy. In M. L. Aronson & L. R. Wolberg (Eds.), *Group and family therapy*. New York: Brunner/Mazel.

Minuchin, S. (1974). *Families and family therapy*. Cambridge, MA: Harvard University Press.

Mischel, W. (1968). Personality and assessment. New York: Wiley.

Mittleman, B. (1944). Complementary neurotic reactions in intimate relationships. *Psychoanalytic Quarterly, 13*, 479–491.

Mittleman, B. (1948). The concurrent analysis of marital couples. *Psychoanalytic Quarterly, 17*, 182–197.

Nisbett, R. E., & Ross, L. (1980). *Human inference: Strategies and shortcomings of social judgment*. Englewood Cliffs, NJ: Prentice-Hall.

Oberndorf, C. P. (1938). Psychoanalysis of married couples. *Psychoanalytic Review, 25*, 453–475.

O'Leary, K. D., & Arias, I. (1983). The influence of marital therapy on sexual satisfaction. *Journal of Sex and Marital Therapy, 9*, 171–181.

O'Leary, K. D., & Turkewitz, H. (1978). Marital therapy from a behavioral perspective. In T. J. Paolino & B. S. McCrady (Eds.), *Marriage and marital therapy: Psychoanalytic, behavioral and systems theory perspectives*. New York: Brunner/Mazel.

Patterson, G. R. (1971). *Families: Applications of social learning to family life*. Champaign, IL: Research Press.

Patterson, G. R. (1974). Interventions for boys with conduct problems: Multiple settings, treatments, and criteria. *Journal of Consulting and Clinical Psychology, 42*, 471–481.

Patterson, G. R. (1976). Some procedures for assessing changes in marital interaction patterns. *Oregon Research Institute Bulletin, 16*, No. 7.

Paykel, E. S., Myers, J. K., Dienelt, M. N., Klerman, G. L., Lindenthal, J. J., & Pepper, M. P. (1969). Life events and depression: A controlled study. *Archives of General Psychiatry, 21*, 753–760.

Prochaska, J., & Prochaska, J. (1978). Twentieth century trends in marriage and marital therapy. In T. J. Paolino & B. S. McCrady (Eds.), *Marriage and marital therapy: Psychoanalytic, behavioral and systems theory perspectives*. New York: Brunner/Mazel.

Raush, H. L. (1965). Interaction sequences. *Journal of Personality and Social Psychology, 2*, 487–499.

Robinson, E. A., & Price, M. G. (1980). Pleasurable behavior in marital interaction: An observational study. *Journal of Consulting and Clinical Psychology, 48*, 117–118.

Roffe, M. W., & Britt, B. C. (1981). A typology of marital interaction for sexually dysfunctional couples. *Journal of Sex and Marital Therapy, 7*, 207–222.

Rounsaville, B. J., Weissman, M. M., Prusoff, B. A., & Herceg-Baron, R. L. (1979). Marital disputes and treatment outcome in depressed women. *Comprehensive Psychiatry, 20*, 483–490.

Sager, C. (1966). The development of marriage therapy: An historical review. *American Journal of Orthopsychiatry, 36*, 458–467.

Sager, C. J. (1976). The role of sex therapy in marital therapy. *American Journal of Psychiatry*, *133*, 555–558.

Satir, V. (1967). *Conjoint family therapy*. Palo Alto, CA: Science & Behavior Books.

Schindler, L. & Vollmer, M. (1984). Cognitive perspectives in behavioral marital therapy: Some proposals for bridging theory, research, and practice. In K. Hahlweg & N. S. Jacobson (Eds.), *Marital interaction: Analysis and modification*. New York: Guilford Press.

Seligman, M. E. P. (1975). *Helplessness*. San Francisco: W. H. Freeman.

Sluzki, C. E., & Ransom, D. C. (Eds.). (1976). *Double bind: The foundation of the communicational approach to the family*. New York: Grune & Stratton.

Smith, M. L., & Glass, G. V. (1977). Meta-analysis of psychotherapy outcome studies. *American Psychologist*, *32*, 752–760.

Snyder, D. K. (1979). *Marital satisfaction inventory*. Los Angeles: Western Psychological Services.

Spanier, G. B. (1976). Measuring dyadic adjustment: New scales for assessing the quality of marriage and similar dyads. *Journal of Marriage and the Family*, *38*, 15–28.

Steinglass, P. (1978). The conceptualization of marriage from a systems theory perspective. In T. J. Paolino & B. S. McCrady (Eds.), *Marriage and marital therapy: Psychoanalytic, behavioral and systems theory perspectives*. New York: Brunner/Mazel.

Stuart, F. M., & Hammond, D. C. (1980). Sex therapy. In R. B. Stuart (Ed.), *Helping couples change: A social learning approach to marital therapy*. New York: Guilford Press.

Stuart, R. B. (1969). Operant interpersonal treatment for marital discord. *Journal of Consulting and Clinical Psychology*, *33*, 675–682.

Stuart, R. B. (1976). An operant-interpersonal program for couples. In D. H. Olson (Ed.), *Treating relationships*. Lake Mills, IA: Graphic Publishing Co.

Stuart, R. B. (1980). *Helping couples change: A social learning approach to marital therapy*. New York: Guilford Press.

Stuart, R. B., & Stuart, F. (1973). *Marital Precounseling Inventory*, Champaign, IL: Research Press.

Terman, L. M. (1938). *Psychological factors in marital happiness*. New York: McGraw-Hill.

Thibaut, J. W., & Kelley, H. H. (1959). *The social psychology of groups*. New York: Wiley.

Turkewitz, H., & O'Leary, K. D. (1981). A comparative outcome study of behavioral marital therapy and communication therapy. *Journal of Marital and Family Therapy*, *7*, 159–170.

Tversky, A., & Kahneman, D. (1973). Availability: A heuristic for judging frequency and probability. *Cognitive Psychology*, *5*, 207–232.

Vincent, J. P., Weiss, R. L., & Birchler, G. R. (1975). A behavioral analysis of problem solving in distressed and nondistressed married and stranger dyads. *Behavior Therapy*, *6*, 475–487.

Watzlawick, P., Beavin, J. H., & Jacobson, D. D. (1967). *Pragmatics of human communication*. New York: Norton.

Weiss, R. L., & Aved, B. M. (1978). Marital satisfaction and depression as predictors of physical health status. *Journal of Consulting and Clinical Psychology*, *46*, 1379–1384.

Weiss, R. L., & Birchler, G. R. (1975). *Areas of change*. Unpublished manuscript, University of Oregon.

Weiss, R. L., Birchler, G. R., & Vincent, J. P. (1974). Contractual models for negotiation training in marital dyads. *Journal of Marriage and the Family, 36*, 321–331.

Weiss, R. L., & Cerreto, M. (1975). *Marital status inventory*. Unpublished manuscript, University of Oregon.

Weiss, R. L., Hops, H., & Patterson, G. R. (1973). A framework for conceptualizing marital conflict, a technology for altering it, some data for evaluating it. In L. A. Hamerlynck, L. C. Handy, & E. Mash (Eds.), *Behavior change: Methodology, concepts, and practice*. Champaign, IL: Research Press.

Weiss, R. L., & Margolin, G. (1977). Marital conflict and accord. In A. R. Ciminero, K. S. Calhoun, & H. E. Adams (Eds.), *Handbook for behavioral assessment*. New York: Wiley.

Weissman, M. M., & Paykel, E. S. (1974). *The depressed woman: A study of social relationships*. Chicago: University of Chicago Press.

Wills, I. A., Weiss, R. L., & Patterson, G. R. (1974). A behavioral analysis of the determinants of marital satisfaction. *Journal of Consulting and Clinical Psychology, 42*, 802–811.

Zilbergeld, B., & Evans, M. (1980). The inadequacy of Masters and Johnson. *Psychology Today, 14*(3):29–43.

Author Index

Subject Index

Springer Series in Social Psychology

Attention and Self-Regulation: A Control-Theory Approach to Human Behavior
Charles S. Carver/Michael F. Scheier

Gender and Nonverbal Behavior
Clara Mayo/Nancy M. Henley (Editors)

Personality, Roles, and Social Behavior
William Ickes/Eric S. Knowles (Editors)

Toward Transformation in Social Knowledge
Kenneth J. Gergen

The Ethics of Social Research: Surveys and Experiments
Joan E. Sieber (Editor)

The Ethics of Social Research: Fieldwork, Regulation, and Publication
Joan E. Sieber (Editor)

Anger and Aggression: An Essay on Emotion
James R. Averill

The Social Psychology of Creativity
Teresa M. Amabile

Sports Violence
Jeffrey H. Goldstein (Editor)

Nonverbal Behavior: A Functional Perspective
Miles L. Patterson

Basic Group Processes
Paul B. Paulus (Editor)

Attitudinal Judgment
J. Richard Eiser (Editor)

Social Psychology of Aggression: From Individual Behavior to Social Interaction
Amélie Mummendey (Editor)

Directions in Soviet Social Psychology
Lloyd H. Strickland (Editor)

Sociophysiology
William M. Waid (Editor)

Compatible and Incompatible Relationships
William Ickes (Editor)

Facet Theory: Approaches to Social Research
David Canter (Editor)

Action Control: From Cognition to Behavior
Julius Kuhl/Jürgen Beckmann (Editors)

Springer Series in Social Psychology

The Social Construction of the Person
Kenneth J. Gergen/Keith E. Davis (Editors)

Entrapment in Escalating Conflicts: A Social Psychological Analysis
Joel Brockner/Jeffrey Z. Rubin

The Attribution of Blame: Causality, Responsibilty, and Blameworthiness
Kelly G. Shaver

Language and Social Situations
Joseph P. Forgas (Editor)